MW01470821

PSYCHOTHERAPEUTIC DRUG MANUAL

COMMITTEE ON THERAPEUTICS
NEW YORK STATE
OFFICE OF MENTAL HEALTH

Julie Magno Zito, Editor

THIRD EDITION
Revised

A Wiley-Interscience Publication
JOHN WILEY & SONS, INC.
New York / Chichester / Brisbane / Toronto / Singapore

Copyright © 1994 by John Wiley & Sons, Inc.
Copyright © 1989 by Research Foundation for Mental Hygiene, Inc.

Library of Congress Cataloging in Publication Data:

New York (State). Office of Mental Health. Committee on
  Therapeutics.
    New York State Office of Mental Health psychotherapeutic drug
  manual / Committee on Therapeutics. Office of Mental Health : Julie
  Magno Zito, editor. — 3rd ed., rev.
      p.   cm. — (Wiley series in general & clinical psychiatry)
    Includes bibliographical references.
    ISBN 0-471-30530-8 (cloth : alk. paper)
    1. Mental illness—Chemotherapy—Handbooks, manuals, etc.
  2. Psychotropic drugs—Effectiveness—Handbooks, manuals, etc.
  3. Psychotropic drugs—Side effects—Handbooks, manuals, etc.
  I. Zito, Julie Magno. II. Title. III. Title: Psychotherapeutic
  drug manual. IV. Series: Wiley series in general and clinical
  psychiatry.
      [DNLM: 1. Psychotropic Drugs—therapeutic use. 2. Psychotropic
  Drugs—administration & dosage. 3. Mental disorders—drug therapy.
  QV 77 N5329n 1994]
  RC483.N48   1994
  615'.788—dc20
  DNLM/DLC
  for Library of Congress   93-17909

For our patients who make us aware
of the need for a patient-oriented,
longitudinal model for psychopharmacology

New York State Office of Mental Health
Committee on Therapeutics

John Oldham, M.D.
Chief Medical Officer
NYS Office of Mental Health
Director of NYS Psychiatric Institute
Department of Psychiatry, Columbia Presbyterian Medical
    Center, NY

Kurt Patton, M.S., R.Ph.
Director of Health Policy and Services
NYS Office of Mental Health

Zebulon Taintor, M.D.
Vice-Chairman, Department of Psychiatry
New York University Medical Center, NY

Herman M. van Praag, M.D., Ph.D.
Silverman Professor and Chair, Department of Psychiatry
Albert Einstein College of Medicine, NY

Jan Volavka, M.D., Ph.D.
Chief of Clinical Research Division
Nathan S. Kline Institute for Psychiatric Research
Professor, Department of Psychiatry, New York University, NY

Preface to the Revised Third Edition

The enthusiastic response to the third edition of the *Psychotherapeutic Drug Manual* since its publication in 1989 has been gratifying. To make the manual available to residency training, prescribing physicians, and clinical administrators in the United States and abroad, the Committee on Therapeutics authorized this revised edition. The new pocket style of the manual is designed to be more readable and convenient for busy professionals.

The *Psychotherapeutic Drug Manual* is not an exhaustive text on the principles of prescribing psychotherapeutic drugs. There are numerous texts available that provide greater detail and they are cited throughout the manual. Instead, the aim of this manual is to provide relevant, documented information on the effectiveness and safety of the most frequently prescribed psychotherapeutic agents. It emphasizes the benefit-to-risk relationship for prescribing each agent as well as for the use of these agents in combination. We hope that psychiatry residents and others new to psychopharmacology who use this manual will come to a deeper appreciation of the complexity of psychopharmacotherapy and will choose to adopt a long-term effectiveness and safety model. The *Manual* emphasizes such an approach.

In this revision, chapters have been updated to include newer agents, such as clozapine and clomipramine. Collectively, the chapters provide a current knowledge base in psychopharmacology so that prescribing physicians, residents in training, nurses, pharmacists, and other professionals charged with responsibility for overseeing the quality of drug therapy will have a common reference point. Controversial issues are amply documented and rely on well-known North American and international experts in psychopharmacology.

The drug dosage and interaction guidelines listed in Part II have been revised based on the pilot experience of the past two years. As we progress toward the year 2000, systematic drug monitoring continues to grow in importance for establishing effective and safe drug therapy. Along with monitoring, pharmacoepidemiologic methods for the evaluation of drug therapy in large populations in the clinical setting are a next step toward a more systematic clinical science of psychotherapeutic agents. It is hoped that the revised third edition of the *Psychotherapeutic Drug Manual* will assist large systems such as the Health Maintenance Organization (HMO), the Veterans Administration, and other state mental health systems in accomplishing this important goal.

JULIE M. ZITO, PH.D.
EDITOR

Orangeburg, New York
November 1993

Preface to the Third Edition

The New York State Office of Mental Health is unique among American state mental health systems because it is charged with the care of a very large proportion of our nation's severely mentally ill. With this large population comes the challenge for care that is not only humane, but which meets modern standards of excellence in clinical practice.

To achieve excellence in meeting our goals, we rely on many talented and dedicated professionals. Among these individuals, I am happy to acknowledge the Committee on Therapeutics, a group of prominent university and public psychiatry leaders. The Committee has served for the past 13 years as consultants to the state on psychopharmacologic issues. Their task has been to develop and revise previous editions of the *Psychotherapeutic Drug Manual.*

Today, I am happy to review the third edition of the manual which represents the product of the Committee's efforts during the past three years. This reference manual is written primarily for prescribing physicians but may be useful to other health care professionals in nursing, pharmacy, psychology, and social work who have clinical responsibilities involving psychopharmacologic drug use. The manual has been considerably broadened to include guidelines that detail the selection, dosing, and side-effect monitoring of psychotropic and other neuroactive agents commonly used in psychiatric patients.

These guidelines will accompany the introduction of a prospective drug-monitoring system. Together with up-to-date drug information, process-oriented drug monitoring and clinical accountability, the prescribing physician should find psychopharmacologic drug dilemmas more understandable and easier to resolve. We believe that constant assessment by these longitudinal monitoring methods will lead to safer and more effective drug therapy and overall, to better outcome for those we serve.

RICHARD C. SURLES, PH.D, COMMISSIONER
NEW YORK STATE OFFICE OF MENTAL HEALTH

April 1989

Acknowledgments

The task of developing the third edition of the Psychotherapeutic Drug Manual and its present revision evolved over several years. Aside from adding new drugs to the guidelines, the Committee's goal was to develop consensus on current psychopharmacologic practice. The need for consensus in areas of clinical practice is not unique to this field. Today, the clinical sciences often are faced with controversies because of discrepant findings and the need to act in behalf of patients despite insufficient information. Thus, the Committee decided to summarize the principles of pharmacotherapy they believe to be pertinent today. The chapters devoted to these issues were derived from a broad range of textbooks, journals, and clinical experience that the Committee then reviewed and approved.

Many individuals contributed to this task by sharing their clinical and research experience, critical review of previous drafts and by kind and supportive acts. Adult guidelines received scrutiny from a number of outside consultants. First among these is Dr. Ross Baldessarini, noted textbook author and professor of psychiatry, who patiently revised the chapter on antidepressants. Expert neurology reviewers included Dr. Stanley Resor, Director of Seizure Clinic, Columbia-Presbyterian Hospital, and Dr. Ilo Leppik of the University of Minnesota and the Comprehensive Epilepsy Program. Among Nathan Kline Institute researchers, Dr. Richard Squires, noted for his contributions to benzodiazepine research, carefully reviewed and revised the draft on anxiety and sleep disorders. Mr. Thomas Cooper, Chief of the Psychopharmacology Laboratory at Nathan Kline and New York Psychiatric Institute reviewed the lithium guidelines and offered thoughtful comments. Dr. Istvan Bitter, Visiting Professor from Hungary, reviewed several chapters in detail and offered insightful changes. Dr. James Chou provided information on benzodiazepines in clinical usage.

All of the committee reviewers were helpful. Special thanks to Dr. Donald Klein who offered detailed comments for each of the adult chapters of the Manual and to Dr. Heinz Lehmann for a historical perspective.

Dr. Thomas Craig has contributed much to the pharmacoepidemiology of psychiatric disorders, and generously critiqued the chapters on antipsychotics and neuroactive agents used for the control of their adverse effects.

Very special thanks to Dr. Magda Campbell and Dr. Lawrence Greenhill, Professor of Psychiatry, Columbia University, and Dr. Richard Reuben, Professor of Clinical Neurology, NYU Medical Center, for assistance in writing the children's guidelines. Other members of Dr. Campbell's subgroup included Dr. Gloria Faretra and Dr. S. Aluwalia.

Critical reading of many sections of the third edition was generously done by my collaborators, Dr. Maurice R. Green and Dr. Jules Ranz. Dr. Green also enthusiastically assisted with this revision as well. A special note of gratitude to Kurt Patton, M.D. R.Ph., for his help in developing these most recent editions. Herb Reich, Senior Editor at Wiley, guided the task to fruition. Elizabeth Eaton, M.A., provided energetic assistance with the revision. As always, Professor Sandy Zito and Sandra and David Zito were supportive and generous.

JULIE M. ZITO, PH.D.
SECRETARY AND EDITOR

Contents

Introduction

For any medication, the potential benefit of improved treatment must be counterbalanced by acceptable risks of adverse effects. While this is true for the use of any medication, the situation for the persistently mentally ill is often complicated by medical problems with the end result of complex multi-drug regimens.

To assist the New York State prescribing physician in the task of longitudinal monitoring of symptoms and side effects of commonly used agents, this edition of the *Psychotherapeutic Drug Manual* has been prepared.

The *Manual* is one responsibility of the Committee on Therapeutics which was established in 1975 and charged with the following:

1. Establishing clinical policy on the appropriate methods of prescribing and administering drugs for patients in facilities within the jurisdiction of the Office of Mental Health and periodically updating these guidelines to reflect changes in knowledge and practice.

2. Integrating specific guidelines for appropriate drug prescribing within the drug ordering and monitoring system.

3. Developing standards and policies for the drug review process to be established in each psychiatric facility.

4. Assisting in the design and implementation of a continuing education program for medical staff and allied health professionals, supplemental to the review process, on the psychopharmacological treatment of mental disorders and on issues in drug prescribing.

5. Recommending to OMH clinical pharmacoepidemiologic studies to evaluate the effectiveness and safety of marked medications in problem areas as identified by the statewide drug review process.

This revision of the *Manual* is a substantial departure from the brief format of the previous editions. In this edition, we have attempted to provide the epidemiologic and clinical research basis for the Committee's recommendations. This information is necessary to develop a better understanding of the broad clinical and scientific framework in which drug therapy recommendations are made.

The interpretation of drug therapy guidelines needs some clarification. Slavish adherence to these guidelines was never intended. Only in rare instances is rigid adherence to the guidelines necessary. Rather, clinicians are asked to determine how an individual patient's clinical characteristics fit the benefit-to-risk analysis of a current drug use issue and then to act accordingly. These actions include: detailed written medical record notes, documentation of peer or supervisory review, patient consent, specific monitoring protocols for lab values, symptom and side effect clinical ratings, and treatment outcome. When the justification is supported by the clinical factors of the case and written in the medical record as suggested, the clinician who departs from the guidelines will be practicing systematic clinical psychopharmacology.

The *Manual* is divided into four parts: Part I details the principles of psychotherapeutic drug use in seven chapters, each of which is devoted to a major diagnostic category for which psychotropic or neuroactive agents are the major therapy. Part II reviews New York State clinical policies and clinical review procedures for the prospective clinical monitoring program. Part III lists the psychotherapeutic drug formulary and includes both psychotropic and ancillary drugs so that specific information needed for medication decisions will be readily available. Part IV is a quick reference section with lists of important laboratory and plasma level guides. In addition, it contains sample patient information sheets for major psychotropic drugs. These sheets are useful in promoting more informed patient participation in drug decision-making.

Last, it is our hope that the *Manual* will be used in the training of professionals, particularly those who are new to public psychiatry and to the unique psychopharmacologic challenges presented by severe mental illness. We are entering an era of unusual political change in the delivery of health care. Psychiatry will not be spared the costs and benefits of such attention. Clinicians will be well-served by improving their skills in the psychopharmacologic management of the seriously ill patient.

ROBERT CANCRO, M.D., CHAIRMAN
COMMITTEE ON THERAPEUTICS

PART I

Principles of Psychotherapeutic Drug Use

CHAPTER 1

Psychotic Disorders and the Antipsychotic Agents

INTRODUCTION

DRUG SELECTION

DOSING CONSIDERATIONS

3

INTRODUCTION

Psychoses defined in DSM-III-R include organic mental syndromes, schizophrenia, mood disorders, and paranoid states. Medications used to treat patients during hospitalization and in their outpatient follow-up care vary depending on target symptoms, length of treatment, and individual response. General principles for dosing with antipsychotics are presented in this chapter. Chapter 2 will consider the use of neuroactive agents, such as anticholinergic agents, to treat the extrapyramidal effects of antipsychotics.

The antipsychotics (neuroleptics, major tranquilizers) have been used extensively for the past 40 years in the treatment of acute psychotic episodes associated with schizophrenia and major affective disorders as well as for the long-term management of chronic organic and schizophrenic psychoses. The antipsychotics are the mainstay of drug therapy in schizophrenia and are among the least expensive and most effective treatment modalities.

In Table 1.1, frequently used antipsychotics are listed according to their chemical classification. Pharmacologic effects of these compounds are exerted on the dopaminergic, alpha-adrenergic, cholinergic, and histaminergic systems. The effects are observed clinically as reductions in psychomotor function that are reflected in changes in cognition, affect, and behavior. The efficacy of the antipsychotics in the treatment of acute psychotic episodes is well established by double-blind controlled clinical trials that have demonstrated significant reductions in target symptoms (e.g., disordered thinking, anxiety, delusions, hallucinations and social withdrawal). The medications are used to control symptoms so that additional therapeutic measures in psychosocial rehabilitation (e.g., vocational and social relations) can be introduced.

DRUG SELECTION

Recent reviews of efficacy studies and the published reports of experience in clinical settings suggest that among the dozen or more agents currently available pronounced differences in clinical response do not exist.[1] However, side effect profiles differ among the chemical classes available. In the list of relative effects, Table 1.1 provides estimates of side effects in terms of the degree of anticholinergic, sedative, adrenergic blocking (usually observed as orthostatic hypotension), and extrapyramidal effects.[2] Depending on the symptoms presented, some side effects can be used for beneficial effect. For example, an agitated patient's psychosis may be well controlled with a sedating agent, for example, an aliphatic or piperidine phenothiazine (such as chlorpromazine or thioridazine). The use of more than one antipsychotic simultaneously is not recommended because it makes clinical dosing decisions more difficult while exposing the patient to a greater range of side effects.[3]

TABLE 1.1. Relative effects of commonly used antipsychotic drugs.*

Class	Generic Name (Brand Name)	Potency	Anticholinergic**	Sedative	Hypotensive	EPSE
Phenothiazines, Aliphatic	Chlorpromazine (Thorazine)	Low	Moderate	Strong	Oral:Moderate IM:Strong	Moderate
Phenothiazines, Piperidine	Mesoridazine (Serentil)	Low	Moderate	Moderate	Moderate	Weak
	Thioridazine (Mellaril)	Low	Strong	Moderate	Moderate	Weak
Phenothiazines, Piperazine	Fluphenazine (Prolixin)	High	Weak	Weak	Weak	Strong
	Perphenazine (Trilafon)	Moderate	Weak	Weak	Weak	Strong
	Trifluoperazine (Stelazine)	High	Moderate	Weak	Weak	Strong
Thioxanthenes	Thiothixene (Navane)	High	Weak	Weak	Moderate	Moderate
Dihydroindolones	Molindone[†] (Moban)	Moderate	Weak	Weak	Weak?	Weak
Dibenzoxazepines	Loxapine (Loxitane)	Moderate	Moderate	Moderate	Weak	Moderate
Debenzodiazepines	Clozapine[††] (Clozaril)	Low	Strong	Moderate?	Weak?	Unknown
Butyrophenones	Haloperidol (Haldol)	High	Weak	Weak	Weak	Strong
Diphenylbutyldelpiperidines	Pimozide[††] (Orap)	High	Weak	Weak	Weak	Strong

* Adapted from reference 1.
** Adapted from reference 2.
[†] Questionable efficacy.
[††] Indication limited by FDA.

Because of the large patient variability in clinical response, the past medication experience of the patient should be the first source of information in selecting an antipsychotic drug. If this is lacking, general principles should be used. These principles, based on structure-activity relationships and expected response, are outlined in the following section. Finally, the greater the clinician's familiarity with a given agent, the more likely that clinical experience will enter into the process of achieving optimal dosing.

DOSING CONSIDERATIONS

Estimated Equivalent Dosage

Although most commonly used antipsychotics are considered to have comparable therapeutic effect, they differ greatly in potency. Therefore, comparisons among these agents must be made based on equivalent doses, that is, relative potency. Table 1.2 lists approximate dose equivalents of commonly used agents based on a standard dose of 100 mg chlorpromazine.[4] For example, a 2 mg dose of fluphenazine has a therapeutic effect with an approximate equivalence of 100 mg of chlorpromazine, although the two drugs differ in side effects. Comparisons between drugs that ignore relative potency can result in erroneous clinical deductions about relative effectiveness.

Antipsychotics can be grouped into low-dose and high-dose agents. Low-dose treatment strategies involve high potency agents such as fluphenazine and haloperidol in relatively small dosages (for example, 5–10 mg per day). When the patient's symptoms can be controlled with a low dose, the long-term advantage of minimizing the risk of adverse long-term effects is achieved. The low-dose (high-potency) agents[5] include fluphenazine, haloperidol, thiothixene, and trifluoperazine while high-dose (low-potency) agents include chlorpromazine, thioridazine, mesoridazine, loxapine, and molindone. A low dose can be achieved with a low-potency agent by selecting a dose comparable to the high-potency agent.

Pharmacokinetic Factors

To optimize dosage adjustment, several pharmacokinetic principles of the antipsychotic drugs should be considered. These include:

TABLE 1.2. Antipsychotic drug dosing information.

Class	Generic Name	Adult Oral Daily Dosage Range (mg)			Single IM Dose[1]		Dosage Forms[2]	CPZ-EQ[3] Dose	CPZ-EQ Multiplier
		Maintenance	Acute, Severe	65+	Adult	65+			
1. Phenothiazines									
Aliphatic	Chlorpromazine	up to 800	up to 2000	up to 300	25–30	12.5–25	OS, OL, I	100	1
Piperidine	Mesoridazine	up to 300	up to 400	up to 200	25	12.5	OS, OL, I	50	2
	Thioridazine	up to 600	up to 800	up to 300	—	—	OS, OL	100	1
Piperazine	Fluphenazine HCl	up to 20	up to 40	up to 10	1.25–5.0	up to 2.5	OS, OL, I	2	50
	Fluphenazine Decanoate[6]	up to 25 q wk	—	up to 12.5 q wk	N/A	N/A	I	1.25 q wk	80
	Perphenazine	up to 32	up to 64(96)[4]	up to 32	4–10	2–6	OS, OL, I	10	10
	Trifluoperazine	up to 20	up to 60	up to 20	1–2	0.5–1	OS, OL, I	5	20
2. Thioxanthenes	Thiothixene	up to 30	up to 60(90)[4]	up to 30	2–4	1–2	OS, OL, I	5	20
3. Dihydroindolones	Molindone	up to 100	up to 225	up to 100	—	—	OS, OL	10	10
4. Dibenzoxazepines	Loxapine	up to 100	up to 250	up to 100	12.5–25	6.25–12.5	OS, OL, I	10	10
5. Dibenzodiazepines	Clozapine	up to 600	up to 900	—	N/A	N/A	OS	50	2
6. Butyrophenones	Haloperidol	up to 20	up to 40(100)[5]	up to 20	2–5	0.5–2.5	OS, OL, I	2	50
	Haloperidol	up to 300	—	up to 150	N/A	N/A	I	20	5
	Decanoate[6]	q month		q month	—	—	—	q month	—
7. Diphenylbutylpiperidines	Pimozide	.1–4 mg (child & adoles.) equivalent to 0.75–6.75 Haloperidol			—	—	OS	1.3[7]	77

[1] To control agitation, usually administered in 6-hour intervals.
[2] OS = oral solid, OL = oral liquid, I = injectable.
[3] Modified from reference 4. Estimated equivalent of a 100 mg dose of chlorpromazine.
[4] Dosages in parentheses have been used in selected severely ill patients but lack efficacy based on clinical trial data.
[5] Doses above 40 mg per day (2000 CPZ-EQ per day) should be closely monitored for behavioral toxicity in conjunction with plasma levels (range 5–15 ng/ml).
[6] Refer to Table 1.3 for Fluphenazine Decanoate and Table 1.4 for Haloperidol Decanoate conversions. Long-acting Decanoate products are only indicated for stabilized chronic psychosis.
[7] Data from study of Naruse et al., *Acta Paedopsychiatrica 48*: 173–184, 1982.

1. The high lipid solubility that permits passage across the blood-brain barrier
2. The relatively long elimination half-life $(t_{1/2})$. For example, chlorpromazine requires about 30 hours, on the average, for its plasma level to fall to one-half its level
3. The high apparent volume of distribution (e.g., about 20 L/kg for chlorpromazine) which correlates with the high brain concentrations that have been documented. Brain levels of some antipsychotics, for example, haloperidol, are ten to thirtyfold greater than concentrations in blood. Variation among antipsychotics is supported by brain/plasma ratios ranging from 1–2 : 1 for mesoridazine and thioridazine to 22–34 : 1 for haloperidol[6]
4. High binding to plasma albumin; for example, chlorpromazine is approximately 85% plasma bound.

Collectively, these factors predict that many antipsychotic agents have a relatively long duration of action and will be stored in body tissues for significant periods of time after dosing has stopped.

Plasma Level Monitoring

The use of plasma levels of the antipsychotics in routine clinical practice has been limited by:

1. The low plasma concentrations of these drugs necessitating sensitive detection methods;
2. The number of active metabolites that many agents produce; and
3. The poor correlation between plasma level and therapeutic response and the large interpatient variation.

The large interpatient variability is illustrated by the range of effective levels of chlorpromazine—from 30 to 350 ng/ml. This represents more than ten-fold variation in plasma concentration and makes plasma level monitoring a highly individualized process. Haloperidol assays (optimal levels of approximately 5–15 ng/ml) may hold greater promise because its single active metabolite offers greater specificity.[7] However, studies to indicate plasma level/response correlations in large populations of patients are needed before routine plasma level monitoring will be useful in optimizing drug therapy. Plasma levels can be effectively used to document noncompliance with a prescribed regimen, to rule out malabsorption (rare) when a patient requires large oral doses, and to rule out drug toxicity.[8] For example, to avoid drug toxicity for chlorpromazine and thioridazine, levels should be below 1000 ng/ml. For these purposes and for individual patient monitoring of clinical response, plasma level, and drug dose, the therapeutic ranges of selected agents that are recommended by the New York State Psychiatric Institute and Nathan Kline Institute Psychopharmacology Analytical Laboratories are presented under the specific drug information (by generic drug name) in Part III. For a listing of the drugs with available assays and their usually effective plasma level ranges see Part IV.

Dosing Guidelines

The protocol as outlined is based on general rules for dosing with the antipsychotics.

Initiate dosage* at the low end of the range, for example, 25 or 50 mg p.o. (25 mg IM) of chlorpromazine or the equivalent of another antipsychotic. Typical daily dose upper limits for the management of the chronic and acute, severe psychotic episode are listed in Table 1.2. With the chlorpromazine-equivalent (CPZ-EQ) multiplier list in the last column, one can calculate that a 20 mg fluphenazine HCl dose is approximately 20(50) or 1000 mg chlorpromazine equivalents. This allows an estimate of relative antipsychotic drug exposure. The patient is then observed for symptom control and side effects. Dosage is adjusted by regular assessment of the target symptoms. The length of the time between assessments for the nonemergency situation should reflect the time to steady state of the drug in question. A reasonable interval is 7 days for haloperidol ($t_{1/2}$, 24 hours) and chlorpromazine ($t_{1/2}$, 30 hours) based on their respective average half-lives.[9] However, more recent evidence indicates that the $t_{1/2}$ of haloperidol increases to 70 hours at 7 days[10] and may explain the past tendency to overshoot the optimal dose.

---

* Patients with no history of clinical exposure to the antipsychotics should receive a test dose. A test dose is defined as a single dose (initiated at the low end of the dose range) followed by close observation for 2–4 hours for the appearance of an allergic or other adverse reaction.

Acute Psychosis

Acute symptom control varies with the individual patient. Table 1.2 lists general guidelines for those less severely ill (generally outpatient) and those more severely ill (generally hospitalized), although these distinctions may blur. The more relevant issue concerns the degree of close monitoring and safety available for patients who may require protection from postural hypotensive, fainting or falling episodes, and excessive sedation. For each antipsychotic listed in Part III, a recommended dosage for adults is indicated. These dosages follow FDA package insert recommendations and reflect well documented clinical experience. However, in specific instances, doses above these guidelines are sometimes tried upon the review and approval of the facility's Medical Director. OMH guidelines provide general rules for dosing up to 2000 mg CPZ-EQ per day. Data from clinical investigations do not support consistently greater efficacy in doses exceeding 1800 mg CPZ-EQ per day,[2] although the most recent review of previous studies suggests lower doses: daily doses above 600 CPZ-EQ (10–12 mg of haloperidol) are not consistently associated with clinical improvement.[7] Two recent studies, one an open study in VA inpatients[11] and the second a rigorous, double-blind study in NYS OMH inpatients[12] offer specific support for reduced dosing of haloperidol. In the latter study of 111 patients, there was no consistent relationship between low, intermediate, or high plasma levels of haloperidol and clinical improvement. Patients in the high haloperidol plasma range tended to have more side effects. Similarly, in the VA study of 80 men with a DSM-III diagnosis of schizophrenia, patients did not respond better to 20 mg per day after two weeks than those receiving 5 or 10 mg per day. In addition, the elopement rate was 35% of the 20 mg per day group versus only 4% of those given the lower doses. Both studies concluded that the dosage of haloperidol should be lower than suggested by previous studies and current clinical practice.

Rapid neuroleptization is a technique introduced during the 1970s to shorten the time interval needed to control acute psychotic symptoms. Recent findings do not support its usefulness because efficacy (measured by decreased symptoms or hospital days) is not improved[13] and safety (measured by the frequency of serious adverse events) is considerably lessened.[14] Focal neuroleptization has been suggested as an alternative.[15] In this approach, a newly admitted psychotic patient who requires rapid intervention would receive an antipsychotic according to the following regimen:

Phase I: Introduce injectable low-dose antipsychotic (e.g., 2–5 mg haloperidol IM or other agent) in small rapid doses until the target symptoms are controlled, the patient is sedated or becomes cooperative with the treatment program. Control is usually achieved in 2 to 4 doses although doses up to 30 mg IM in 24 hours have been documented as safe in terms of EKG and blood pressure monitoring. Close patient observation during Phase I consists of pulse, blood pressure, and acute dystonic reaction monitoring. Close monitoring for other serious adverse reactions, for example, neuroleptic malignant syndrome and drug-induced catatonia, is also warranted.

Phase II: 12 to 24 hours after the symptom control is achieved, there is a switch to the same daily dose of medication by oral administration, although, strictly speaking, these are not pharmacologically equivalent doses.

Chronic Psychosis

For the chronic patient, dosage adjustment may be based on an estimate of the time required to achieve a plasma level concentration at steady state. Steady state is defined as approximately 5 times the elimination half-life of the drug. For chlorpromazine, intervals of 150 hours (about 6 days) would be needed to monitor the drug effect appropriately. This approach is particularly useful in the management of chronic psychotic disorders where the goal of current practice is to achieve symptom control at the lowest possible dosage to minimize long-term drug exposure (see tardive section next). Titrating the chronic patient's dose upward in 5 to 7 day intervals allows the maximum clinical response to emerge before the dose is increased. Daily doses exceeding 1000 mg CPZ-EQ show no advantage for most patients.[4] Doses in the range of 300–900 mg per day of chlorpromazine or its equivalent reflect an effective range for most chronic patients based on previous clinical investigations. The more recent review of Baldessarini et al.[7] found maintenance daily doses not greater than 600 mg of chlorpromazine (or 10 to 15 mg of haloperidol or fluphenazine) per day were likely to produce maximum beneficial effects.

Based on an approximate elimination half-life of 24 to 70 hours for haloperidol, a low-dose strategy for the chronic patient with less severe symptoms can be achieved without intramuscular injections. This approach consists of starting with oral low doses, for example,

5 mg of haloperidol (or other agent in equivalent dosage) repeated every hour until the patient's florid symptoms are controlled which often occurs well below 40 mg daily. Following stabilization for several days at this dosage range, a downward adjustment is started in 5 mg increments every 5 days until the patient is controlled at a reasonable maintenance level, typically 10 or 20 mg at bedtime. Some patients may not require continuous maintenance medication and alternative approaches include intermittent or targeted approaches such as those of Carpenter,[16] Herz,[17] and Davis.[18] Identifying schizophrenic patients who do not benefit from maintenance treatment is discussed by Buckley.[19]

Long-Acting Dosage Formulations

Fluphenazine decanoate and haloperidol decanoate are products in which an antipsychotic is esterified and suspended in sesame oil. The resulting depot injectable is long-acting and can provide a therapeutic response in patients for weeks or months. The advantages of this drug formulation include reduced patient and staff time devoted to drug administration and assured dosage in the patient who does not adhere to the prescribed medication regimen. Only patients who have been stabilized on a short-acting antipsychotic drug regimen are candidates for conversion to the long-acting formulation. To simplify the process further, the short-acting formulation should be of the same parent drug. Patients who have been stabilized on other short-acting agents can be converted to approximate chlorpromazine-equivalent doses of the parent drug, monitored for stable dosage and then switched to the long-acting form. In a series of studies evaluating the role of drug therapy in chronic schizophrenia, Hogarty et al.[20] illustrated the effectiveness of the combined role of long-acting neuroleptic along with social therapy in reducing relapse over time. At the same time, the research shows that drug noncompliance is not sufficient, by itself, to explain relapse among schizophrenic outpatients. Drug and social therapy are viewed as enabling fewer relapses than if the patient were deprived of both treatments.

Fluphenazine Decanoate. There is considerable controversy about the therapeutic plasma level-dose relationship of fluphenazine decanoate[21,22,23] and a lack of sufficient empirical data to clarify the conversion from oral fluphenazine doses to the long-acting form. Based on the findings of a 1976 multicenter, double-blind controlled study, the following rule was suggested for conversion of fluphenazine hydrochloride to decanoate:[24] 20 mg fluphenazine HCl are roughly equivalent to 25 mg fluphenazine decanoate every three weeks. This rule replaced other rules[25] and resulted in a considerably greater potency of the decanoate form than previously accepted. In several of the old rules, 25 mg weekly is equivalent to 1000 CPZ-EQ per day, while Chien and Cole published the least potent rule based on 17.3 mg fluphenazine enanthate weekly equivalent to 388 mg chlorpromazine.[26]

Because of the wide variation in the published conversion estimates, a survey of specialists in psychopharmacology was undertaken. Again, there was no clear consensus on the relationship between fluphenazine hydrochloride and decanoate. However, there was concordance on a relationship between the extremes of the earlier published rules. The fluphenazine hydrochloride to decanoate conversion rule suggested by Kane[27] (25 mg every 3 weeks of decanoate is equivalent to 665 CPZ-EQ per day) and the chlorpromazine-equivalent conversion rules of Davis[28] have been applied to develop Table 1.3.

To facilitate adaptation of clinical practice to the newer rule, doses should be restricted to smaller amounts or to longer time intervals between injections wherever clinically possible. As a guide to newer dosing, Table 1.3 lists the relative potency (expressed in chlorpromazine-equivalents) for the various dosing schedules of fluphenazine decanoate that are frequently encountered. These are theoretically determined values and should be interpreted as an approximation. Definitive values await more rigorously designed research studies. Single doses above 50 mg are no longer recommended and doses in the shaded portion of the table reflect high-dose exposures of equivocal efficacy.[22] Higher doses may be required for individuals who fail to be managed at lower doses and should be justified on an individual case basis. To use the table, locate a dose of oral fluphenazine in column 2 (e.g., 20 mg) and 3 (1000 CPZ-EQ mg) which is currently being used to control the patient's psychosis. Then read the weekly decanoate dose from column 1 (12.5 mg). This dosage would be administered every week. To lengthen the interval between doses to every 3 weeks, locate the CPZ-EQ dose in column 7 (1000) and read the decanoate doses in column 1 (37.5 mg). Thus, one can give 12.5 weekly or 37.5 mg every three weeks.

Haloperidol Decanoate.   The recommended conversion from oral haloperidol to decanoate is the following: 5 mg oral haloperidol per

TABLE 1.3. Equivalency table for fluphenazine decanoate (FPZ DEC) and fluphenazine hydrochloride (FPZ HCl) expressed in chlorpromazine equivalents (CPZ-EQ) according to the rule suggested by Kane.

(1) FPZ DEC	Dosing Schedule: Weekly		Q 2 Weeks		Q 3 Weeks		Monthly	
	(2) Oral FPZ HCl	(3) CPZ-EQ*	(4) Oral FPZ HCl	(5) CPZ-EQ	(6) Oral FPZ HCl	(7) CPZ-EQ	(8) Oral FPZ HCl	(9) CPZ-EQ
6.25 (.25 cc)	10	500	5	250	3.3	165	2.5	125
12.5 (.50 cc)	20	1000	10	500	6.6	333	5.0	250
18.75 (.75 cc)	30	1500	15	750	10	500	7.5	375
25 (1.00 cc)	40	2000	20	1000	13.3	665	10	500
37.5 (1.50 cc)	*60*	*3000*	30	1500	20	1000	15	750
50 (2.00 cc)	*80*	*4000*	40	2000	26.3	1315	20	1000
62.5 (2.50 cc)	*100*	*5000*	*50*	*2500*	33.3	1665	25	1250
75 (3.00 cc)	*120*	*6000*	*60*	*3000*	40	2000	30	1500
87.5 (3.50 cc)	*140*	*7000*	*70*	*3500*	*46.6*	*2330*	35	1750
100 (4.00 cc)	*160*	*8000*	*80*	*4000*	*53.3*	*2665*	40	2000

* FPZD mg doses in column 1 are converted to estimated equivalent daily oral fluphenazine doses (column 2) and to estimated daily chlorpromazine-equivalent doses (column 3) by using the empirical rule suggested by Kane and the chlorpromazine equivalents of Davis. Doses in italicized area are *not* recommended.

day is equivalent to 50 mg haloperidol decanoate every month. A ten-fold increase is suggested for the initial conversion from oral to long-acting haloperidol injected at monthly intervals. Short-acting oral or injectable haloperidol can be used for additional symptom control during the initial three month period before it is reasonable to assume that a steady state dosing pattern is achieved. Maximum doses of 300 mg per administration are suggested because of the limited clinical experience above this dose[29] and doses above 200 mg should be cautiously used with close monitoring. In Table 1.4 a list of commonly used haloperidol decanoate doses and approximate equivalent doses of oral haloperidol and chlorpromazine are provided.

In 1993, the maximum monthly dose of haloperidol decanoate was raised from 300 to 450 mg per month. The new maximum dose assumes that a stabilized patient is receiving this amount as the *sole* antipsychotic agent. Combinations of this high maximum dose with oral daily doses is not intended by researchers advocating this dose. Furthermore, high combined dosing contradicts recent rigorous studies, and, until further efficacy supports the need for high combined usage, it is not recommended. Consequently, for patients receiving more than one psychotropic (excluding an antiparkinson agent), the better-established maximum dose of 300 mg per month is advised.[30]

Clozapine for Treatment-Resistant Schizophrenia

In February 1990, clozapine was made available in the United States for the management of severely ill schizophrenic patients. The FDA-approved package insert guidelines state that because of the significant risk of agranulocytosis and seizures associated with its use,

TABLE 1.4. Equivalency table for haloperidol decanoate and oral haloperidol expressed as actual and chlorpromazine-equivalent doses.

HPL Dec	Q Monthly	HPL Q Day	CPZ-EQ
50 mg	(1.0 cc)	5 mg	250 mg
100	(2.0 cc)	10	500
150	(2.5 cc)	15	750
200	(3.0 cc)	20	1000
250*	(3.5 cc)	25	1250
300*	(4.0 cc)	30	1500

* Most patients can be managed with doses of 200 mg or less per month.[31] Dose above 200 mg require cautious, close monitoring. Severe parkinsonism was observed in a clinical trial of doses of 200 mg per injection.[32]

clozapine should be used only when the available antipsychotics are insufficient either because of lack of response or intolerable side effects at the doses that are needed.

Clozapine is an atypical antipsychotic of the dibenzodiazepine type and has weak dopamine-blocking activity in addition to antiadrenergic, antihistaminic, antiseritonergic, and potent anticholinergic effects. The elimination half-life is estimated at 12 hours and twice a day dosing is suggested. The information on relative potency of clozapine to existing antipsychotics is limited at this time to the suggestion of a 1:2 ratio.[53] Thus, patients being switched from 1200 mg per day of chlorpromazine should receive approximately 600 mg per day clozapine, assuming equivalent clinical response.

There is a 1 to 2% incidence of agranulocytosis with clozapine in comparison to the 1 in 10,000 (0.01%) risk with other antipsychotics. This risk prompted the FDA to require assurance that adequate clinical laboratory monitoring is provided during clozapine therapy. To meet this need the manufacturer developed the Clozaril Patient Management System (CPMS) and required weekly WBC counts for as long as clozapine treatment continues. An unbundling of laboratory and drug prices occurred in the spring of 1991 and various alternative monitoring programs have been developed. Regardless of how the monitoring occurs, weekly review is mandated. When WBC counts fall below 3500/mm or there is a substantial drop below baseline, even though the count is above 3500/mm, or if immature forms are present, a CBC and differential count should be done immediately. Results of this testing will determine if continuation of clozapine is appropriate. If the total WBC count falls below 3000/mm or the granulocyte count below 1500/mm, clozapine therapy must be interrupted immediately.

Indications.   Clozapine is indicated **only** for patients with severe schizophrenia who have failed to respond adequately to a series of other antipsychotic medications. Severity has been defined in terms of both symptoms and functional capacity.

Guidelines for Administration

Patient selection: Before applying to the Drug Monitoring Committee for approval to use clozapine, patient consent should be sought. The patient and family should be engaged in a discussion of the benefits and risks of clozapine. The Clozapine Screening Form (see Part IV) has operational criteria for patient selection. These criteria are: confirmed diagnosis of schizophrenia, evidence of failure of previous antipsychotic drug trials (at least three trials of antipsychotics of at least 1000 CPZ-EQ per day in two classes for six weeks each) and severity of symptoms (BPRS greater than 45) and dysfunctioning (previous admissions and length of hospitalizations). In addition, clozapine can be considered for those patients for whom an effective dose of existing antipsychotics cannot be achieved due to intolerable adverse effects. The effect of clozapine on existing tardive dyskinesia remains to be determined.[34]

Exclusion criteria: Among those who should not receive clozapine are patients who have certain medical problems, particularly blood and myeloproliferative disorders, AIDS-related complex (ARC) or AIDS, severe CNS depression from any cause, and concurrent medications known to suppress bone marrow functioning, such as carbamazepine or zidovudine (AZT). Conditions requiring medical clearance are seizure disorders, cardiac, hepatic, renal disorders, narrow-angle glaucoma, and prostatic hypertrophy.

Dosing: There is considerable experience of successful clinical management with average daily doses of approximately 400 mg.[35] Initial doses of 25 mg 1 to 2 times a day are continued with daily dose increments of 25 to 50 mg until a target dose of 300 to 450 mg is achieved by the end of two weeks. Subsequent dosage increments should be made no more than 1 or 2 times a day in increments of 25 mg to minimize the risk of hypotension, seizure, and sedation. The dose range is 300 to 900 mg and doses above 600 mg per day are a Severity level 2 exception. The rationale for justifying doses above 600 mg per day is based on empirical data indicating that increased seizures are associated with doses exceeding 600 mg per day.[36] Discontinuation of the drug should be done in gradual decrements over a period of not less than two weeks. For example, from 600 to 450 on day 1, 300 on day 5, 150 on day 10 and discontinue on day 14.

Response: The clinical and economic issues surrounding this drug require that the decision to continue its use should be made at six weeks, to justify entering a period of increased risk of agranulocytosis.[37] To insure that favorable patient response is not missed, evaluation may be continued through 12 weeks of treatment. Response to clozapine is measured by the change from baseline symptom and side effect scores. (See Part IV for Clozapine Evaluation Form.) Clozapine should be continued beyond 12 weeks only when documented improvement occurs. Benefit should be assessed by control of positive and negative symptoms or control of violence as well as social and vocational functioning and readiness for discharge. Drug discontinuation may be warranted due to side effects or adverse events. Finally, patient cooperation factors such as refusing phlebotomy and intolerance of side effects may result in the decision to discontinue the drug.

Side effect monitoring: Regular observation for the following major reported side effects is required: seizures, sedation, anticholinergic effects, hypotension, tachycardia, fever, and hypersalivation.

Reported clinical experience with clozapine emphasizes the need for intensive side effect monitoring. Of particular concern are the risk of sudden hypotensive episodes which may result in falls, excessive secretion (salivary and bronchial, possibly contributing to respiratory infections), and hyperthermia. Clozapine may elicit delirium. This is particularly likely to occur in older patients on higher dosages.[38]

Clozapine drug interactions: Although the safety of clozapine in combination with other drugs has not been systematically evaluated, it should *not* be used with other agents having a known potential to suppress bone marrow function (e.g., carbamazepine). Other interactions involve additive CNS depressant and anticholinergic effects and protein binding displacement effects. Recent reports of two deaths in America[39] and the previous report of severe, life-threatening respiratory arrests in Europe[40] have led to an FDA approved box warning on the combination of benzodiazepines with clozapine. To avoid unnecessary risk, benzodiazepines should be avoided and alternatives (e.g., chloral hydrate (oral) or sodium amytal (injections)) are recommended for periodic management of acute agitation or aggressive behavior. Because of the limited information on the safety of this combination and the availability of suitable alternatives, benzodiazepines and clozapine are listed as a Severity 1 drug interaction.

Augmentation of Antipsychotic Treatment

Clozapine's marketing for treatment-resistant schizophrenia is reflective of a trend in recent years related to the growing pool of psychotic patients described as resistant to standard antipsychotics. Estimates of 10 to 20% have been given[41] and have led to protocols for augmentation of standard antipsychotic with benzodiazepines and other psychotropics. A discussion of antipsychotic augmentation is located in

Chapter 5, pp. 155, 161. The role of lithium to augment antipsychotics for treatment-resistant schizophrenia is not well established because the data are sparse. A recent study[42] reported no benefit from a 4-week single-blind randomized study of lithium augmentation of antipsychotic. The two study groups did not differ in age, gender, severity of symptoms, length of hospitalization, or concurrent antipsychotic dosage.

Antipsychotic Drug Discontinuation

Because of the long half-life and extensive body storage of the antipsychotics, abrupt drug withdrawal may not produce symptoms for weeks for short-acting agents or months for depot formulations. However, clinical reports of serious, usually transient adverse effects after abrupt discontinuation are known and the possibility of receptor disuse supersensitivity has been suggested. Whatever the mechanism, some time is needed for neurotransmitters and drug receptors to readjust to pre-drug level of function. The patient must also adjust to physiological, psychological, and behavioral functioning at reduced or pre-drug levels.

   Clinical reports[43] of withdrawal symptoms include: (a) transient flu-like symptoms, dysphoria, and dyskinesias that may disappear after four to six weeks. Cholinergic rebound including symptoms of nausea, vomiting, and perspiration is one suggested mechanism;[44] (b) The unmasking of tardive dyskinesia which is frequently observed; and (c) an increase in psychotic and behavioral symptoms (behavioral toxicity or psychotoxicity) which has been described more elaborately as supersensitivity psychosis[45] and disputed.[46] Debating the concept and its mechanism is, perhaps, less important than recognizing the importance of this problem to patients and clinicians. Differentiating these behavioral symptoms from clinical decompensation is challenging and requires careful attention to the nature of the symptoms and to their temporal pattern. Tapering, that is, a gradual reduction of medication, at a rate of about 25% every 5 to 7 days, may minimize these problems. Changing no more than one drug at a time also aids this process of ruling out behavioral change due to drug therapy. See Part IV for a sample longitudinal monitoring form.

Tardive Dyskinesia Monitoring

A detailed analysis of the research findings and clinical experience on drug-induced tardive dyskinesia was published by the American Psychiatric Association in 1980 and updated in 1992.[47] A summary of the APA position is reproduced below. The selection and dosing of antipsychotic drugs should be guided by efforts to relieve symptoms at the lowest effective dose.

American Psychiatric Association Task Force Summary on Tardive Dyskinesia Monitoring

Tardive dyskinesia (TD) is a syndrome of choreoathetoid and/or other involuntary movements that may affect mouth, lips, tongue, arms, legs or trunk; TD is associated with the long-term (usually greater than six months) use of neuroleptics (antipsychotics).

The proportion of patients developing abnormal involuntary movements is believed to increase with increasing length of treatment or total exposure to neuroleptics. The syndrome can develop after relatively brief (3 to 6 months) treatment periods at low dosages. However, it is impossible at present to identify which patients are at risk.

In cross-sectional studies, the majority of cases are judged to be mild (i.e., not obvious to the untrained observer or subjectively troublesome to the patient).

Identification and diagnosis are complicated by the fact that neuroleptic drugs may mask TD symptoms. Drug discontinuation or dosage reduction may reveal previously masked symptoms.

Although there are few long-term follow-up studies, the condition does not appear to be generally progressive. The prevalence of tardive dyskinesia increases with age.

The course of the condition is difficult to predict in individual patients. Though some cases will have symptoms resolved, a proportion of patients will show persistent dyskinesias even after drug discontinuation.

There is no established treatment for tardive dyskinesia.

Recommendations for the use of neuroleptics

Long-term use of neuroleptics is primarily indicated in schizophrenia, paranoia, childhood psychoses, and certain neuropsychiatric disorders such as Gilles de La Tourette's syndrome and Huntington's disease. Short-term administration (less than six months) is justifiable in many cases of acute psychotic episode, severe mania or agitated depression and certain organic mental disorders. Rarely, patients with other conditions who have not responded to alternative treatment may benefit from the use of neuroleptics.

All patients receiving long-term treatment require periodic evaluation and documentation of continued need and benefit. Along with monthly evaluations, a more careful review of changes over longer periods, e.g., 3 to 6 months, is useful.

The benefits and risks of long-term neuroleptic treatment should be discussed with patients and families and their informed consent to treatment documented.

Patients should be examined routinely (at least quarterly) for signs of tardive dyskinesia.

Neuroleptic drugs should be administered at the lowest effective dosage. Attempts at dosage reduction and in some cases (depending upon clinical state, past history, etc.) drug discontinuation should be considered.

Additional Pharmacodynamic and Clinical Principles

Factors related to the absorption, distribution, metabolism, and elimination of the antipsychotics are known to alter the dose-response pattern. In this section, the following factors are discussed: age, pregnancy and lactation, and additional factors such as smoking, dosing schedules, noncompliance, missed doses, cost considerations, and informed consent.

Liver and Kidney Function as a Dosing Factor

Since the antipsychotics are liver metabolized and extensively plasma bound, patients with either compromised liver function or those in renal failure require reduced doses. Therefore, an assessment of the patient's liver and kidney function should be made before treatment begins by reviewing hepatic function tests (e.g., SGOT, SGPT, bilirubin) and kidney function tests (e.g., BUN and creatinine). (See Part IV for Automated Chemistry—20 Laboratory Reference Values.)

Age as a Dosing Factor

Children and Adolescents.   Children and adolescents require specialized pharmacotherapeutic consideration. Chapter 7 provides a detailed review of dosing considerations in this patient population. Dosing guidelines for children and adolescents are provided for those agents for which there is sufficient clinical experience. These dosing and plasma level guidelines are also listed in the formulary section by generic drug name.

Geriatric Patients. Impaired psychotropic drug metabolism with advancing age has been reported. The reduced rate of metabolism is presumed to be due in large part to a gradual decline in the activity of the microsomal drug metabolizing enzymes as well as to the loss of liver mass in relation to body size. Impaired liver function accompanying congestive heart failure and reduced renal function also may contribute to a slowing of the biotransformation of drugs. In addition, increased receptor sensitivity has been hypothesized as a possible explanation for the need for dosage reductions in the aging patient.[48]

Specific dosing recommendations are provided for some agents listed in the formulary section. Moreover, a general principle followed by many experts in psychogeriatrics is to initiate dosage at one-third to one-half that of younger adults. Pharmacokinetic factors play a role in optimal dose selection for the elderly patient.[49] If an increase in dose is necessary, it should be made gradually at intervals that are much longer than the five half-lives suggested for younger adults. For example, if the average adult patient required 150 hours (30 multiplied by 5) to reach steady state, the geriatric patient would be expected to require many more hours for the same dose because of the longer time to metabolize the drug. In addition, the possibility of reduced kidney and liver function, reduced lean body mass, along with the general fragility of the elderly, can increase the half-life of a drug in an elderly person leading to an augmented clinical response and more severe side effects.

Safety during Pregnancy and Lactation

The antipsychotic drugs are not established as safe and efficacious for the pregnant or lactating patient. Since the drugs cross the blood brain barrier and the blood-placental barrier, there is a risk of fetal malformation.[50] Two cases of severe limb malformation have been reported following maternal use of haloperidol early in the first trimester of pregnancy. Clinical use in pregnant patients for whom nondrug alternatives are not sufficient, should be restricted to low, divided doses and avoided during the first trimester and last weeks of pregnancy and during lactation. Since patients are unaware of the exact time a pregnancy starts, counseling women of child-bearing age to avoid pregnancy while receiving haloperidol is suggested. At the time of admission, pregnancy status should be noted on the Admission Assessment form.

Medication Administration Factors

Smoking. Clinical investigations have demonstrated that the dominant effect of smoking on tissue is enhanced drug metabolism caused by induction of hepatic microsomal enzymes.[51] However, wide interindividual variability exists and thus it remains a selective and unpredictable effect. In one study, age was factored into the relationship between drug/liver metabolism and smoking. The findings suggest that the enhanced liver metabolizing ability of smokers was not sustained with increasing age.[52]

Although widespread smoking is observed among hospitalized mentally ill patients, there are no empirical data to suggest altering the dosage of antipsychotic or other liver-metabolizing drugs according to the patient's smoking habits. Recent work on the antidepressant plasma levels of smokers versus nonsmokers is discussed in Chapter 4.

Dosing Schedules. The relatively long half-life of the antipsychotic drugs makes possible once- or twice-a-day dosing schedules unless specific effects, for example, daytime sedation of a low-potency agent, are desired. The reduced number of administrations per day is associated with increased compliance and cost savings in terms of drug dollars and nursing administration. The reduction in medication errors has been documented. Another advantage of single bedtime dosing is that it may permit the peak plasma level to occur during sleep, thereby reducing patient discomfort associated with side effects.

Route of Administration. The dosing relationship between an injectable short-acting agent and its oral counterpart is based on the bioavailability of the drug. Bioavailability refers to the proportion of an oral dose available after the absorption phase has occurred. For example, 60 to 70% of an oral dose of haloperidol is estimated to be absorbed. This empirically-derived relationship is similar to the clinical rule of thumb that the injectable short-acting dose should be about one-third less than the oral dosage.[53]

Noncompliance. Antipsychotic drug noncompliance is a significant problem, particularly in the long-term management of chronic psychotic patients. Increasing the patient's role in drug decision-making is an approach that may reduce covert noncompliance in the apparently cooperative patient.[54] If the patient's cooperation can be gained in determining past and current experience with dysphoria and other unsatisfactory drug-related effects, a therapeutic alliance may lead to an improved drug dosing/compliance pattern. Together, the physician and the patient may be able to produce a longitudinal record of dose-response that will optimize drug dose and minimize the need for the patient to refuse medication. Written drug information sheets which are designed for the patient or caregiver can assist in longitudinal monitoring. Sample sheets are included in Part IV.

Given the wide interpatient variability in dose-response, it is difficult to estimate the pharmacologic effect of missed doses. Falloon described satisfactory drug compliance for outpatients in the maintenance phase of treatment as two-thirds of the intended doses.[55] From a psychodynamic standpoint, the refusing patient may be expressing dissatisfaction with the treatment program manifested as simply "forgetting."

Informed Consent and the Involuntary Patient.   Until the recent past, the psychotic patient was presumed to be unable to make informed decisions about treatment. However, since the 1970s, a number of court decisions have upheld the right of the involuntarily committed psychiatric patient to refuse antipyschotic drug treatment in nonemergency situations.[56] In June 1986, in the *Rivers vs. Katz* decision,[57] the right to refuse treatment for hospitalized patients in New York State was affirmed. Assuming nonemergency conditions, that is, when the patient is not in imminent danger of harm to self or others, the refusing patient who requires antipsychotic medication must undergo a court hearing to determine competency to refuse treatment.

Cost Considerations.   Table 1.5 lists the prices for comparable doses (relative to 100 mg of chlorpromazine) of commonly used antipsychotics based on a study in a New York State facility.[58] Short-acting injectable dosage forms are considerably more costly than oral forms in terms of drug product prices, staff time and patient comfort. Long-acting fluphenazine and haloperidol formulations vary considerably in price and must be considered separately. For a patient receiving 5 mg per day oral maintenance fluphenazine HCl, the price is approximately $9.75 per month compared with $0.68 per fluphenazine decanoate injection (12.5 mg per 4 weeks) from a multidose vial or $7.20 from a unit dose syringe.

A 5 mg per day oral dosage of haloperidol at a cost of approximately $8.40 per month is nearly doubled ($14.30) when converted to haloperidol decanoate (50 mg per month). Long-acting haloperidol is nearly twice the price of long-acting fluphenazine. The most costly

TABLE 1.5. Relative cost of frequently used antipsychotic drugs.[4]

	Oral Solid	Oral Liquid	Injection
Chlorpromazine HCl	100 mgUD = .05	.09	25 mg = .96
Clozapine[4]	50 mgUD = 2.26	—	—
Fluphenazine HCl	2 mgUD = .48[1]	.16	1 mg = .53
Fluphenazine Decanoate[2]	—	—	5 mg q 4 wk = 2.62
Haloperidol	2 mgUD = .02 (1.6 equivalents rounded to 2)	.08	1 mg = .15
Haloperidol Decanoate[3]	—	—	20 mg q 4 wk = 20.19
Loxapine	10 mgUD = .23	.61	5 mg = .75
Mesoridazine	50 mgUD = .64	.62	12.5 mg = 1.46
Molindone	10 mgUD = .54	.33	—
Perphenazine	10 mgUD = .34	.65	2.5 mg = 2.28
Thioridazine	100 mg = .11	.09	—
Thiothixene	5 mg = .12	.07	1.25 mg = .36
Trifluoperazine	5 mg = .22	.38	1.25 mg = 2.29

[1] Multiple dosage units to make the total dose indicated.

[2] Oral to depot equivalence may vary depending on conversion rule used. Theoretical dose based on equivalence rule: 20 mg/d HCl equivalent to 12.5 mg Decanoate q 1 wk.[27] Multidose vial price was used to calculate this cost. If the unit dose product is used the cost is $14.61 for any amount up to 25 mg.

[3] Oral to depot equivalence is based on the rule: 5 mg oral equivalent to 50 mg Decanoate q 4 wk.[31] Table of Equivalence from JM Davis, defined as the dose required to achieve therapeutic efficacy of 100 mg of chlorpromazine. See Kaplan and Sadock's Textbook of Psychiatry, 4th edition, Vol. 2, p. 1495–1498.

[4] New York state OMH prices for both contract and non-contract items effective February 1993.

antipsychotic to date is clozapine which is currently marketed at a price 10 times standard antipsychotic agents without including the cost of weekly laboratory services to monitor hematologic lab values.

SIDE EFFECT MONITORING

Monitoring patients for side effects of the psychotropic agents is complicated by the difficulty of behavioral toxicity. Behavioral toxicity refers to an adverse behavioral symptom produced by a drug. For example, at toxic doses phenytoin is known to cause mental confusion and delirium. In the psychiatric patient, these symptoms are often indistinguishable from symptoms (e.g., agitation and disordered thinking) that may be target symptoms of the underlying psychotic illness.

To assist in differentiating drug and illness-based symptoms the following rules are recommended:

1. Reduce medication regimens to the fewest drugs possible
2. Make one drug dose change at a time whenever possible
3. Make a review of body systems at each clinical assessment in which a dosage change is made.

In this way, symptom changes may be more easily associated with dosage changes and behavioral toxicity may become apparent.

Side effects may be classified into patient-specific, class-specific, and drug-specific. Patient-specific undesired effects are usually rare events reported in a particular patient. Class-specific effects are commonly reported side effects associated with a class of drugs. Many of these effects are dose-dependent side effects (i.e., as the dose increases the side effect increases). Drug-specific effects are observed with a single agent in a class.

The FDA provides a reporting form (FDA 1639) to detect new serious adverse reactions or drug-drug interactions during the postmarketing surveillance of drugs. A sample form is provided in Part IV.

Patient-Specific Adverse Reactions

Allergic reactions and individual case reports fall into this category. Rash, fevers, and decreased WBC are examples of allergic reactions. In the past, allergic reactions involving hepatotoxicity were frequently associated with chlorpromazine. Typically, obstructive jaundice, fever, and eosinophilia were reported. Patients who are given an antipsychotic for the first time should be carefully monitored at the beginning of treatment for these rare but serious reactions. In addition to pretreatment laboratory tests for hepatic and renal function, a CBC should be obtained to monitor for allergic reactions involving the hematologic and immunologic systems.

Class-Specific Side Effects

The major categories of frequently occurring side effects of the antipsychotic agents are presented next to serve as a checklist of major effects that are associated with these drugs. A full discussion of the prevalence, pathophysiology, and treatment of these effects is available in the textbooks of Kaplan and Sadock[4] and Baldessarini.[59]

Neurologic Effects

1. Extrapyramidal Side Effects (EPSE) and Neuroleptic Malignant Syndrome
   - Acute dystonic reactions: torticollis, retrocollis, opisthotonus, oculogyric crisis, laryngospasm[60]
   - Drug-induced parkinsonism: tremor, festinating gait, rigidity, hypokinesia, drooling
   - Akinesia, classically defined as stupor or extreme hypokinesia, is commonly used to refer to hypokinesia[61]
   - Akathisia, the subjective feeling of inner restlessness, or inability to sit still. Akathisia is often mistaken for new symptoms of anxiety, insomnia, irritability and agitation
   - Tardive dyskinesia, defined as abnormal involuntary movements of face, mouth, lips, tongue and extremities usually after long-term (greater than six months) antipsychotic exposure
2. Neuroleptic Malignant Syndrome (NMS). See discussion in Chapter 2.
3. Seizure-Threshold Lowering. Clozapine-treated patients were reported to have a 2.8% incidence of seizures and life-table analysis predicted a cumulative 10% risk of seizures after 3.8 years of treatment.[62] This incidence is twice as high as was found in a similar retrospective review of standard antipsychotics (1.2%).[63] Both studies found a dose effect (i.e., as dosage increased the incidence of seizures increased).

Anticholinergic Effects

These may be divided into acute and chronic effects.

1. Acute: Acute anticholinergic poisoning can be a life-threatening event that involves both central and peripheral blockade of cholinergic receptors. Among the symptoms are restless agitation, confusion, perhaps seizures, hyperthermia, dry and sometimes flushed skin, tachycardia, sluggish, perhaps dilated pupils, decreased bowel sounds and often acute urinary retention (Baldessarini[59] (p. 74)).

Other acute effects:
   - Reactions in patients with narrow angle glaucoma (rare form of glaucoma)
   - Acute reactions in patients with prostatism

- Acute reactions in patients susceptible to decreased gastrointestinal functioning can lead to paralytic ileus and fatalities have occurred
2. Chronic:
   - Blurred vision, loss of accommodation
   - Gastrointestinal effects of decreased bowel function and constipation
   - Genito-urinary effects of urinary retention, altered ejaculatory function, and priapism
   - Dry mouth, nasal congestion
   - Decreased sweating
   - Cardiac effects: commonly, tachycardia, hypotension

Endocrine Effects

1. Hyperprolactinemia
2. Galactorrhea
3. Gynecomastia
4. Amenorrhea
5. Sexual dysfunction: reduced libido, impotence
6. Weight gain
7. Glucose metabolism disturbances e.g., high or prolonged glucose tolerance test curves

Hematologic Effects

1. Leukopenia
2. Agranulocytosis: incidence <.01%, associated more frequently with low potency phenothiazines; 1–2% prevalence reported for clozapine

Central Depressant Effects

1. Lethargy. Lethargy progressing to loss of consciousness as the dose is increased has been observed. Akinesia is often mistaken for new symptoms of lethargy, withdrawal and depression or the "negative syndrome."
2. Anxiety and Akathisia. These drug-induced symptoms are difficult to distinguish from an exacerbation of the underlying illness. Dosage reduction is the first consideration in treating drug-induced anxiety and akathisia. Ancillary drug treatment of this problem is discussed in Chapter 2.

3. Depressed Mood. Depressive symptoms (syndrome) and suicide[64,65] are reported in schizophrenia patients who receive antipsychotics. There is controversy about whether these symptoms are (1) part of the underlying acute phase of the schizophrenic disorder; (2) emerge in the postpsychotic period; (3) are part of the "negative syndrome" or (4) are induced by antipsychotic drugs or doses which exceed the patient's need. This issue presents a considerable challenge for clinicians and researchers.

Cardiovascular Effects

1. Alpha-adrenergic blocking (orthostatic hypotension)
2. Cardiotoxic effects: sudden death (see below: Other)
3. Conduction defects

Thermoregulatory Dysfunction

Heat stroke

Dermatologic and Ophthalmic Reactions with Phenothiazines

1. Phototoxicity (severe sunburn)
2. Lens and cornea pigmentation (prevalence of 27% was reported for phenothiazines in a clinical study[66])

Other

1. Sudden unexplained deaths in young psychiatric patients receiving antipsychotics have been reported sporadically since the 1960s. There are plausible hypotheses related to (1) the sudden cessation of cardiovascular competence on an arrhythmogenic or hypotensive basis or both cardiovascular effects[67] of the drugs, (2) the anticholinergic effect of loss of the gag reflex, choking, and subsequent asphyxia and (3) seizure-threshold lowering. Research design difficulties and the varying validity and reliability of the autopsy reports as the primary source of information on unobserved deaths are partly responsible for a paucity of systematic study. Study findings supporting both increased[64] and decreased[65] mortality rates in psychiatric patients, in general, compared with an age- and sex-matched general population sample, serve as a reminder of the need for further research on a serious, unresolved question.
2. Laryngeal edema, laryngospasm,[60] bronchospasm, angioedema.
3. Asphyxia: loss of gag reflex.

Drug-Specific Adverse Reactions

Thioridazine

The reports of pigmentary retinopathy associated with thioridazine at doses greater than 1000 mg per day led to a package insert warning and a maximum daily dose of 800 mg. Since mesoridazine is the active metabolite of thioridazine but has been used less extensively than the parent compound, a comparable dosage ceiling is recommended (maximum daily dose of 400 mg).

DRUG-DRUG INTERACTIONS

Within-Class Interactions

Drug interactions can be divided into *within-* and *between-* class types. Within class drug interactions are combinations of 2 or more antipsychotics. The practice is not recommended because the desired clinical effects (reduction of psychotic symptoms) do not differ among the antipsychotics although patients on 2 drugs are subjected to a wider range of side effects. Also, the use of drug combinations makes dose optimization more difficult.

Between-Class Interactions

Between class drug interactions involving the antipsychotic agents typically involve additive effects (e.g., central depressant effects with combinations involving the benzodiazepines, other sedatives, or hypnotics). However, in recent years, there is evidence of additional mechanisms that may be responsible for drug toxicity. Some of these effects are believed to occur by increasing the plasma level of the antipsychotic (e.g., addition of high dose propranolol, which is *not* recommended).[68, 69] For these reasons, longitudinal monitoring of combinations should be assessed by sequential evaluation periods. Period 1 should consist of baseline single drug (plasma level) and behavior ratings followed by period 2 ratings for the addition of a second agent to the drug regimen. The inclusion of patient ratings of satisfaction in this model would better establish dose ranges that are safe, effective, and acceptable to the patient. See Part IV for a sample longitudinal monitoring form.

Specific Between-Class Interactions

A review of common drug-drug interactions and their clinical significance in psychiatric disorders is provided by Glassman and Salzman[70] and their mechanisms are detailed in Hansten and Horn's textbook.[71] The major drug interactions in which the antipsychotics are involved include the following classes of drugs:

Antacids, Antidiarrheals.   Delayed absorption; avoid co-administration within a 2-hour interval.

Lithium.   Case reports of severe neurotoxicity in combination with antipsychotics have been reported. Nevertheless, the use of antipsychotics, especially haloperidol, with lithium remains one of the most controversial issues. Despite widespread use, there are reports of drug intoxication on doses that separately are within the therapeutic range.[72] Evidence is accumulating from experimental animal studies that supports a drug interaction for antipsychotics and lithium. These studies indicate an increase in brain tissue levels of the primary drug after addition of the second agent. For example, the addition of lithium to a haloperidol regimen resulted in significantly higher levels of haloperidol than before the lithium was added.[73] Similarly, the *in vitro* addition of thioridazine and other phenothiazines to a lithium regimen produced increased intracellular lithium levels.[74]

Tricyclic Antidepressants.   Combined use with antipsychotics has produced increased serum levels of each drug presumably due to competitive inhibition of liver metabolizing enzymes.

Barbiturates, Phenytoin, and Carbamazepine.   Combined use with antipsychotics may produce decreased serum levels of the individual antipsychotics due to liver enzyme induction. However, reductions of haloperidol plasma levels on the order of 50%[75] and 60% were accompanied by clinical deterioration in only a minority ($\frac{1}{6}$) of patients. Thus, the clinical significance of this interaction is mixed. It is possible that "clinical improvements" that are anecdotally reported when ancillary agents such as carbamazepine are added to the regimen of patients receiving high doses of antipsychotics may be explained by the decreased serum level of the antipsychotic agent,[75,76,77] an effect which could more easily and safely be achieved by an antipsychotic dose reduction.

Benzodiazepines. The combination with antipsychotics has been used for short-term (less than 4 months) relief of anxiety and insomnia in patients with psychotic disorders. Sedating antipsychotics administered at night may avoid the use of this combination which becomes a problem for some patients when attempts are made to discontinue the benzodiazepine. Recent advocacy of the intermittent use of oral or injectable benzodiazepine (such as lorazepam) in acute psychosis is based on an attempt to reduce the overall antipsychotic dose exposure. The use of this approach should be justified on the basis of reduced, low-dose antipsychotic management.[78] For further discussion of combined antianxiety-antipsychotic therapy see Chapter 5.

Alcohol. Combined use of alcohol with antipsychotics increases central depressant effects.

REFERENCES

1. Baldessarini RJ: Drugs and the treatment of psychiatric disorders, in Goodman and Gilman's Pharmacological Basis of Therapeutics, 8th ed. Edited by Gilman AG, Rall TW, Nies AS, Taylor P. New York, Pergamon Press, 1990

2. Shader RI (ed): Manual of Psychiatric Therapeutics. Boston, Little Brown, 1975

3. Ayd FJ, Jr.: Rational pharmacotherapy: Once-a-day drug dosage. Dis Nerv Sys 1973; 34:371–378

4. Davis JM: Antipsychotic drugs, in Comprehensive Textbook of Psychiatry/IV, 4th ed, vol 2. Edited by Kaplan HI, Sadock BJ. Baltimore, Williams & Wilkins, 1985

5. Baldessarini RJ, Katz B, Cotton P: Dissimilar dosing with high-potency and low-potency neuroleptics. Am J Psychiatry 1984; 141:748–752

6. Sunderland T, Cohen BM: Blood to brain distribution of neuroleptics. Psychiatry Research 1987; 20:299–305

7. Baldessarini RJ, Cohen BM, Teicher M: Significance of neuroleptic dose and plasma level in the pharmacological treatment of psychoses. Arch Gen Psychiatry 1988; 45:79–91

8. Rivera-Calimlim L, Hershey L: Neuroleptic concentrations and clinical response. Ann Rev Pharmacol and Toxicol 1984; 24:361–386

9. Cooper TB: Plasma level monitoring of antipsychotic drugs. Clinical Pharmacokinetics 1978; 3:14-38

10. Froemming JS, Lam YWF, Jann MW, Davis CM: Pharmacokinetics of haloperidol. Clin Pharmacokinet 1989; 17:396–423

11. Van Putten T, Marder SR, Mintz J: A controlled dose comparison of haloperidol in newly admitted schizophrenic patients. Arch Gen Psychiatry 1990; 47:754–760

12. Volavka J, Cooper TB, Czobor P, Bitter I, Meisner M, Laska E, Gastanega P, Krakowski M, Chou JC-Y, Crowner M, Douyon R: Haloperidol blood levels and clinical effects. Arch Gen Psychiatry 1991; 49:354–361

13. Ericksen SE, Hurt SW, Chang S: Haloperidol dose, plasma levels and clinical response: A double-blind study. Psychopharm Bull 1978; 14:15–16

14. Bollini P, Andreani A, Colombo F, Bellantuono C, Beretta P, Arduini A, Galli T, Tognoni G: High-dose neuroleptics: Uncontrolled clinical practice confirms clinical trials. Brit J Psychiatry 1984; 144:25–27

15. Tupin J: Focal neuroleptization: An approach to optimal dosing for initial and continuing therapy. J Clinical Psychopharmacology 1985; 5:15S–21S

16. Carpenter WT, Heinrichs DW: Intermittent pharmacotherapy of schizophrenia, in Drug Maintenance Strategies in Schizophrenia. Edited by Kane J. Washington DC, American Psychiatric Press, 1984, pp 69–82

17. Herz M, Melville C: Relapse in schizophrenia. Am J Psychiatry 1980; 137:801–805

18. Davis JM, Andriukatis S: The natural course of schizophrenia and effective maintenance drug treatment. J Clin Psychopharmacology 1986; 6:2S–10S

19. Buckley P: Identifying schizophrenia patients who should not receive medication. Schizophrenia Bull 1982; 8:429–432

20. Hogarty GE, Schooler NR, Ulrich R, Mussare F, Ferro P, Herron E: Fluphenazine and social therapy in the aftercare of schizophrenic patients. Arch Gen Psychiatry 1979; 36:1283–1294

21. Glazer WM: Depot fluphenazine: Risk/benefit ratio. J Clin Psychiatry 1984; 45:28–35

22. Brown WA, Silver MA: Serum neuroleptic levels and clinical outcome in schizophrenic patients treated with fluphenazine decanoate. J Clin Psychopharmacology 1985; 5:143–147

23. Marder SR, Hawes EM, van Putten T, Hubbard JW, McKay G, Mintz J, May PR, Midha KK: Fluphenazine plasma levels in patients receiving low and conventional doses of fluphenazine decanoate. Psychopharmacology 1986; 88:480–483

24. Schooler NR, Levine J: The initiation of long-term pharmacotherapy in schizophrenia: Dosage and side effect comparisons between oral and depot fluphenazine. Pharmakopsych Neuro-Psychopharm 1976; 9:159–169

25. Ereshefsky L, Saklad SR, Davis CM, Jann MW, Burch NC, Richards A: Clinical implications of fluphenazine pharmacokinetics. Paper presented at 1984 American Psychiatric Association meeting

26. Chien C, Cole JO: Depot phenothiazine treatment in acute psychosis: A sequential comparative clinical study. Am J Psychiatry 1973; 130:13–18

27. Kane JM: Personal communication, 1987

28. Davis JM: Comparative doses and costs of antipsychotic medication. Arch Gen Psychiatry 1976; 33:858–861

29. Gelders YG, Reyntjens AJM, Ash CW, Aerts TJ: 12-month study of haloperidol decanoate in chronic schizophrenic patients. Intl Pharmacopsychiatry 1982; 17:247–254

30. Ereshefsky L, Toney G: What are the recently approved dosing guidelines for haloperidol decanoate and how will they affect clinical practice? Relapse Summer 1993; 3:1

31. Kane JM: Dosage strategies with long-acting injectable neuroleptics, including haloperidol decanoate. J Clin Psychopharmacology 1986; 6:20S–23S

32. Magyar I, Bitter I: Periodische dosierung der depot neuroleptika: Prophylaxe dir nebenwirkungen? in Problematik und Behandlung Psychotisch Kranker. Edited by Haase JH. Perimed, Erlangen, 1987

33. Kane JM, Honigfeld G, Singer J, Meltzer H, Clozaril Collaborative Study Group: Clozapine for the treatment-resistant schizophrenic. Arch Gen Psychiatry 1988; 45:789–796

34. Naber D, Lepping M, Grohmann R, Hippius H: Efficacy and adverse effects of clozapine in the treatment of schizophrenia and tardive dyskinesia—a retrospective study of 387 patients. Psychopharmacology 1989; 99:S73–S76

35. Marder SR, VanPutten T: Who should receive clozapine? Arch Gen Psychiatry 1988; 45:865–867

36. Lieberman JA, Kane JM, Johns CA: Clozapine: Guidelines for clinical management. J Clin Psychiatry 1989; 50:329–338

37. Honigfeld G, Patin JR, Singer J: The Clozaril Monograph Vol 1. Sandoz Pharmaceuticals, East Hanover NJ, August, 1987

38. Bitter I: Personal communication, 1990

39. Citizens Health Research Interest Group, Washington, DC: Personal Communication, 1991

40. Sassim N, Grohmann R: Adverse drug reactions with clozapine and simultaneous application of benzodiazepines. Pharmacopsychiatry 1988; 21:306–307

41. Davis JM, Schaffer CB, Killian GA, Kinard C, Chan C: Important issues in the drug treatment of schizophrenia. Schizophrenia Bull 1980; 6:70–87

42. Collins PJ, Larkin EP, Shubsachs AP: Lithium carbonate in chronic schizophrenia—a brief trial of lithium carbonate added to neuroleptics for treatment of resistant schizophrenic patients. Acta Psychiatr Scand 1991; 84:150–154

43. Gardos G, Cole JO, Tarsy D: Withdrawal syndromes associated with antipsychotic drugs. Am J Psychiatry 1978; 135:1321–1324

44. Lieberman J: Cholinergic rebound in neuroleptic withdrawal syndromes. Psychosomatics 1981; 22:253–254

45. Chouinard G, Jones BD: Neuroleptic-induced supersensitivity psychosis: Clinical and pharmacological characteristics. Am J Psychiatry 1980; 137:16–21

46. Palmstierna T, Wistedt B: Tardive psychosis: Does it exist? Psychopharmacology 1988; 94:144–145

47. American Psychiatric Association: Tardive Dyskinesia, Task Force Report 18. Washington DC, APA Press, 1980; Tardive Dyskinesia: A Task Force Report of the American Psychiatric Association. Washington, DC, American Psychiatric Association, 1992

48. Ban TA: Psychopharmacology for the Aged. Basel, S. Karger, 1980

49. Greenblatt DJ, Abernathy DR, Shader RI: Pharmacokinetic aspects of drug therapy in the elderly. Therapeutic Drug Monitoring 1986; 8:249–255

50. Kopelman AE, McCullar FW, Heggeness L: Limb malformations following maternal use of haloperidol. JAMA 1975; 231:62–64

51. Jusko WJ: Role of tobacco smoking in pharmacokinetics. J Pharmacokinetics and Biopharmaceutics 1978; 6:7–39

52. Vestal RE, Wood AJ: Influence of age and smoking on drug kinetics in man: Studies using model compounds. Clin Pharmacokinetics 1980; 5:309–319

53. Forsman A, Ohman R: Applied pharmacokinetics of haloperidol in man. Curr Therapeutic Research 1977; 21:396–411

54. Blackwell B: Treatment adherence: A contemporary overview. Psychosomatics 1979; 20:27–35

55. Falloon IR, Boyd JL, McGill CW, Razani J, Moss HB, Gilderman AM: Family management in the prevention of exacerbations of schizophrenia: A controlled study. New Eng J Med 1982; 306:1437–1440

56. Brooks AD: The consitutional right to refuse antipsychotic medications. Bull Am Acad Psychiatry and Law 1980; 8:179–221

57. Zito JM, Craig TJ, Wanderling JS: New York under the *Rivers* decision: An epidemiologic study of drug treatment refusal. Am J Psychiatry 1991; 148:904–909

58. Zito JM, Craig TJ, Wanderling JA, Siegel C: Pharmaco-epidemiology in 136 hospitalized schizophrenic patients. Am J Psychiatry 1987; 144:778–782

59. Baldessarini RJ: Antipsychotics, in Chemotherapy in Psychiatry: Principles and Practice, 2nd ed. Cambridge, Harvard University Press, 1985

60. Koek RJ, Pi EH: Acute laryngeal dystonic reactions to neuroleptics. Psychosomatics 1989; 30:359–364

61. Rifkin A, Quitkin F, Klein DF: Akinesia. Arch Gen Psychiatry 1975; 32:672–674

62. Devinsky O, Honigfeld G, Patin J: Clozapine-related seizures. Neurology 1991; 41:369–371

63. Logothetis J: Spontaneous epileptic seizures and electroencephalographic changes in the course of phenothiazine therapy. Neurology 1967; 17:869–877

64. Achté KA, Lönnquist J, Piirtola O, Niskasen P: Verlauf and prognose schizophrener psychosen in Helsinki, in Psychiatrische Verlaufsforschung. Edited by Schwimmelpennig H. Huber, Bern, Stuttgart, Wien, 1980

65. Drake RE, Ehrlich J: Suicide attempts associated with akathisia. Am J Psychiatry 1985; 142:499–501

66. Barsa JA, Newton JC, Saunders JC: Lenticular and corneal opacities during phenothiazine therapy. JAMA 1965; 193:10–12

67. Zugibe FT: Sudden death related to the use of psychotropic drugs, in Legal Medicine. Edited by Wecht CH. Philadelphia, Saunders WB, 1980, pp 75–90

68. Peet M, Bethell MS, Coates A, Khamnee AK, Hall P, Cooper SJ, King DJ, Yates RA: Propranolol in schizophrenia I. Comparison of propranolol, chlorpromazine and placebo. Brit J Psychiatry 1981; 139:105–111

69. Silver JM, Yudofsky SC, Kogan M, Katz BL: Elevation of thioridazine plasma levels by propranolol. Am J Psychiatry 1986; 143:1290–1292

70. Glassman R, Salzman C: Interactions between psychotropic and other drugs: An update. Hosp and Community Psychiatry 1987; 38:236–242

71. Hansten PD, Horn JR: Drug Interactions and Updates, 6th ed. Philadelphia, Lea and Febiger, 1990

72. Miller F, Menninger J: Correlation of neuroleptic dose and neurotoxicity in patients given lithium and a neuroleptic. Hosp and Community Psychiatry 1987; 38:1219–1221

73. Nemes ZC, Volavka J, Lajtha A, Cooper TB, Sershen H: Concurrent lithium administration results in higher haloperidol levels in brain and plasma of guinea pigs. Psychiatry Research 1987; 20:313–316

74. Pandey GN, Goel I, Davis JM: Effect of neuroleptic drugs on lithium uptake by the human erythrocyte. Clin Pharmacol Therapeutics 1979; 26:96–102

75. Kahn EM, Schulz SC, Perel JM, Alexander JE: Change in haloperidol level due to carbamazepine—a complicating factor in combined medication for schizophrenia. J Clin Psychopharmacol 1990; 10:54–57

76. Arana GW, Goff DC, Friedman H, Ornsteen M, Greenblatt DJ, Black B, Shader RI: Does carbamazepine-induced reduction of plasma haloperidol levels worsen psychotic symptoms? Am J Psychiatry 1986; 143:650–651

77. Kidron R, Averbuch I, Klein E, Belmaker RH: Carbamazepine-induced reduction of blood levels of haloperidol in chronic schizophrenia. Biol Psychiatry 1985; 20:219–222

78. Arana GW, Ornsteen ML, Kanter F, Friedman HL, Greenblatt DJ, Shader RI: The use of benzodiazepines for psychotic disorders: A literature review and preliminary clinical findings. Psychopharm Bull 1986; 22:77–87

CHAPTER 2

Neuroactive Agents for the Management of Antipsychotic-Related Effects

INTRODUCTION

Adverse neurological effects following the use of an antipsychotic were recognized soon after the introduction of chlorpromazine in the early 1950s and led to frequent use of anticholinergic agents to reduce the acute and gradually emergent extrapyramidal side effects (EPSE). The partial mechanism of these effects is believed to involve antipsychotic drug blockade of nigrostriatal dopamine receptors inducing a dopamine deficiency that leads to imbalance in the dopaminergic-cholinergic system.[1] EPSE once were thought to signal an effective dose of the antipsychotic but clinical studies have shown that clinical efficacy is not dependent on the production of EPSE.[2]

Routine Usage: Pro and Con

There has been considerable controversy[3] during the past thirty years over the need for routine use of the antiparkinson agents due to: (1) variable occurrence of the EPSE; (2) questions about the need for continuous long-term usage; (3) questions about the validity of withdrawal studies; (4) clinical reports and studies suggesting a reduction in effectiveness of the antipsychotic by the addition of an anticholinergic agent; (5) conflicting studies on the physicochemical basis for the putative drug interaction between antipsychotics and anticholinergic agents; (6) concerns about the safety of routine anticholinergic agents. Each of these topics will be described in further detail.

1. Variable occurrence of the EPSE. The reported incidence of antipsychotic-induced EPSE varies from 4 to 50% according to the definition of the EPSE, type, and dose of antipsychotic and patient population.[4] Lehmann[5] reported a 30% prevalence of EPSE with aliphatic and piperidine phenothiazines (low-potency agents) and up to 50% with other (high-potency) antipsychotics. In another early study, a significantly higher incidence of EPSE

occurred with higher dosage of antipsychotic alone compared with lower dosed combination treatment of an antipsychotic and barbiturate.[6] Among recent studies, the prevalence of dystonic reactions was shown to be lower as the dose exposure of the antipsychotic decreased. Whereas high doses of haloperidol, for example, produced a 38% incidence of dystonia, lower doses (mean of 558 mg per day) of chlorpromazine produced no reactions.[7] Rapidly administered high doses of antipsychotics have been recognized as risk factors for EPSE.[8]

2. Need for continuous usage.

PRO: Klein[9] is a strong proponent of the initial use of antiparkinson agents at the time of antipsychotic initiation as well as continuous usage beyond the two weeks suggested by Baldessarini[10] or the alternative, treatment-emergent approach of Simpson and colleagues.[11] Baldessarini indicates that treatment for up to two weeks offers protection against the risk of dystonia in 90% of cases. The arguments for routine, continuous use are based on: (1) concerns about under-recognition of behavioral symptoms such as akinesia. For example, a placebo controlled withdrawal study of procyclidine resulted in a significant increase in akinesia among the placebo-treated patients after three weeks of treatment;[12] (2) the belief that antiparkinson agents do not interfere with antipsychotic drug effects, including plasma level changes; and (3) continuation avoids the risk of a reduction in compliance that might follow from a frightening adverse drug experience.

CON: This view is based on an individualized decision to continue anticholinergics based on the benefits of routine antiparkinson agents, favored for those with known risk factors such as young male patients, as against the risks of cognitive dysfunction and unnecessary usage. In this view, routine initiation and continuous prophylaxis is thought to be unnecessary except in high-risk patients and specific situations. It is expected that in the future, antiparkinson use will be even less necessary because antipsychotic dosing patterns are changing. Thus, the popularity of high-potency antipsychotic agents and rapid neuroleptization (now obsolete) may partly explain the past trend toward increased usage of anticholinergic agents. The current emphasis on low-dose treatment strategies will probably lead to reduced need for antiparkinson drug, particularly if strategies for conservative antiparksinsonian drug usage are adopted.[13]

It is also important to recognize that the antiparkinson agent may not be effective in relieving EPSE. For example, in the study of Smarek,[7] 12% of those treated with high doses of an antipsychotic and an antiparkinson given in combination failed to be protected against dystonia. The control of akathisia is even lower.

3. Study confounder. In antiparkinson withdrawal studies such as that of Rikfin et al.[12] which support the continuing use of antiparkinson agents during antipsychotic maintenance therapy, the question of confounding of results due to withdrawal effects limits their validity. Short-term effects (cholinergic rebound) due to withdrawal of the antiparkinson agents may be misinterpreted as a continuing need for relief of the EPSE.

4. Reduced effectiveness of the combination. European clinical reports suggested that the therapeutic effect of the antipsychotic was counteracted by the antiparkinson agent.[14] This practical approach was followed by more rigorous studies[15, 16] that further supported the reduction in effectiveness of the antipsychotic by the addition of an anticholinergic agent.

5. Drug interaction. Following initial reports of antipsychotic plasma level lowering by anticholinergic,[17] 2 studies with a more rigorous design reported no significant decrease in chlorpromazine[18] or butaperazine[19] levels with antiparkinsonian agents. In the latter study, radioimmunoassay procedures were used to measure anticholinergic activity after a 2-week drug exposure period.

In a recent example of a more definitive study of the anticholinergic interaction with antipsychotics, procyclidine was shown to significantly reduce plasma levels of chlorpromazine ($p < .005$), haloperidol ($p < .0005$), and fluphenazine decanoate ($p < .01$) in chronic psychotic patients and to be reversed upon withdrawal of the anticholinergic agent.[20] Moreover, contrary to the expectation that this might reduce clinical response, no changes in BPRS were noted. This suggests that the more parsimonious alternative approach of reducing the dosage of antipsychotic agent might be achieved in some of these chronically medicated patients who receive both agents.

It is plausible that both a receptor effect and a plasma level effect are responsible for the clinical effects of anticholinergics on antipsychotic-treated patients. Until this theory is ultimately validated, the recent interaction findings supporting antipsychotic dosage reduction as the *first* consideration in reducing EPSE, deserve clinical consideration.

Further research using controlled, crossover designs in both acute and chronic patients who exhibit EPSE at baseline must be done before a definitive relationship between plasma level, clinical response and EPSE symptom control for these 2 drug classes emerges.

6. Safety concerns. Perhaps most important are the concerns about safety. For example, the additive effects of these agents in producing central anticholinergic toxicity,[21] the impairment of swallowing that may produce choking, asphyxia, and death[21] and deficits such as memory impairment that may result from chronic anticholinergic therapy[22] and from antipsychotics with anticholinergic activity.[23] Emergency, life-threatening central anticholinergic intoxication has occurred at usual doses of an antipsychotic, antiparkinson, and tricyclic antidepressant—presumably due to additive effects.[24]

Prevalence of Antiparkinson Agents

Studies on the extent of antiparkinson usage that were conducted a decade ago estimated that the prevalence of anticholinergic usage was 30 to 40% of antipsychotic-treated patients.[25, 26] Continuous usage for more than six months has been documented in 50% of long-term patients.[25] In a similar population, computerized monitoring and educational feedback to prescribers was shown to significantly reduce the usage of these agents.[27]

Anticholinergic drug overuse has been suggested by the findings from clinical studies of successful anticholinergic drug withdrawal from chronic psychiatric populations.[28] Unnecessary usage was inferred from the finding that there was less than 10% recurrence of EPSE after withdrawing an anticholinergic agent from patients receiving a combined anticholinergic-antipsychotic regimen for more than 3 months. Similarly, in a 4-week double-blind study of chronic schizophrenic patients, 28 patients matched on age, sex, WAIS

Vocabulary score, and the antimuscarinic potency of their psychoactive drugs were randomized to benztropine or placebo and observed for 4 weeks after a 2-week adjustment period on the study drug.[29] Improved memory after withdrawal of anticholinergic was inferred from the increased Wechsler Memory Scale scores in the placebo group. Only 14% of the patients who demonstrated signs of clinical decompensation (measured by BPRS ratings) along with increased EPSE (measured by Simpson Angus Rating Scale for EPSE) required resumption of the benztropine. These findings assumed that a difference in akinesia was detectable based on Simpson Angus clinical rating scores. The studies support the benefit of trial discontinuations in patients receiving antiparkinson agents continuously for more than 12 weeks.

Half to two-thirds of patients receiving anticholinergic agents with antipsychotics probably do not require them, although it is not clear who those patients are. Therefore, identifying characteristics that increase the risk of EPSE, such as previously having a dystonic reaction, male gender, younger age group, high potency antipsychotic and relatively high dosage, would help to justify their use. On the other hand, groups at high risk for adverse anticholinergic effects, such as the elderly and those receiving a low-potency agent, are less justifiable for co-administration at the time an antipsychotic is initiated.

In summary, until further evidence supports the case for routine antiparkinson agent use, routine prophylactic use in not recommended. Reducing routine prophylactic prescribing is advocated because of complexities with somatic and behavioral toxicity, the latter being particularly difficult in the psychiatric patient who is not well-known to the prescribing physician.[30] Secondly, there are difficulties of discontinuation after continuous use for periods of more than 12 weeks.[10] Such problems make systematic evaluation of drug therapy very complicated.

Extrapyramidal Side Effects (EPSE) and Anticholinergic Agents

Before presenting specific drug selection information (see next section), this section will present definitions and general information relevant to prescribing neuroactive agents. Extrapyramidal side effects are common to all the antipsychotics but low-potency agents (chlorpromazine, thioridazine, mesoridazine) have a balance of weak D-2 receptor blocking effect plus high cholinergic receptor blocking that tends to reduce the incidence of EPSE and obviate the need for extrinsic anticholinergic medication. High-potency agents (fluphenazine, haloperidol, thiothixene) have high D-2 receptor blocking effect and low intrinsic anticholinergic activity and therefore are more likely to produce EPSE. EPSE risk increases with increasing dose regardless of potency type and with the rate of dosing changes.

Typically there are 3 major categories of extrapyramidal effects produced by antipsychotic-induced imbalance in the dopaminergic-cholinergic brain pathways for which anticholinergic drug therapy is used. These are dystonia, parkinsonism, and akathisia, in order of decreasing efficacy.

Acute Dystonic Reactions

Acute dystonic reactions may be manifested as the following: (a) oculogyric crisis—defined as rolling of the eyes upward, (b) opisthotonus—arching of the back, (c) torticollis—neck twisting sidewards, and (d) retrocollis—neck twisting backwards. These acute reactions tend to occur early in treatment, are dramatic in onset and may be very frightening to the uninformed patient or family observer. Fortunately, these reactions respond rapidly to injections of an anticholinergic agent. Patient and family education regarding the possibility of these reactions eliminates the fright from unexpected effects.

Parkinsonism

Parkinsonian symptoms consist of bradykinesia, rigidity, and resting tremor which may progress to akinesia, gait disturbances (shuffling), and drooling. A late onset type of EPSE is rabbit syndrome which is characterized by perioral movements and was estimated to occur in 2.3% of a chronically medicated psychiatric inpatient population.[31] Antipsychotic agent without an anticholinergic drug therapy was responsible for the effect that disappeared upon procyclidine administration (dechallenge) and reappeared upon readministration (challenge). Rabbit syndrome is differentiated from tardive dyskinesia by its favorable response to anticholinergic agents. Dysphagia, or difficulty swallowing, is a symptom of Parkinsonism and may be caused by antipsychotic-induced blockade of the proximal pharyngeal and esophageal musculature. A guide for evaluating antipsychotic-induced dysphagia has been developed.[32]

Akinesia is defined as decreased spontaneity in movement and speech. In the 1970s, it was identified as an under-recognized drug-induced symptom that is often relieved in nonchronic patients by an antiparkinson agent.[33] Antipsychotic-induced akinesia is difficult to distinguish from negative symptoms of schizophrenia and depression.[34] Negative symptoms include alogia, amotivation, social withdrawal, flattened affect, and attentional dysfunction. The syndrome, described as "akinetic depression in schizophrenia"[35] may be misdiagnosed as post-psychotic depression, a new illness symptom that would lead to additional psychotropic medication—typically a tricyclic antidepressant with strong additive anticholinergic activity in itself.[36] Thus, if the anticholinergic used to reduce antipsychotic-induced akinesia is not successful, there may be further anticholinergic effects from the tricyclic agent that sets up a risk of central anticholinergic toxicity. To avoid this difficulty, protocols for systematic drug changes are needed.

To answer this need, one approach suggests that whenever the clinical symptoms permit, trial reductions in the antipsychotic should be made in gradual decrements of, say, not more than 25% at intervals of not less than 5 to 10 days. For depot products, the time interval for adjustments is considerably longer and 4-month intervals for haloperidol decanoate and 6-month periods for fluphenazine decanoate are suggested as averages for time to re-establish steady state after a dosage change is made. When dosage reduction fails to control EPSE, efforts are then directed at assessing the benefits and risks of anticholinergic therapy in the individual patient.[9]

On a research level, criteria for differentiating negative symptoms, depression and antipsychotic-induced side effects must be worked out and then applied to practice settings before a straightforward approach occurs. Several authors[34, 37] discuss differentiation of akinesia, depression, and negative symptoms. Interpreting their approach regarding drug therapy, it appears that antidepressant usage is reserved for the patient whose "depressive" symptoms are improved with antidepressant drug usage *after ruling out* (1) the option of a dose lowering of the antipsychotic, and (2) improvement by adding anticholinergic. The symptoms that are unimproved by antidepressant become categorized as negative symptoms by exclusion.

Akathisia

Akathisia, which is defined as motor restlessness and anxiety, and may manifest itself as pacing to relieve the sensation, is often accompanied by dysphoria—sometimes profound. The increased risk of violence and suicide emphasizes the importance of this drug-induced symptom. There have been efforts to diagnose this subjective effect in a structured manner with increased validity and reliability.[38] This approach has led to distinctions between the voluntary movements of akathisia and the involuntary leg movements of tardive dyskinesia.[39] Akathisia usually occurs early in treatment and may follow rapid increases in dose.[40] Akathisia usually is only partly relieved by drugs with anticholinergic activity such as benztropine and diphenhydramine. It is relatively common, occurring in at least 20% of antipsychotic-treated patients. When anticholinergics fail and the severity of the akathisia cannot be controlled by changes of antipsychotic drug or dose, other agents such as benzodiazepines,[41] propranolol, a beta-adrenergic blocking agent[42,43] and clonidine, an alpha$_2$ adrenergic agonist,[44] have been tried.

Clinical investigators emphasize the need for distinctions between akathisia, which requires dose reduction of the antipsychotic or addition of an anticholinergic or other agent, and increased anxiety, agitation, and uncooperative behaviors, which suggests the need for increased antipsychotic dosing.[41] When perceived as increased symptoms of anxiety and resistance to treatment, akathisia leads to increased antipsychotic dosing and further misery for the patient. Akathisia, measured by independent assessment with structured EPSE rating scales, was prevalent in 74% of 27 patients receiving high-dose antipsychotic ($\geq$ 1700 CPZ-EQ per day). Akathisia should be considered when there is an increase in aggressive, uncooperative behaviors coincident with increased antipsychotic dosage.[45] Acute akathisia can be so disabling that attempted suicide was reported as an effort to relieve it.[46] The misery of akathisia is further underscored by the experience of antipsychotic drug volunteers.[47,48] Reductions in patient compliance associated with EPSE, particularly akathisia are well-documented.[49]

Neuroleptic Malignant Syndrome and Other Severe Neurological Effects

Among the more severe neurological effects associated with antipsychotic drug usage there is pharyngo-laryngeal spasm[50] which can be life-threatening. There is a small but growing experience with the severe thermoregulatory dysfunction which is called neuroleptic malignant syndrome (NMS).[51,52] Whereas 60 cases had been reported worldwide by 1980, there were an additional 53 cases reported in the subsequent five years. This suggestion of its increasing occurrence has led to retrospective estimates of its prevalence. For example, Pope et al.[53] found 1.4% one year-prevalence of definite or probable NMS in a review of 500 antipsychotic-treated patients in a large psychiatric hospital. Overall these studies argue for an increasing trend in NMS wherever high-potency agents are used in high doses, although definitive studies require prospective study of a large cohort and consistency in the operational definition of NMS.

NMS is a life-threatening event and the currently reported mortality estimate is 22%.[54] The major manifestations are rigidity, altered consciousness, elevated creatine phosphokinase (CPK) levels and sometimes fever. Minor manifestations include fluctuating tachycardia, altered blood pressure, tachypnea, sweating, coarse tremor or rigor and leukocytosis. Immediate emergency supportive care including discontinuation of antipsychotics is standard practice. Anticholinergic agents fail to relieve the syndrome. There are reports that abrupt withdrawal of high dose multiple anticholinergics precipitated an NMS-like crisis in Parkinsonian patients.[55] Thus, immediate discontinuation of the antipsychotic and gradual discontinuation of the anticholinergic is appropriate. More heroic drug interventions that have been partially successful include dopamine agonists such as bromocriptine up to 20–60 mg per day[56] and dantrolene.[51]

The current literature emphasizes appropriate dosing of antipsychotic agents as a means of avoiding the risk of NMS. This perspective is partly based on viewing NMS as the most extreme type of extrapyramidal toxicity. Thus, the NMS risk may be increased by initiating very high doses or by rapid neuroleptization, especially if given intramuscularly.[54] Beside the risks associated with rapid neuroleptization, the practice is not recommended (see Chapter 1) because there is no greater efficacy than with conventional dosing.[8] As an alternative, the protocol suggested by Tupin[57] utilizes small doses of injectable haloperidol adjusted to a satisfactory clinical response (maximum of 30 mg) during the first 24 hours and then converted to the same oral dose for daily administration beginning on the following day.

Individuals with a history of NMS require extreme caution in future drug dosing. Depot formulations are not suggested and lithium should be used cautiously.[58] Succinylcholine and drugs with anticholinergic properties such as tricyclic antidepressants have been shown to provoke or worsen NMS or the related syndrome called malignant hyperthermia.[59]

DRUG SELECTION

Frequently Used Agents

Table 2.1 lists the commonly used agents along with product formulations available and the usual dose range. Anticholinergic agents are synthetic analogs of the atropine-type alkaloids and are comparable in pharmacologic effect. Selection is empirical since there are no efficacy studies comparing the various classes or agents for the treatment of antipsychotic-induced neurological effects. Anticholinergic agents such as benztropine have been most often used for EPSE, extending their use beyond the treatment of idiopathic parkinsonism.[60] Effectiveness of the anticholinergics for EPSE was demonstrated by the inverse correlation of plasma anticholinergic activity (measured by radioimmune activity assay) and EPSE.[61] In recent years, diphenhydramine, originally introduced as an antihistamine and also used as a sedative-hypnotic, was recognized to have some anticholinergic activity and has been successfully used instead of the more potent anticholinergic agents. In psychiatry, diphenhydramine usage has greatly expanded based on this single effect.

Currently, the studies of other pharmacologic agents to relieve EPSE mainly involve case reports and small samples and generally lack rigor. Propranolol is being increasingly used in clinical practice

TABLE 2.1. Agents frequently used in the management of the extrapyramidal side effects of antipsychotic agents and atypical agents for use when common agents are not indicated.

Primary Action	Generic Name	Brand Name	Product Form[a]	Daily Dose Range (mg) 18–64 Yr	65+ Yr
Anticholinergic	benztropine	Cogentin	O,I	1–8	1–4
	biperiden	Akineton	O,I	2–6	1–4
	procyclidine	Kemadrin	O	6–20	3–10
	trihexyphenidyl	Artane	O,L	5–15	2–6
Antihistaminic	diphenhydramine	Benadryl	O,L,I[b]	25–100	25–50
Beta-blocker	propranolol[c]	Inderal	O	20–120	10–60
Dopaminergic	amantadine	Symmetrel	O,L	100–300	100–200

[a] Product forms: Oral solid (O), liquid (L), and injectable (I).

[b] Both IM and IV dosing are used to control acute dystonic reactions. See text for injectable dosing guidelines.

[c] For akathisia only; also, IV benzodiazepines have been used.

for akathisia and tremor yet the data supporting its use are meager. Racemic (d,l) propranolol blocks both β_1 and β_2 receptors and was shown to be superior to β_2 selective blockers (e.g., metoprolol[62]). D-propranolol lacks β-adrenergic receptor blockade and was studied to determine the role of β-blockade in alleviating neuroleptic-induced akathisia. A crossover, double-blind study[63] of d-propranolol versus placebo in 11 patients resulted in no change of scores for either group. When subsequently treated with racemic-propranolol, 8 of the 11 patients showed improvement in akathisia scores. The authors concluded that β-receptor blockade contributes to the effect of propranolol in akathisia. Overall, the evidence supporting the efficacy for this FDA unlabeled indication of propranolol is based largely on unblinded observation in small samples. For example, there is an open (unblinded) study[43] of 14 patients evaluated for a short duration. The positive improvement in akathisia was counterbalanced by the lack of effect against parkinsonism. Propranolol treatment of akathisia is a situation that introduces the complexity of managing a 3-drug class combination consisting of antipsychotic, antiparkinson agent and beta-blocker. In addition, the risk of propranolol-induced depression, a well-known problem in the medical literature, may be increased[64] and produce behavioral toxicity that cannot be easily identified in the psychiatric patient. Until further clinical efficacy and safety data emerge on propranolol, these regimens should be reserved for the severely disabled patient who fails to be managed by dose reductions or addition of anticholinergic or benzodiazepine. Additional double-blind comparative data with baseline measures of akathisia and comparable antipsychotic dosage, perhaps conducted in a naturalistic setting, would help to answer questions about the efficacy of propranolol for EPSE. Long-term safety questions, particularly in combination with multiple psychotropic agents, await further usage. If propranolol is added to a patient's regimen, close pulse and blood pressure monitoring is indicated. Intravenous diazepam was reported to be as effective as intravenous diphenhydramine in relieving acute dystonia and akathisia in 27 patients. It is reserved for patients who cannot be treated with anticholinergic agents.[42]

Amantadine is an antiviral agent that has been used by neurologists for parkinsonian patients who develop tolerance to regular use of other agents. The use of amantadine in drug-induced EPSE was evaluated in a double-blind comparison with benztropine and while fewer anticholinergic side effects (dry mouth, constipation, blurred vision, difficulty in urination, etc.) were reported for the amantadine-treated patients, there was more excitement reported among them.[65] Comparable efficacy was reported for the two agents. However, despite its potency, neurologists report that amantadine produces only limited, short-term efficacy in parkinsonism and is considerably more expensive than the first-choice agents.[60] Most limiting of amantadine's side effects (and of other dopamine agonists (for example, L-dopa and bromocriptine) is the production of psychosis in the nonpsychiatric Parkinson Disease patient[60] and the exacerbation or recurrence of psychosis in psychiatric patients.[66] In an open trial of 30 patients[67] treated with neuroleptic and benztropine, BPRS ratings were significantly elevated after switching patients from benztropine to amantadine. The most severely disturbed patients were likely to have worsening psychotic symptoms. Usual routine clinical monitoring is inadequate for distinguishing drug-induced increases in psychotic behavior and therefore these agents are of limited use in psychiatric populations. Until there is further evaluation of the advantages, amantadine should be reserved for those with severe EPSE in whom anticholinergics are not indicated (e.g., those with narrow angle glaucoma, reduced GI motility, and urinary retention).

Anticholinergic toxicity (confusion, dependent edema, hot dry skin, dilated pupils) was reported in Parkinson's Disease patients upon introduction of amantadine to the regimen of ineffective anticholinergic drug.[68] The combination is not recommended in psychiatric patients without intensive side effect monitoring of anticholinergic effects and evidence of the failure of simpler regimens to successfully treat the EPSE.

Dopamine Agonists

Table 2.2 lists dopamine agonists that are reserved for severe neurological crises particularly neuroleptic malignant syndrome. These agents present special problems in psychiatric patients because they produce psychosis in themselves. In high doses, bromocriptine is frequently associated with nightmares, hallucinations and paranoid delusions.[69] Even at low doses, acute psychiatric hospitalization has been reported.[70] Upon discontinuation of the drug the episode resolved with no sequelae.

Levodopa (L-dopa), the most powerful antiparkinson agent introduced for idiopathic parkinsonism, has been estimated to produce

TABLE 2.2. Agents generally reserved for NMS.

Primary Pharmaco'l Action	Generic Name	Brand Name	Product Form*	Daily Dose Range (mg)	
				18–64 Yr	65+ Yr
Dopamine agonist	bromocriptine	Parlodel	O	5–60	not reported
	dantrolene	Dantrium	O	60–600	not reported

* Product forms: Oral solid (O), liquid (L), and injectable (I).

psychiatric symptoms in 20% of Parkinsonian patients.[71] In addition, it has been reported to produce pronounced psychogenic effects,[72] including hypersexuality and agitation[73] and, consequently, is not used for antipsychotic-induced parkinsonism. Among 5 chronic schizophrenic patients receiving neuroleptics, the addition of levodopa at approximate doses of 1 gram per day produced worsening of paranoia in two, and hallucinations in three, one of whom did not have such symptoms at baseline. These symptoms resolved upon discontinuation of levodopa.[74] In a second study, at doses greater than 1 gram per day, 4 chronic schizophrenic patients had "marked deterioration" in behavioral status with no reduction of EPSE.[75] Additional negative experience with levodopa includes reports of confusional states[76] and mania.[77] When administered in doses of 3–6 grams per day to 10 chronic schizophrenic patients who were not receiving neuroleptics, all patients were reported as having behavioral worsening.[78] In addition to its potential for acute psychosis, lack of efficacy, agitation, and on-off performance effects (i.e., rapid oscillation in motor performance) suggest that L-dopa is not a useful treatment for neuroleptic-induced parkinsonism.

DOSING CONSIDERATIONS

Initiation

As discussed earlier (p. 40, Routine Usage), distinctions have been made between initiating the antiparkinson agent to treat emergent symptoms (i.e., following the antipsychotic) and routine co-administration to prevent or reduce the symptoms that may emerge. Anticholingeric agents are used to treat the symptoms *if* they occur. Consequently, routine prescribing at the time an antipsychotic is initiated is not recommended unless specific criteria are met.[10, 13] Among the specific situations in which an anticholinergic is useful at the start of antipsychotic treatment are the following: (1) those with no history of antipsychotic drug response who require moderate to substantial doses and who cannot be closely monitored and treated if an acute EPSE occurs; (2) those requiring relatively high doses of high-potency agents especially if rapid injectable administration is used; (3) those with a personal or family history of antipsychotic-induced EPSE. The effectiveness of the anticholinergic agents was reported to reduce the risk of dystonia by 1.9-fold in all patients treated with different neuroleptics and by 5- to 8-fold in patients treated with high-potency agents.[79] The authors concluded that the anticholinergics were effective in preventing neuroleptic-induced dystonia, particularly in young male patients treated with high-potency neuroleptics.

Treatment of Acute Dystonic Reactions

Immediate treatment of an acute dystonic reaction usually consists of an injection (IM or IV) of benztropine (1–2 mg IV, up to 8 mg in 24 hours) or diphenhydramine (25 mg IV or 25–50 mg IM up to a maximum of 400 mg in 24 hours).

Treatment of Gradually Emerging EPSE

In response to clinical signs of parkinsonism, an oral anticholinergic agent is introduced and monitored for its effect during the initial 2 weeks of treatment.[10] As the psychotic episode resolves (typically 4 to 6 weeks following onset, although this may take as long as 12 to 24 weeks in some cases) antipsychotic dose reductions may be considered. These should be gradual dose reductions with the goal of eventual discontinuation. Successful discontinuation may be more readily achieved after short-term than long-term use due to anticholinergic withdrawal phenomena.[80,81]

Maintenance

If a switch to maintenance therapy with a long-acting injectable antipsychotic is intended, the role of anticholinergic agent depends on the individual patient's experience with recurrent EPSE. Sometimes EPSE recur regularly for a few days following depot injections and are treated with several days of anticholinergic agent. Gradual withdrawal from this protocol would allow continual assessment of the need for ongoing anticholinergic therapy as well as avoid the difficulties associated with long-term continuous usage.

Withdrawal

In medical conditions such as idiopathic parkinsonism, abrupt withdrawal of anticholinergics is associated with a rebound exacerbation of symptoms.[67] Similarly, withdrawal effects occur in psychiatric patients. Numerous authors report withdrawal effects following the discontinuation of anticholinergic agents used to treat antipsychotic-induced parkinsonism[80,81] as well as when the antipsychotic drug itself, with its intrinsic anticholinergic effect, is withdrawn.[82,83,84]

When chronic psychiatric patients were withdrawn from anticholinergic agents, they demonstrated transient withdrawal symptoms (increased anxiety, insomnia, increased psychotic symptoms, physical complaints such as flu-like symptoms, and increased autonomic effects such as pulse, orthostatic hypotension, and tachycardia). These effects reduced to baseline levels after 6 weeks of a double-blind, placebo-controlled withdrawal of anticholinergic agent.[81] Baker et al.[29] showed improved memory in chronic psychiatric patients who were withdrawn from anticholinergic agents.

A suggested protocol for gradual withdrawal in patients who have been exposed continuously to prophylactic anticholinergics for months or longer consists of a 25% dose reduction the first week and if uneventful, a repeat 25% reduction weekly until the drug is discontinued at 6 weeks. If adverse symptoms are noted the process is stopped until their transient nature is determined or a "floor" (lowest effective dose) is reached.

Additional Factors

Abuse by Patients with Drug-Seeking Behaviors

Anticholinergic agents have been associated with abusive use for their euphorigenic effect.[85,86,87,88] In one estimate, 7% of psychiatric outpatients were seeking and selling them for euphoric and hallucinogenic effects.[89] By contrast, schizophrenic patients have reported their use to alleviate negative symptoms (social withdrawal, anergy and fatigue) that may be antipsychotic drug-induced.[90] Avoiding unnecessary antiparkinson agents is one approach to reducing the availability of these agents. However, abusive use is generally recognized to be present in a distinct subpopulation and the inference that patients are "faking" when they seek medication is inappropriate unless there is a documented history of abusive drug use involving anticholinergics. Nevertheless, if the EPSE can be minimized by reducing the antipsychotic dosage and by conservative use of anticholinergic in response to specific patient symptoms, the availability of these drugs for abusers would be reduced. The larger question regarding their use to reduce negative symptoms poses a research challenge since recent studies suggest a worsening of positive symptoms[16,91,92] while treating the negative symptoms with anticholinergic agents.

Anticholingeric Agents and Tardive Dyskinesia

Tardive dyskinesia is a well-known syndrome of abnormal involuntary movements that is currently estimated to occur in 15–20 percent of antipsychotic-treated patients who receive medication for more than one year. The presence of anticholinergic agents in the drug regimen of such patients is postulated to lower the threshold of tardive and to increase the severity of movements[93] and is consistent with overactivity in the dopamine system as the hypothesized etiology of tardive dyskinesia.[10] Improvement was demonstrated in a controlled discontinuation of anticholinergics in 10 chronic schizophrenic patients with tardive dyskinesia[94] although Cole[80] reported no change. Trial reductions and discontinuation of anticholinergics in these patients are topics for further systematic study. The relationship between tardive dyskinesia, impaired gag reflex and anticholinergic drug usage was studied by Craig and Richardson.[95] Patients with tardive dyskinesia receiving anticholinergics were significantly more likely to have gag reflex impairment. In clinical practice, tardive patients who can be managed without anticholinergics would benefit from the reduced risk of impaired gag reflex.

Sensitivity in the Elderly

Age is a risk factor for memory impairment with anticholinergic agents in normal volunteers[96] and particularly in the elderly patient with an organic diagnosis such as dementia of the Alzheimer type.[97] Also, decreased self-care skills in the elderly have been reported.[98] Cautious dosing in the elderly for the following anticholinergic-acting drugs is advised: anticholinergics, diphenhydramine, tricyclic antidepressants and antipsychotics. Outpatients and unrestricted inpatients should be advised to avoid over-the-counter sleep products. These products may have a scopolamine-related compound as their major ingredient, although recently some companies have revised the formulations to omit these agents.

A 6-fold risk of toxic delirium associated with strongly anticholinergic antidepressants in the elderly compared with younger patients was observed in a large drug surveillance system.[99] These findings support the general caution on anticholinergic usage in the elderly.

ANTICHOLINERGIC SIDE EFFECT MONITORING

Common Side Effects

Routine side effect monitoring of the anticholinergics requires assessment for the following frequently occurring side effects:

Oral: Dry mouth, difficulty swallowing.

Eye: Blurred vision due to mydriasis and cycloplegia (avoid use in narrow (closed) angle glaucoma—injections have produced this effect but it is rare in orally treated patients).

GI: Constipation and gastrointestinal slowing (close monitoring in patients with GI disorders is needed to avoid intestinal obstruction). Infrequently, fatal adynamic ileus has been reported in patients receiving combinations of drugs with anticholinergic effects.

GU: Urinary retention; use in prostatic hypertrophy is generally avoided.

Cardiac effects: Tachycardia with hypotension, increased pulse, and orthostatic hypotension.

Psychiatric Symptoms: Psychological and behavioral disturbances related to anticholinergic use are a particular problem for the psychiatric patient population. These effects include mental confusion, excitement, agitation, delirium, paranoid reactions and hallucinations. They are presumed to increase with dose since they are most dramatic in acutely intoxicated individuals. The elderly are among the most susceptible individuals for these effects particularly those over 70 and with dementia. Memory deficits have been reported in experimentally designed studies of psychogeriatric patients who received anticholinergics[100] and these findings have been observed in younger volunteers as well.[101] Thus, considerable care in dosing psychotropics agents which have anticholinergic activity is emphasized. Overall, the difficulty in distinguishing symptoms of psychiatric illness from drug-induced side effects is a serious challenge to effective and safe drug therapy in patients chronically medicated with agents from several psychotropic classes each of which contributes to the overall anticholinergic drug load.

Antihistamines such as diphenhydramine have additional side effects such as drowsiness and dizziness, euphoria and paradoxical excitation (describes unexpected excitation when most individuals experience CNS depressant effects such as drowsiness). This effect is particularly evident in children.

Acute Intoxication

Central and peripheral cholinergic blockade following acute intoxication can be life-threatening and involve many vital centrally-mediated effects. Among these effects are: agitation, disorientation, sleep disturbances, grand mal seizures, increased body temperature, dry, flushed skin, tachycardia, sluggish, and at least moderately dilated pupils,[10] as well as decreased bowel sounds and acute urinary retention. Progression to coma occurs in severe intoxication. Emergency supportive care is required; there is limited experience with the use of an injectable anticholinesterase agent such as physostigmine (Eserine) to increase metabolism of the anticholingeric agents. This approach requires expert management.

DRUG-DRUG INTERACTIONS

Within-Class Interactions

The combination of two or more anticholinergic agents for control of EPSE should be avoided since there is no data to support these combinations and the effective dosing of two agents is more difficult than one.

Between-Class Interactions

The three classes of psychotropics with anticholinergic effects are the antiparkinson agents (anticholinergic and other agents with anticholinergic activity such as diphenhydramine), the tricyclic antidepressants and the antipsychotic agents. While combinations of these agents may be unavoidable, constant monitoring for increases in anticholinergic effects and lack of efficacy should be used to determine dosage changes once complete avoidance of the anticholinergic agent has been ruled out. Introduction of an anticholinergic at the start of antipsychotic therapy should be based on the patient meeting criteria for high risk of EPSE. Similarly, continuous use beyond three months should be accompanied by indications that gradually titrated trial reductions were accompanied by nontransient symptoms which could not be tolerated by the patient.

REFERENCES

1. Klawans HL, Jr.: The pharmacology of extrapyramidal movement disorders, in Monographs in Neural Sciences 2. Edited by Cohen M. Basel, Karger, 1973, pp 7–47, 117–133

2. Chien CP, DiMascio A: Drug-induced extrapyramidal symptoms and their relations to clinical efficacy. Am J Psychiatry 1967; 123:1490–1498

3. Ayd FJ, Jr.: Prophylactic antiparkinson drug therapy: Pros and cons. Intl Drug Therapy Newsletter 1986; 21:5–6

4. DiMascio A, Demirgian E: Antiparkinson drug overuse. Psychosomatics 1970; 11:596–601

5. Lehmann HE: Psychopharmacological treatment of schizophrenia. Schizophrenia Bull 1975; 13:27–45

6. Hanlon TE, Schoenrich C, Freinek W, Turek I, Kurland AA: Perphenazine-benztropine mesylate treatment of newly admitted psychiatric patients. Psychopharmacologia 1966; 9:328–339

7. Sramek JJ, Simpson GM, Morrison RL, Heiser JF: Anticholinergic agents for prophylaxis of neuroleptic-induced dystonic reactions: A prospective study. J Clin Psychiatry 1986; 47:305–309

8. Bollini P, Andreani A, Colombo F, Bellantuono C, Beretta P, Arduini A, Galli T, Tognoni G: High dose neuroleptics: Uncontrolled clinical practice confirms clinical trials. Brit J Psychiatry 1984; 144:25–27

9. Klein DF, Gittelman R, Quitkin F, Rifkin A: Diagnosis and Drug Treatment of Psychiatric Disorders: Adults and Children. 2nd ed. Baltimore, Williams and Wilkins, 1980

10. Baldessarini RJ: Chemotherapy in Psychiatry: Principles and Practice. 2nd ed. Cambridge, Harvard University Press, 1985

11. McEvoy JP, Simpson GM: Dystonia, neuroleptic dose, and anticholinergic drugs [letter]. Am J Psychiatry 1987; 144:393–394

12. Rifkin A, Quitkin F, Kane J, Strure F, Klein DF: Are prophylactic antiparkinson drugs necessary? A controlled study of procyclidine withdrawal. Arch Gen Psychiatry 1978; 35:483–489

13. Lake CR, Casey DE, McEvoy JP, Siris SG, Boyer WF, Simpson G: Anticholinergic prophylaxis in young adults treated with neuroleptic drugs. Psychopharm Bull 1986; 22:981–984

14. Haase HJ, Janssen PAJ: The Action of Neuroleptic Drugs. A psychiatric, neurologic, and pharmacological investigation. Amsterdam, North-Holland Publ Co, 1985:178

15. Singh MM, Kay SR: A comparative study of haloperidol and chlorpromazine in terms of clinical effects and therapeutic reversal with benztropine in schizophrenia. Theoretical implications for potency differences among neuroleptics. Psychopharmacologia 1975; 43:103–113

16. Johnstone EC, Crow TJ, Ferrier IN, Frith CD, Owens DG, Bourne RC, Gamble SJ: Adverse effects of anticholinergic medication on positive schizophrenic symptoms. Psychol Med 1983; 13:513–527

17. Rivera-Calimlin L, Castañeda L, Lasagna L: Effects of mode of management on plasma chlorpromazine in psychiatric patients. Clinical Pharmacol Therapeutics 1973; 14:978–986

18. Simpson GM, Cooper TB, Bark N, Sud I, Lee JH: Effects of antiparkinsonian medication on plasma levels of chlorpromazine. Arch Gen Psychiatry 1980; 37:205–208

19. Hitri A, Craft RB, Fallon J, Sethi R, Sinda D: Serum neuroleptic and anticholinergic activity in relationship to cognitive toxicity of antiparkinsonian agents in schizophrenic patients. Psychopharm Bull 1987; 23:33–37

20. Bamrah JS, Kumar V, Krska J, Soni SD: Interactions between procyclidine and neuroleptic drugs. Some pharmacological and clinical aspects. Brit J Psychiatry 1986; 149:726–733

21. Craig TJ: Medication use and deaths attributed to asphyxia among psychiatric patients. Am J Psychiatry 1980; 137:1366–1373

22. Tune LE, Strauss ME, Lew MF, Breitlinger E, Coyle JT: Serum levels of anticholinergic drugs and impaired recent memory in chronic schizophrenic patients. Am J Psychiatry 1982; 139:1460–1462

23. Perlick D, Stastny P, Katz T, Mayer M, Mattis S: Memory deficits and anticholinergic levels in chronic schizophrenia. Am J Psychiatry 1986; 143:230–232

24. Hvisdos AJ, Bennett JA, Wells BG, Rappaport KB, Mendel SA: Anticholinergic psychosis in a patient receiving usual doses of haloperidol, desipramine, and benztropine. Clin Pharm 1983; 2:174–178

25. Schroeder NH, Caffey EM, Lorei TW: Antipsychotic drug use: Physician prescribing practices in relation to current recommendations. Dis Nerv Syst 1977; 38:114–116

26. Mason AS, Nerviana V, DeBurger RA: Patterns of antipsychotic drug use in four Southeastern state hospitals. Dis Nerv Syst 1977; 38:541–547

27. Craig TJ, Behar RJ: Changes in the prescription of anticholinergic drugs (1970–1977) in a state hospital. Intl Pharmacopsychiatry 1981; 16:84–91

28. Orlov P, Kasparian G, DiMascio A, Cole JO: Withdrawal of antiparkinson drugs. Arch Gen Psychiatry 1971; 25:410–412

29. Baker LA, Cheng LY, Amara IB: The withdrawal of benztropine mesylate in chronic schizophrenic patients. Brit J Psychiatry 1983; 143:584–590

30. DiMascio A, Shader RI: Clinical Handbook of Psychopharmacology. New York, Science House, 1970

31. Yassa R, Lal S: Prevalence of the rabbit syndrome. Am J Psychiatry 1986; 143:656–657

32. Weiden P, Harrigan M: A clinical guide for diagnosing and managing patients with drug-induced dysphagia. Hosp and Community Psychiatry 1986; 37:396–398

33. Prosser ES, Csernansky JG, Kaplan J, Thiemann S, Becker TJ, Hollister LE: Depression, parkinsonian symptoms, and negative symptoms in schizophrenia treated with neuroleptics. J Nerv Mental Dis 1987; 175:100–105

34. Rifkin A, Quitkin F, Klein DF: Akinesia. Arch Gen Psychiatry 1975; 32:672–674

35. Van Putten T, May PRA: "Akinetic depression" in schizophrenia. Arch Gen Psychiatry 1978; 35:1101–1107

36. McGlashan TH, Carpenter WT, Jr.: Postpsychotic depression in schizophrenia. Arch Gen Psychiatry 1976; 33:231–239

37. Bartels SJ, Drake RE: Depressive symptoms in schizophrenia: comprehensive differential diagnosis. Comprehensive Psychiatry 1988; 29:467–483

38. Braude WM, Barnes TR, Gore SM: Clinical characteristics of akathisia. A systematic investigation of acute psychiatric inpatient admissions. Brit J Psychiatry 1983; 143:139–150

39. Munetz MR: Akathisia variants and tardive dyskinesia (letter). Arch Gen Psychiatry 1986; 43:1015

40. Van Putten T: The many faces of akathisia. Comprehensive Psychiatry 1975; 16:43–47

41. Gagrat D, Hamilton J, Belmaker RH: Intravenous diazepam in the treatment of neuroleptic-induced acute dystonia and akathisia. Am J Psychiatry 1978; 135:1232–1233

42. Lipinski JF, Jr., Zubenko GS, Cohen BM, Barreira PJ: Propranolol in the treatment of neuroleptic-induced akathisia. Am J Psychiatry 1984; 141:412–415

43. Adler L, Angrist B, Peselow E, Corwin J, Maslansky R, Rotrosen J: A controlled assessment of propranolol in the treatment of neuroleptic-induced akathisia. Brit J Psychiatry 1986; 149:42–45

44. Adler L, Angrist B, Peselow E, Reitano J, Rotrosen J: Clonidine in neuroleptic-induced akathisia. Am J Psychiatry 1987; 144:235–236

45. Weiden PJ, Mann JJ, Haas G, Mattson M, Frances A: Clinical nonrecognition of neuroleptic-induced movement disorders: A cautionary study. Am J Psychiatry 1987; 144:1148–1153

46. Drake RE, Ehrlich J: Suicide attempts associated with akathisia. Am J Psychiatry 1985; 142:499–501

47. Belmaker RH, Wald D: Haloperidol in normals (letter). Brit J Psychiatry 1977; 131:222–223

48. Anderson BG, Reder D, Cooper TB: Prolonged adverse effects of haloperidol in normal subjects (letter). New Eng J Med 1981; 305:643–644

49. Van Putten T: Why do schizophrenic patients refuse to take their drugs? Arch Gen Psychiatry 1974; 31:67–72

50. Garcia MM, Mercer PR: A case of neuroleptic-induced laryngospasm. West J Med 1990; 153:438–439

51. Kellam AM: The neuroleptic malignant syndrome, so-called. A survey of the world literature. Brit J Psychiatry 1987; 150:752–759

52. Levenson JL: Neuroleptic malignant syndrome. Am J Psychiatry 1985; 142:1137–1145

53. Pope HG, Jr., Keck PE, Jr., McElroy SL: Frequency and presentation of neuroleptic malignant syndrome in a large psychiatric hospital. Am J Psychiatry 1986; 143:1227–1233

54. Sternberg DE: Neuroleptic malignant syndrome: The pendulum swings [editorial]. Am J Psychiatry 1986; 143:1273–1275

55. Toru M, Matsuda O, Makiguchi K, Sugano K: Neuroleptic malignant syndrome-like state following withdrawal of antiparkinson drugs. J Nerv Ment Dis 1981; 169:324–327

56. Dhib-Jalbut S, Hesselbrock R, Mouradian MM, Means ED: Bromocriptine treatment of neuroleptic malignant syndrome. J Clin Psychiatry 1987; 48:69–73

57. Tupin JP: Focal neuroleptization: An approach to optimal dosing for initial and continuing therapy. J Clin Psychopharmacology 1985; 5:15S–21S

58. Susman VL, Addonizio G: Reinduction of neuroleptic malignant syndrome by lithium. J Clin Psychopharmacology 1987; 7:339–341

59. Franks RD, Aoueille B, Mahowald MC, Masson N: ECT for a patient with malignant hyperthermia. Am J Psychiatry 1982; 139:1065–1066

60. Anon: Drugs used in extrapyramidal movement disorders, in AMA Drug Evaluations, 5th ed. Chicago, American Medical Association, 1983, pp 329–351.

61. Tune L, Coyle JT: Serum levels of anticholinergic drugs in treatment of acute extrapyramidal side effects. Arch Gen Psychiatry 1980; 37:293–297

62. Zubenko GS, Lipinski JF, Cohen BM, Barreira PJ: Comparison of metoprolol and propranolol in the treatment of akathisia. Psychiatry Research 1984; 11:143–148

63. Adler LA, Angrist B, Fritz P, Rotrosen J, Mallya G, Lipinski JF, Jr.: Lack of efficacy of d-propranolol in neuroleptic-induced akathisia. Neuropsychopharmacology 1991; 4:109–115

64. Parker WA: Propranolol-induced depression and psychosis. Clin Pharmacy 1985; 4:214–218

65. DiMascio A, Bernardo DL, Greenblatt DJ, Marder JE: A controlled trial of amantadine in drug-induced extrapyramidal disorders. Arch Gen Psychiatry 1976; 33:599–602

66. Nestelbaum Z, Siris SG, Rifkin A, Klar H, Reardon GT: Exacerbation of schizophrenia associated with amantadine. Am J Psychiatry 1986; 43:1170–1171

67. Wilcox JA, Tsuang J: Psychological effects of amantadine on psychotic subjects. Neuropsychobiology 1990; 23:144–146

68. Schwab RS, Poskanzer DC, England AC, Jr., Young RR: Amantadine in Parkinson's disease. Review of more than two years' experience. JAMA 1972; 222:792–795

69. Anon: Drugs for parkinsonism. The Medical Letter on Drugs and Therapeutics 1986; 28:62–64

70. Taneli B, Ozaskinli A, Kirli A, Erden G, Bora I: Bromocriptine-induced schizophrenic syndrome (letter). Am J Psychiatry 1986; 143:935

71. Brogden RN, Speight TM, Avery GS: Levodopa: A review of its pharmacological properties and therapeutic use with particular reference to Parkinsonism. Drugs 1971; 2: 262–400

72. Angrist B, Thompson H, Shopsin B, Gershon S: Clinical studies with dopamine-receptor stimulants. Psychopharmacologia (Berl.) 1975; 44: 273–280

73. Angrist B, Gershon S: Clinical effects of amphetamine and L-DOPA on sexuality and aggression. Comprehensive Psychiatry 1976; 17:715–722

74. Yaryura-Tobias JA, Diamond B, Merlis S: The action of L-DOPA on schizophrenic patients (a preliminary report). Current Therapeutic Research 1970; 12:528–531

75. Yaryura-Tobias JA, Wolpert A, Dana L, Merlis S: Action of L-DOPA in drug-induced extrapyramidalism. Dis Nerv Syst 1970; 31:60–63

76. Goodwin FK: Behavioral effects of L-DOPA in man. In: Psychiatric Complications of Medical Drugs, pp. 149–174. RI Shader (ed.). New York, Raven Press, 1972

77. Goodwin FK, Murphy DL, Brodie HK, Bunney WE, Jr.: Levodopa: Alterations in behavior. Clin Pharmacol Therapeutics 1971; 12:383–396

78. Angrist B, Sathananthan G, Gershon S: Behavioral effects of L-DOPA in schizophrenic patients. Psychopharmacologia (Berl.) 1973; 31:1–12

79. Arana GW, Goff DC, Baldessarini RJ, Keepers GA: Efficacy of anticholinergic prophylaxis for neuroleptic-induced acute dystonia. Am J Psychiatry 1988; 145:993–996

80. Jellinek T, Gardos G, Cole JO: Adverse effects of antiparkinson drug withdrawal. Am J Psychiatry 1981; 138:1567–1571

81. McInnis M, Petursson H: Withdrawal of trihexyphenidyl. Acta Psychiatr Scand 1985; 71:297–303

82. Lieberman J: Cholinergic rebound in neuroleptic withdrawal syndromes. Psychosomatics 1981; 22:253–254

83. Lacoursier RB, Spohn HE, Thompson K: Medical effects of abrupt neuroleptic withdrawal. Comprehensive Psychiatry 1976; 17:285–294

84. Gardos G, Cole JO, Tarsy D: Withdrawal syndromes associated with antipsychotic drugs. Am J Psychiatry 1978; 135:1321–1324

85. Jellinek T: Mood elevating effect of trihexyphenidyl and biperiden in individuals taking antipsychotic medication. Dis Nerv Syst 1977; 38:353–355

86. Sofair J, Campion J, Angrist B: High dose trihexyphenidyl abuse with psychological dependence. J Clin Psychopharmacol 1983; 3:263–264

87. Dilsaver SC: Antimuscarinic agents as substances of abuse: A review. J Clin Psychopharmacol 1988; 8:14–22

88. MacVicar K: Abuse of antiparkinsonian drugs by psychiatric patients. Am J Psychiatry 1977; 134:809–811

89. Kaminer Y, Munitz H, Wijsenbeck H: Trihexyphenidyl (Artane) abuse: Euphoriant and anxiolytic. Brit J Psychiatry 1982; 140:473–474

90. Fisch RZ: Trihexyphenidyl abuse: Therapeutic implications for negative symptoms of schizophrenia? Acta Psychiatr Scand 1987; 75:91–94

91. Tandon RM, Greden JF, Silk KR: Treatment of negative schizophrenic symptoms with trihexyphenidyl. J Clin Psychopharmacol 1988; 8:212–215

92. Singh MM, Kay SR, Opler LA: Anticholinergic-neuroleptic antagonism in terms of positive and negative symptoms of schizophrenia: Implications for psychological subtyping. Psychol Med 1987; 17:39–48

93. Klawans HL, Jr.: The pharmacology of tardive dyskinesias. Am J Psychiatry 1973; 130:82–86

94. Greil W, Haag H, Rossnagl G, Rüther E: Effect of anticholinergics on tardive dyskinesia. A controlled discontinuation study. Brit J Psychiatry 1984; 145:304–310

95. Craig TJ, Richardson MA: Swallowing, tardive dyskinesia, and anticholinergics (letter). Am J Psychiatry 1982; 139:1083

96. McEvoy JP: A double-blind crossover comparison of antiparkinson drug therapy: Amantadine versus anticholinergics in 90 normal volunteers, with an emphasis on differential effects on memory function. J Clin Psychiatry 1987; 48:9(Suppl)20–23

97. Sunderland T, Tariot PN, Cohen RM, Weingartner H, Mueller EA, Murphy DL: Anticholinergic sensitivity in patients with dementia of the Alzheimer type and age-matched controls. A dose-response study. Arch Gen Psychiatry 1987; 44:418–426

98. Rovner BW, David A, Lucas-Blaustein MJ, Conklin B, Filipp L, Tune L: Self-care capacity and anticholinergic drug levels in nursing home patients. Am J Psychiatry 1988; 145:107–109

99. Schmidt LG, Grohmann R, Strauss A, Spiess-Kiefer C, Lindmeier D, Müller-Oerlinghauser B: Epidemiology of toxic delirium due to psychotropic drugs in psychiatric hospitals. Comprehensive Psychiatry 1987; 28:242–249

100. Potamianos G, Kellett JM: Anti-cholinergic drugs and memory: The effects of benzhexol on memory in a group of geriatric patients. Brit J Psychiatry 1982; 140:470–472

101. Crow TJ, Grove-White IF: An analysis of the learning deficit following hyoscine administration to man. Brit J Pharmacology 1973; 49:322–327

CHAPTER 3

Bipolar Disorder and Lithium

INTRODUCTION

Lithium in Bipolar Disorder

Lithium is indicated to control symptoms during the acute phase of manic episodes. Maintenance therapy is used to prevent or diminish the intensity of subsequent episodes. Sufficient efficacy was established to gain FDA indications for these uses in 1970.

The treatment of acute mania typically requires a 5 to 14-day latency period from the start of drug therapy before the onset of effect. During this time, severe symptoms are usually treated with an antipsychotic agent or a potent benzodiazepine.[1] A longer latency may be needed in some patients [periods up to 21 days have been observed[2]] and necessitates lengthening the period of antipsychotic drug use.

Several reviews[3, 4] document the relative efficacy of lithium in the maintenance phase of Bipolar Affective Disorder, although many patients have an imperfect response and an estimated 20 to 30% of patients are treatment-resistant. Variable control of recurrences, intolerable side effects and noncompliance account for some of the poor response to treatment.

The mechanism of action of the mood-stabilizing effect of lithium is not established. It has a postulated effect in reducing intracellular sodium concentrations. Another effect concerns the antagonism of synaptic transmission mediated by catecholamines which is related to a theory of mania. However, this theory is inconsistent with its effect during the depressive phase of bipolar illness. More recently, there is evidence of blockade of phosphatidyl inositol synthesis at muscarinic (and possibly alpha$_1$-adrenergic receptors).[5]

Other Clinical Usage

There are extensive clinical reports and experience in patients with psychiatric diagnoses other than bipolar disorder who fail to respond to established drug therapy. However, there are insufficient data derived from rigorously conducted double-blind randomized, controlled clinical trials to support these uses. Modest beneficial effects have been reported in some treatment-resistant patients with schizophrenia,[6,7,8] schizoaffective disorder,[9] and unipolar depression in both the acute and maintenance phases.[10] A more recent study of lithium augmentation in schizophrenia had negative findings (see Chapter 1, ref. 42). Among the least studied uses of lithium, which should be considered speculative at this time, are the control of aggressive behaviors, alcoholism, and other behaviors (e.g., obsessive compulsive disorder and phobias). In regard to emotionally unstable character disorders, (referred to as borderline personality disorder in DSM-III), lithium was more effective than placebo in a double-blind crossover controlled study (N = 21).[11]

DOSING CONSIDERATIONS

Acute Mania

Initiating lithium therapy requires a thorough history especially in regard to past experience with lithium and medical conditions that may affect lithium usage (e.g., renal, cardiovascular, and thyroid function). A typical initial dosage is 300 mg 3 times a day. However, because of the narrow therapeutic index, lithium dosing requires plasma level monitoring. One possible approach has been developed by Simpson and Cooper[12] consisting of a single 600 mg dose followed by a 24-hour plasma level. A high correlation between this level and the steady state level obtained when patients were placed on a fixed-dose regimen of 600 mg 3 times a day was reported.

The generally accepted therapeutic plasma range for acute mania is 0.8 to 1.5 mEq/L[13] although a level greater than 1.2 warrants close observation.[14] These levels usually are achieved with doses of 1200 to 1800 mg per day although considerable variability exists. New York State guidelines suggest a dosage maximum of 2400 mg per day unless consistent low-plasma levels and/or symptoms justify greater doses. Each dosage adjustment requires a period equivalent to 5 times the half-life of the drug (in this case, 5 times the half-life of 24 hours or 5 days is suggested) before a plasma level is likely to reflect the steady state serum level of the drug. One or 2 weeks of treatment may be more realistic. The time to steady state is lengthened when the patient has diminished renal function as may often occur in the elderly. Therefore, the initial dosing is based on the assumption of a normal individual's renal capacity to excrete the drug. Individualized dosage titration requires that side effect monitoring accompany plasma level monitoring. (See next section.) A list of minimum standards for monitoring patients at baseline, 3 months and for continuing follow-up of lithium treatment is provided in Part IV.

Maintenance Therapy

The therapeutic range suggested for the maintenance phase of lithium treatment is 0.6 to 1.2 mEq/L although there is evidence of adequate control at 0.4 to 0.6 mEq/L in some patients. The lowest effective dose is the guiding principle and requires individual trials of reduced dosage. Maintenance treatment may be required continuously if the acute episodes are severe, abrupt and without warning. Some authors[13] suggest that for the patient with a gradual onset of acute symptoms, periods off medication may be considered depending on the severity and time course of cycles. In these cases, gradual tapering is recommended. Others suggest continuous lifetime treatment for the bipolar patient.[15] In a sophisticated approach to this question, a clinical decision analysis[16] was performed to show the costs of various lithium continuation strategies: after the first manic episode, after the second episode, after 2 episodes within two years, or none. After 5 years, the number of days of illness for those receiving no treatment was estimated to be 5 times greater than continuous treatment. The model shows that earlier use of lithium increases the benefits (morbidity avoided) and increases the costs (lithium-associated morbidity). Thus, clinical decisions about lithium prophylaxis are seen to involve tradeoffs between different types of morbidity.

Drug Discontinuation

The situations in which drug discontinuation may be undertaken include cases in which the drug is not effective and those stabilized for more than 6 months and having gradual rather than abrupt onset of symptoms.[13] Ultimately, the primary factors in considering drug discontinuation concern the course, frequency and severity of cyclic episodes.

Although there is not a clear consensus on the presence of a withdrawal syndrome, the limited evidence supports a tapering procedure to avoid the possibility of withdrawal symptoms, some of which are indistinguishable from psychiatric symptoms of illness. Abrupt withdrawal symptoms produced relapse including manic psychotic states in reports by Klein[17] and Christodoulou.[18] Withdrawal symptoms (e.g., hyperactive deep tendon reflexes, tremor of the hands, and fatigue have been reported). Dosage reduction should occur gradually in decrements of one-fourth to one-third the daily dose at the upper end of the range and one-half at the lower end of the dose range. Each decrement should last 5 to 10 days or more. Gradual reductions are aimed at providing time for both behavioral and receptor readjustment. A typical reduction for a starting dose of 1200 mg per day would be:

900 per day	day 1–10
600 per day	day 11–20
300 per day	day 21–30 and discontinue

Pharmacokinetic Factors

Lithium is an inorganic salt that is rapidly and completely absorbed from the gastrointestinal tract. Peak plasma levels occur in 1.5 to 2 hours. The drug passes the blood-brain barrier with difficulty at approximately a 2:1 ratio and equilibration occurs after 24 hours. Because of its inorganic nature, there are no metabolites, the drug is not protein bound and is excreted almost entirely by the kidney. About 70 to 80% of the lithium ion passes into the glomerular filtrate which is reabsorbed by the proximal tubule. Since there is competitive proximal reabsorption between sodium and lithium ions, decreases in the body's sodium concentration (which can occur by restricting salt intake and promoting diuresis), tend to produce decreased lithium excretion and can lead to lithium intoxication. The elimination half-life is estimated at 24 hours, suggesting a period of about 5 days for steady state levels to be achieved.

Plasma Level Monitoring

Because of the narrow therapeutic index, serious toxicity occurs when therapeutic doses of lithium are exceeded. The use of plasma-level monitoring is necessary to reduce the risk of toxic doses. The procedure to monitor lithium levels suggests that the first level be drawn on the second day although this is not likely to be at a steady state concentration. The time interval to achieve steady state is about 5 days after the drug is initiated for the patient with normal renal function. Trough (basal) levels are the most reliable levels for monitoring.[14] A morning trough level is drawn 12 hours following the previous evening dose and before the next morning dose is administered. Sometimes 8- or 10-hour intervals are preferred because of scheduling difficulties. Regardless of the period selected, the failure to follow a consistent time interval, whether 8- or 12-hour periods, leads to transiently inflated levels that occur during the drug's distribution phase. Irregularity in the blood sampling interval makes interpretation of plasma levels meaningless. Levels may be repeated weekly until a stabilized dose is achieved, then monthly for 5 to 6 months and then trimonthly. Each dosage increase requires plasma level monitoring according to this protocol. Dramatic changes in the patient's health status that are likely to affect renal function require lithium monitoring. For example, prolonged hypotension, drug regimen changes (e.g., the addition of diuretics or drugs which cross the blood-brain barrier, require reassessment of the lithium plasma level).

Preliminary Laboratory and Clinical Values

Safe lithium usage requires adequate cardiovascular and renal function. Therefore, before initiating lithium treatment, baseline renal and cardiovascular tests are suggested. The usual baseline renal tests include BUN, serum creatinine, and urine analysis. When abnormal values are obtained, the testing should progress to 24-hour urine volume, creatinine clearance and renal concentrating ability for a complete evaluation. Cardiovascular function tests include an electrocardiogram. Serum electrolytes and complete blood count and a blood sugar also are recommended. Reference values for blood chemistries are found in Part IV.

A baseline thyroid function (T-3, T-4, T-7) is useful to monitor the suppression effect of lithium on thyroid function. Serum TSH is a more sensitive indicator of hypothyroid function.

Additional Pharmacodynamic and Clinical Principles

Child and Adolescent Dosing

The clinical experience regarding lithium in children and adolescents is discussed in Chapter 7.

Geriatric Patient Dosing

Studies of drug clearance in the geriatric patient indicate small decreases in renal clearance of lithium.[13,19] Dosage should be reduced to accommodate this effect. In addition, the geriatric patient is known to be more sensitive to the behavioral effects of psychotropic drugs.[20] A subtle organic mental syndrome can occur in elderly patients on prolonged lithium therapy.[21] In general, one-third to one-half the adult dosage initially should be used with elderly patients to establish plasma levels at the low end of the therapeutic range. More frequent dosing intervals or the use of sustained release tablets may avoid those side effects associated with peak levels.[19]

Safety during Pregnancy and Lactation

Lithium must be avoided during pregnancy and lactation. Women in the child-bearing years should be advised of the need for effective contraception during lithium therapy. Lithium in toxic doses produced teratogenic effects in animals such as fetal wastage and central nervous system abnormalities. Human fetal abnormalities include severe cardiovascular defects.[22] Nursing should be avoided because breast milk contains 30–50% of the mother's plasma lithium levels and presents a risk to the baby who is nursed.

Medication Administration Factors

Dietary and Environmental Factors

Because lithium excretion is influenced by sodium and water changes, patients' dietary and exercise habits should be monitored to prevent fluctuations in the lithium level. Salt restricted diets, increased diuresis, and acute febrile states have led to serious lithium intoxication while exercise and heavy sweating may lead to lowered plasma lithium levels and to diminished effectiveness of the lithium (Jefferson,[13] p. 293).

Dosage Formulations

Table 3.1 lists the commonly used formulations of lithium. The short-acting forms are the solid carbonate (300 mg equivalent to 8 milliequivalents Li) and liquid citrate (300 mg, 8 mEq per 5 ml). These products achieve a peak serum level within 1.5 to 2 hours. Three times a day dosing is the usual initial treatment schedule. Once the dosage is stabilized and if tolerated, 12-hour intervals may be used to provide more convenient dosing. The long-acting formulations (e.g., Lithobid

TABLE 3.1. Lithium products, form, dosage units and relative costs.*

Salt	Brand Names	Form	Dosage Unit	Unit Cost	Relative Cost**
Carbonate	Lithonate	short-acting	300 mg/cap	.07 UD	1.0
	Lithotab	short-acting	300 mg/tab	.05 bulk	0.7
	Eskalith-CR	long-acting	450 mg/tab	.26 bulk	2.5
	Lithobid	long-acting	300 mg/tab	.15 UD	2.1
Citrate	Cibalith-S	short-acting liquid	300 mg/5 ml	—	—
	Lithium Citrate Syrup	short-acting liquid	300 mg/5 ml	.26/5 mlUD	4.1
				.41/10 mlUD	N/A

* OMH facility prices (February 1993).
** Comparison is based on a dose of 900 mg per day.

(300 mg) and Eskalith-CR (450 mg)) gradually release the drug and peak within 4.5 to 5 hours. The convenience of twice a day dosing is possible with these long-acting preparations although the long-term advantages, such as reduced post-absorption peaking, are not yet demonstrated. Long-acting products are more expensive and may not be as well absorbed. They may be a suitable alternative for the patient intolerant of the side effects associated with gastric absorption of the drug, although some clinical experts suggest a greater risk of lower gastrointestinal symptoms (e.g., cramps and diarrhea).

Noncompliance

Noncompliance among long-term lithium users is estimated to be about 20 to 30% of patients according to VanPutten.[23] Reasons for discontinuing the medication include (1) missing the creativity and productivity of the manic state, (2) denial of the existence of a chronic illness, and (3) the belief that medication is no longer needed because the patient feels well and (4) increased denial during early hypomanic stages. Lithium clinics have shown that participation in education and support groups can improve compliance.[24] Family and significant others can be valuable assets in assisting the therapeutic alliance between patient and prescribing physician. Their assistance is needed to help identify a drug compliance pattern that is acceptable to both the patient and physician. A key factor in this process is the monitoring of target symptoms, vocational productivity, and social interactions as well as side effects. Side effects are a major cause of patient dissatisfaction with lithium, alone or in combination with other psychotropics. Higher doses tend to produce more severe patient dysfunctioning. Careful documentation of these side effects and subsequent dosage adjustments or changes in the product formulation may lead to greater cooperation with treatment.

SIDE EFFECT MONITORING

Common Side Effects

The following list of frequently reported side effects are usually considered dose-dependent.[25] To reduce the severity of a side effect a reduction in dose should be tried whenever clinically possible.

Side effects at therapeutic doses (or plasma levels) of lithium:

1. Tremor: A fine rapid hand tremor which does not stop during voluntary movements. It is a resting or essential tremor.
2. Muscular weakness and an increased risk of myasthenia gravis[21] (p. 123) have been reported.
3. Gastrointestinal effects: Nausea, vomiting and diarrhea are associated with peak plasma levels and may be reduced by altering the formulation, frequency, or dosage. Mild dry mouth is also reported.
4. Renal effects: Polyuria up to 5 liters/day and polydipsia (thirst) develop after one or more months in about 10 to 20% of patients. Mild thirst and polyuria develop transiently in the early phase of treatment in most patients. This polyuria/polydipsia may be produced by a relative insensitivity to antidiuretic hormone and has been shown to resolve when the drug is discontinued.
5. Central nervous system effects: Confusion and a dysphoric effect described by patients as a mental dulling are reported.
6. Endocrine effects: Weight gain and edema, especially in females, is reported. Hypothyroidism occurs in about 3% of lithium-treated patients. Supplemental thyroxine is used to treat this disorder. There is some increase in fasting blood sugar values and in insulin requirement occasionally.

7. Cardiovascular effects: Electrocardiographic changes include flattening of T-waves. Rarely, hypotension and arrhythmias are reported.

8. Hematologic effects: White blood cells are increased and this leucocytosis effect has been used to treat WBC-deficiency disorders such as rheumatoid arthritis and Felty's Syndrome.

9. Dermatologic effects: Lichens simplex chronicus, maculopapular rash, exacerbations of psoriasis, acneiform eruptions, and hair loss have been reported[13] (p. 331–333).

Long-Term Effects

Rat studies indicate renal damage at low lithium doses.[13] In humans, however, the morphological kidney changes that may be found in about 6 to 15% of patients[26] on long-term therapy do not appear to seriously interfere with renal function,[27] although appropriate medical consultation and monitoring is indicated in long-term lithium users (i.e., urinalysis, creatinine clearance, and renal consultation).

Recently, Goodnick et al.[28] reported successful withdrawal of long-term patients. Three weeks following discontinuation of lithium the group of six patients had increased T-3 (11% increase), T-4 (11% increase), and free T-4 (25% increase), while calcium (5% decrease), cholesterol (6%), triglycerides (26%) and white cell counts (39%) decreased. These findings were interpreted as indicative of the reversibility of lithium-induced effects of hypothyroidism, leukocytosis and hyperparathyroidism. There were, however, no significant changes in BUN, sodium, and creatinine.

Acute Intoxication

Lithium intoxication in humans is a dose-dependent phenomenon and progresses through the following stages which have been well documented.

Increasing tremor, nausea and vomiting, ataxia, blurred vision, tinnitus, dysarthria (slurred speech), confusion, increased deep tendon reflexes, nystagmus, stupor, coma and sometimes generalized seizures. As the plasma level increases from 1.5 upwards these effects have been observed until fatalities occurred at plasma levels of 5mEq/L.

Acute intoxication is managed as a medical emergency with hospitalization. The drug is discontinued immediately, gastric lavage and supportive care of vital functions is undertaken. Hemodialysis and correction of fluid and electrolyte balance is indicated for severe, chronic intoxication.

DRUG-DRUG INTERACTIONS

Medical Drug Interactions

Most diuretics may increase lithium levels due to the ability of the diuretic to promote the loss of sodium. Renal lithium clearance was reduced by as much as 40% when 500 mg of chlorothiazide per day was added. The reduced clearance led to lithium dose reductions of 50%.[29] Thiazide diuretics have had the most pronounced effects although the use of furosemide and spironolactone and other diuretics also requires intensive lithium monitoring. Whenever diuretics are added or removed the plasma lithium determination should be performed and the lithium reduced as indicated. Additionally, thiazide diuretics may require potassium supplementation.

Lithium is reported to prolong the effect of the neuromuscular blocking agent, succinylcholine chloride, and to produce post-surgical apnea.[30]

Calcium channel blockers such as diltiazem[31] and nifedipine[32] are reported to produce *de novo* mania and psychosis when used in nonpsychiatric patients. Diltiazem and lithium were proposed to have synergistic calcium channel blocking action to explain the development of confusion, forgetfulness, rigidity, ataxia, and depression in a 66-year-old patient with a diagnosis of bipolar affective disorder.[33] When diltiazem was discontinued the lithium was tolerated as previously.

Nonsteroidal antinflammatory agents such as piroxicam and indomethacin produced lithium toxicity perhaps through prostaglandin inhibition of renal excretion.

Potassium iodide and lithium produce additive hypothyroid effects and the combination should be avoided.

Methyldopa and lithium may produce lithium intoxication without increasing plasma levels of lithium. The effect may occur because of increased lithium levels in brain tissue.

Sodium chloride and sodium bicarbonate promote lithium excretion because of the competitive excretion by sodium ions.

Theophylline and its salts increase lithium excretion. The introduction of theophylline to a stabilized lithium regimen may render the lithium less effective.

Tetracycline may increase lithium levels by interfering with renal function.

Psychotropic Drug Interactions

Major reference works[34, 35] on drug-drug interactions discuss the putative mechanisms and clinical significance of the following interactions among neuroactive classes that are frequently prescribed for psychiatric disorders.

Antipsychotics

(See Chapter 1 for a related discussion.) Combinations of lithium and antipsychotics are used frequently to control the early stage of acute mania. In addition, there is some long-term usage in treatment-resistant individuals with typical and atypical psychotic disorders. However, optimal dosing in these patients has not been studied nor has the efficacy of combined therapy for chronic patients been established. In addition, there are concerns about the safety of antipsychotics and lithium. In an early study, chlorpromazine was reported to increase lithium levels by reducing renal clearance.[36] However, later reports of increased lithium levels after withdrawing phenothiazines[35] were postulated to be related to *increased* lithium renal *clearance* in the presence of chlorpromazine.[37] When the phenothiazine was withdrawn, lithium intoxication developed at previously tolerated doses. A more serious question concerns lithium and haloperidol which was reported to produce serious and fatal encephalopathy.[38] These reports are few compared with the considerable usage that is occurring without serious adverse consequences. The limited epidemiologic data[39] available suggest that the drug combination does not produce frequent serious adverse effects. More recent studies[40] suggest that the combination produces additive side effects that can be corrected by dosage reduction. Population studies in large samples of patients who are well-defined clinically and pharmacologically are needed to address the question of lithium-haloperidol interactions. In general, whenever lithium is added to the drug regimen of a patient who is not having an acute manic episode, and the drug regimen consists of agents which cross the blood-brain barrier, a downward adjustment of the additional agents, particularly antipsychotics, is reasonable. Closer monitoring of the blood levels of both lithium and the antipsychotic may be useful. Side effect monitoring should include subjective effects (e.g., dysphoria, and nonspecific complaints that may be related to additive generalized CNS depressant effects).

Antiepileptics

Carbamazepine has been reported to increase lithium levels to toxic levels in several cases. Half of a group of 10 patients receiving chronic lithium treatment developed symptoms of intoxication after the addition of moderate doses of carbamazepine.[41] A similar experience was reported in a patient for whom neither drug alone produced symptoms.[42] These problems occurred at usual plasma lithium levels. Although this combination has been used successfully in several case reports [N = 3],[43] the combined usage has not been reported in sufficient numbers to clarify the benefit to risk assessment. Until more definitive results explain the toxicity in some patients caution is advised in combining these agents in treatment-resistant mania and careful monitoring of dose, plasma levels and side effects should follow the guidelines for longitudinal drug monitoring (see Part IV).

Phenytoin has been reported to increase lithium plasma levels to toxic levels with symptoms of ataxia, tremor, gastrointestinal side effects, polyuria and polydipsia. Individualized longitudinal monitoring of plasma levels, target symptoms and side effects at baseline (before adding the second drug) would make it relatively easy to determine the frequency and severity of this type of interaction. See Part IV for a sample form suggested for general longitudinal monitoring of multiple psychotropic agents.

Benzodiazepines

Alprazolam was reported to increase lithium levels by 28% in normal volunteers and the effect was postulated to be due to decreased urine flow rate.[44] Short-term use of the combination was not shown to be of serious clinical consequence.

Diazepam and lithium produced severe hypothermia in a single case.[45]

Tricyclic Antidepressants

A coarse shaking, parkinsonian symptoms and increased risk of seizures have been reported for combinations with lithium.

REFERENCES

1. Chou JC: Recent advances in treatment of acute mania. J Clin Psychopharmacology 1991; 11:3–21

2. Klein DK: Personal communication

3. Schou M: Problems of lithium prophylaxis: Efficacy, serum lithium, selection of patients. Bibl Psychiatr 1981; 160:30–37

4. Davis JM: Overview: Maintenance therapy in psychiatry: II. Affective disorders. Am J Psychiatry 1976; 133:1–13

5. Baraban JM, Worley PF, Snyder SH: Second messenger systems and psychoactive drug action: Focus on the phosphoinositide system and lithium. Am J Psychiatry 1989; 146:1251–1260

6. Alexander PE, Van Kammen DP, Bunney WE, Jr.: Antipsychotic effects of lithium in schizophrenia. Am J Psychiatry 1979; 136:283–287

7. Growe GA, Crayton JW, Klass DB, Evans H, Strizich M: Lithium in chronic schizophrenia. Am J Psychiatry 1979; 136:454–455

8. Small JG, Kellams JJ, Milstein V, Moore J: A placebo-controlled study of lithium combined with neuroleptics in chronic schizophrenic patients. Am J Psychiatry 1975; 132:1315–1317

9. Biederman J, Lerner Y, Belmaker RH: Combination of lithium carbonate and haloperidol in schizo-affective disorder: A controlled study. Arch Gen Psychiatry 1979; 36:327–333

10. Kane JM, Quitkin FM, Rifkin A, Ramos-Lorenzi JR, Nayak DD, Howard A: Lithium carbonate and imipramine in the prophylaxis of unipolar and bipolar II illness: A prospective, placebo-controlled comparison. Arch Gen Psychiatry 1982; 39:1065–1069

11. Rifkin A, Quitkin F, Carillo C, Blumberg AG, Klein DF: Lithium carbonate in emotionally unstable character disorder. Arch Gen Psychiatry 1972; 27:519–523

12. Cooper TB, Bergner PE, Simpson GM: The 24-hour serum lithium level as a prognosticator of dosage requirements. Am J Psychiatry 1973; 130: 601–603

13. Jefferson JW, Greist JH, Ackerman DL: Lithium Encyclopedia for Clinical Practice, 2nd ed. Washington DC, American Psychiatric Press, Inc., 1987

14. Cooper TB: Pharmacokinetics of lithium, in Psychopharmacology: The Third Generation of Progress. Edited by Meltzer HY. New York, Raven Press, 1987

15. Georgotas A, Gershon S: Lithium in manic-depressive illness: Some highlights and current controversies, in Lithium: Controversies and Unresolved

Issues. Edited by Cooper TB, Gershon S, Kline NS, Schou M. Amsterdam, Excerpta Medica, 1979, pp 57–84

16. Zarin DA, Pass TM: Lithium and the single episode: When to begin long-term prophylaxis for Bipolar Disorder. Medical Care 1987; 25:S76–S84

17. Klein HE, Broucek B, Greil W: Lithium withdrawal triggers psychotic states (letter). Brit J Psychiatry 1981; 139:255–256

18. Christodoulou GN, Lykouras EP: Abrupt lithium discontinuation in manic-depressive patients. Acta Psychiatr Scand 1982; 65:310–314

19. Van der Velde C: Toxicity of lithium carbonate in elderly patients. Am J Psychiatry 1971; 127:1075

20. Jefferson JW: Lithium and affective disorder in the elderly. Comprehensive Psychiatry 1983; 24:166–178

21. Baldessarini RJ: Lithium salts, in Chemotherapy in Psychiatry, Principles and Practice. 2nd ed Cambridge, Harvard University Press, 1985

22. Schou M, Amdisen A, Steenstrup OR: Lithium and pregnancy-II. Hazards to women given lithium during pregnancy and delivery. Brit Med J 1973; 2:137–138

23. VanPutten T: Why do patients with manic-depressive illness stop their lithium? Comprehensive Psychiatry 1975; 16:179–183

24. Volkmar FR, Bacon S, Shakir SA, Pfefferbaum A: Group therapy in the management of manic-depressive illness. Am J Psychotherapy 1981; 35:226–234

25. Vacaflor L, Lehmann HE, Ban TA: Side effects and teratogenicity of lithium carbonate treatment. J Clin Pharmacol 1970; 10:387–389

26. Jenner FA: Lithium and the question of kidney damage. Arch Gen Psychiatry 1979; 36:888–890

27. Vestergaard P, Schou M, Thomsen K: Monitoring of patients in prophylactic lithium treatment. An assessment based on recent kidney studies. Brit J Psychiatry 1982; 140:185–187

28. Goodnick PJ, Fieve RR, Schlegel A: Clinical and chemical effects of lithium discontinuation (letter). Am J Psychiatry 1987; 144:385

29. Himmelhoch JM, Poust RI, Mallinger AG, Hanin I, Neil JF: Adjustment of lithium dose during lithium-chlorothiazide therapy. Clin Pharmacol Therapeutics 1977; 22:225–227

30. Hill GE, Wong KC, Hodges MR: Potentiation of succinylcholine neuromuscular blockade by lithium carbonate. Anesthesiology 1976; 44:439–442

31. Binder EF, Cayabyab L, Ritchie DJ, Birge SJ: Diltiazem-induced psychosis and a possible diltiazem-lithium interaction. Arch Intern Med 1991; 151:373–374

32. Hullett FJ, Potkin SG, Levy AB, Ciasca R: Depression associated with nifedipine-induced calcium channel blockade. Am J Psychiatry 1988; 145:1277–1279

33. Palat GK, Hooker EA, Movahed A: Secondary mania associated with diltiazem. Clin Cardiology 1985; 8:251–252

34. Stockley IH: Drug Interactions. Oxford, Blackwell Scientific Publ, 1981

35. Hansten PD, Horn JR: Drug Interactions and Updates. 6th ed. Philadelphia, Lea and Febiger, 1990

36. Sletten I, Pichardo J, Korol B, Gershon S: The effect of chlorpromazine on lithium excretion in psychiatric subjects. Current Therapeutic Research 1966; 8:441–446

37. Pakes GE: Lithium toxicity with phenothiazine withdrawal (letter). Lancet 1979; 2:701

38. Cohen WJ, Cohen NH: Lithium carbonate, haloperidol and irreversible brain damage. JAMA 1974; 230:1283–1287

39. Goldney RD, Spence ND: Safety of the combination of lithium and neuroleptic drugs. Am J Psychiatry 1986; 143:882–884

40. Miller F, Menninger J: Correlation of neuroleptic dose and neurotoxicity in patients given lithium and a neuroleptic. Hosp and Community Psychiatry 1987; 38:1219–1221

41. Chaudhry RP, Waters BG: Lithium and carbamazepine interaction: Possible neurotoxicity. J Clin Psychiatry 1983; 44:30–31

42. Ghose K: Effect of carbamazepine in polyuria associated with lithium therapy. Pharmakopsychiat Neuro-Psychopharmakologie 1978; 11:241–245

43. Lipinski JF, Pope HG, Jr.: Possible synergistic action between carbamazepine and lithium carbonate in the treatment of three acutely manic patients. Am J Psychiatry 1982; 139:948–949

44. Evans RL, Nelson MV, Melethil S, Townsend R, Hornstra RK, Smith RB: Evaluation of the interaction of lithium and alprazolam. J Clin Psychopharmacol 1990; 10:355–359

45. Naylor GJ, McHarg A: Profound hypothermia on combined lithium and diazepam treatment. Brit Med J 1977; 2:22

CHAPTER 4

Pharmacotherapy of Depressive Disorders

INTRODUCTION

According to the DSM-III-R classification system, mood disorders are divided into bipolar disorder and major depression. These disorders are characterized by severe symptoms and functional incapacity, while the cyclothymic (less severe bipolar disorders) and dysthymic disorders (less severe unipolar disorders) may require similar but less intensive management in terms of drug dosage and type of treatment setting. Lithium and the antipsychotics, the major drug therapy for bipolar disorder have been discussed in previous chapters. This chapter focuses on the treatment of depression.

The widely accepted current model for the treatment of depression reflects a biopsychosocial model with both somatic and psychosocial interventions.[1] Somatic treatments include electroconvulsive treatment and medications. As the severity of symptoms diminishes, individual and group supportive therapy, including cognitive and interpersonal treatment, tend to play a greater role in treatment.[2] Drug therapy plays a greater role in the early phase of treatment (6 to 12 months, perhaps indefinitely), when relief of the vegetative symptoms of sleep and appetite disturbance are likely to occur. Psychotherapy tends to affect mood, suicidal ideation, work, interests and coping patterns, effects that may not emerge until 2 or more months of therapy.

Efforts to evaluate combined drug and psychosocial treatment include the NIMH Treatment of Depression Collaborative Research Program for outpatients with moderate to severe depression.[3,4] The interventions were interpersonal psychotherapy and cognitive behavior therapy in comparison with imipramine and placebo. Data analysis of 250 patients indicated that at the end of 16 weeks, drug response, as measured by reduction of symptoms and overall functioning, was more rapid, but not significantly better than either interpersonal or cognitive behavior therapy.

The drug classes used in the treatment of depression include the tricyclic antidepressants, several newer atypical antidepressants, and the monoamine oxidase inhibitors. More recent additions include compounds that are chemically related to these drug classes such as clomipramine, the 3-chloro analog of imipramine, and experimental compounds of greater specificity (e.g., clorgyline for type A MAO inhibition and deprenyl for type B MAO inhibition). Electroconvulsive therapy continues to play a role for severe depression in which drug therapy does not succeed or presents greater risks.

TRICYCLIC ANTIDEPRESSANTS AND ATYPICAL AGENTS

Introduction

The era of antidepressants began with the serendipitous discovery of the mood-elevating properties of iproniazid, an isoniazid analog that was originally introduced for the treatment of tuberculosis. Nathan Kline was among the first American investigators to corroborate the initial European findings with iproniazid in the mid-1950s.[5] Soon thereafter, Roland Kuhn in Switzerland found the phenothiazine analog to be a poor antipsychotic agent but a useful antidepressant—the first of the tricyclic type. More than 30 years of clinical experience have accumulated in support of the use of the tricyclic antidepressants as first-choice agents for the treatment of the typical neurovegetative symptoms of endogenous (major) depression. In light of the relatively high lifetime prevalence for major depression which is estimated at 18 to 23% of females and 8 to 11% of males, the antidepressants enjoy widespread usage across a wide range of patients. Many patients are treated in medical outpatient settings and nursing homes, while the more severely ill individuals are treated by psychiatrists, sometimes with hospitalization. This spectrum of severity corresponds with the many treatment patterns in use. These patterns are reflected in a wide range of target symptoms and treatment goals, dosages, and durations of treatment (acute vs. maintenance) which carry differences in benefits, risks, and costs.

Chemistry and Structure Activity Relationships

In Table 4.1, the frequently used antidepressants are listed according to their chemical classification. Imipramine, a dibenzazepine, was the first of the tricyclics marketed and it has been followed by 9 chemical analogs. Loxapine and clozapine are analogous dibenzazepines with antipsychotic activity but are not proven to be effective as antidepressants. Doxepin is a tertiary amine of the dibenzoxepine type. In addition to the tertiary amines of the dibenzazepine type such as imipramine, trimipramine, and clomipramine, the chloro-analogue of imipramine, there is desipramine, the secondary amine metabolite of imipramine. Amitriptyline and its demethylated metabolite, nortriptyline, as well as protriptyline are dibenzocycloheptene-derived.

The chemical structure of the tricyclic agent imipramine (A) (Figure 4.1) is similar to the general phenothiazine structure (C) and carbamazepine (B), 2 agents which are primarily used for different clinical disorders, emphasizing the overlap of chemical structure, pharmacologic activity, and clinical outcome among these agents for psychiatric and seizure disorders.

Among newer agents, maprotiline is a secondary amine with a structure often described as "tetracyclic" although it is similar both chemically and pharmacologically to desipramine. Amoxapine (nor-loxapine) carries additional risks of the antipsychotic agents, such as extrapyramidal type neurological impairment. Neither maprotiline nor amoxapine are first-choice drugs because of their increased risk of seizure-threshold lowering in the absence of efficacy greater than that of the earlier tricyclics such as imipramine.[6]

TABLE 4.1. Currently used antidepressant drugs.

	Adult Dosage Range (mg/d)			Form[d]	Plasma Range[c] (ng/ml)	Relative Effects[a]				
	Usual	Extreme	Elderly[b] 65+			Anticholinergic muscarinic	Sedative H$_1$	Seizure Potential	Hypotensive alpha$_1$	Cardiac Depressant
Tricyclic Agents										
Tertiary Amines										
Imipramine	50–200	25–300	25–150	OS,I	150–450(IMI+DMI)[c]	3	3	3	4	4
Amitriptyline	75–100	25–300	25–150	OS,I	100–300(AMI+NT)	4	4	3	3	4
Doxepin	75–200	25–300	25–150	OS,OL	50–200	3	4	4	2	2
Trimipramine	50–150	50–300	25–150	OS		4	4	3	3	4
Clomipramine	50–250			OS		3				
Secondary Amines										
Desipramine	75–200	25–300	25–150	OS	100–250[e]	2	2	2	3	3
Nortriptyline	75–150	20–150	20–100	OS,OL	50–150[e]	3	3	2	1	3
Protriptyline	15–40	15–60	10–20	OS		3	1	2	2	4
Amoxapine	200–300	75–600	75–300	OS		3	2	3	1	2
Maprotiline[f]	75–150	25–225	25–75	OS		3	3	4	2	3
Atypical Agents										
Trazodone	150–400	50–600	50–150	OS		0	3	2	3	1
Fluoxetine	20–40	20–80	20[g]	OS		+/−	+/−		+/−	
Bupropion	300–450	—	150–325	OS		0	+/−		+/−	
MAO Inhibitors										
Isocarboxazid	10–30	10–30		OS						
Phenelzine	45–60	15–90		OS						
Tranylcypromine	20–40	10–60		OS						

[a] Relative clinical effects based on analysis of pooled studies.[7] Scores range from 1 (least) to 4 (greatest) effect.

[b] Low extreme defines elderly dose lower limit; upper extreme defines upper dose limit for treatment-resistant patients.[19]

[c] New York State Analytic Psychopharmacology Laboratory usual ranges.

[d] OS = oral solid, OL = oral liquid, and I = injectable for intramuscular use only.

[e] APA Task Force on laboratory tests in psychiatry endorsement of clinical utility.[74]

[f] Nonformulary status due to greater seizure-threshold lowering potential.

[g] Up to 80 mg/day has been used in one study without age related effects. However, 20 mg/day is recommended until further evaluation.[24]

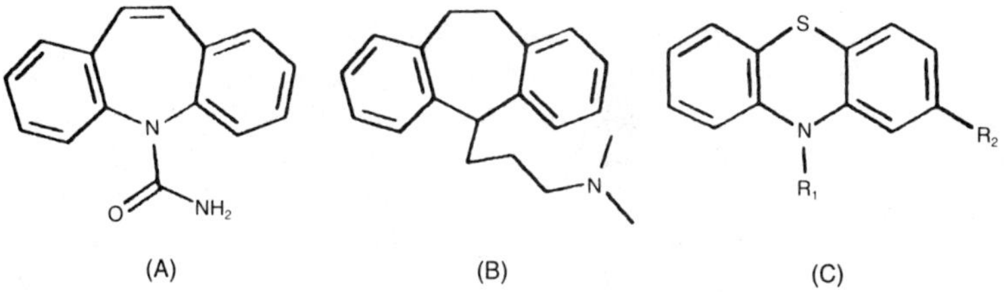

Figure 4.1. Structure of the tricyclic antidepressant imipramine (A), the iminostilbene carbamazapine (B), and the general structure of the phenothiazines.

Drugs marketed since 1980 have sometimes been called "second generation" antidepressants, and several are chemically described as "atypical" antidepressants. These include trazodone, amoxapine, fluoxetine, bupropion, and several others that are no longer available for general use such as nomifensine. Despite the early promise that the newer agents would produce enhanced efficacy and reduce the adverse effects of the older agents, none is better than the tricyclics in efficacy,[8] but some offer a different spectrum of side effects. Drugs recalled from the market or not released in the United States include nomifensine because of hemolytic anemias, and zimelidine because of Guillain-Barré type reactions.

Fluoxetine is an atypical compound of the phenylpropanolamine type and acts as a serotonin re-uptake blocker. In 1988, it was marketed in the United States for the treatment of depression and quickly followed by other SSRIs, e.g., sertraline and paroxetine.

Mechanism of Action

The biogenic amine hypothesis is a widely recognized theory of the mechanism of action of the antidepressants.[9, 10] The theory speculates that depression may be associated with insufficient activity of neurotransmitters, primarily norepinephrine and serotonin (5-hydroxytryptamine) and to a lesser extent, dopamine, in the brain. This activity may be influenced by other amines (e.g., acetylcholine). Mania may be the result of excessive neurotransmission by norepinephrine or dopamine.

The tricyclics are presumed to exert their antidepressant activity by potentiating norepinephrine and other amines through the blockade of re-uptake of the biogenic amines at nerve endings in the brain and subsequent secondary adaptation of amine metabolism and receptors.[11] Despite the widespread acceptance of the theory, numerous inconsistencies remain. First, although uptake sites (transporters) are bound by the drug within hours after a single drug dose, there is a latency period of 2 to 3 weeks or more before clinical antidepressant action occurs. Second, there is a problem related to cause and effect relationships. Although changes in metabolism of biological amine and steroid hormones may be associated with the depression, it does not necessarily follow that these changes cause the depression nor that treating them improves outcome in a simple, direct fashion.

Alternative theories include the amine receptor-sensitivity theory[12] which broadly describes the mechanism of action of the antidepressants as net receptor effects including reduced post-synaptic beta-adrenergic receptor sensitivity and enhanced alpha-adrenergic and serotonergic stimulation. The dysregulation theory[13] refers to a relative failure of one or more of the homeostatic mechanisms which operate to regulate neurotransmitters in affective disorders rather than as simple increases or decreases in the neurotransmitter activity. The antidepressants act to restore equilibrium by altering receptor sensitivities. The process involves a downregulation (desensitization) of presynaptic $alpha_2$ receptors in conjunction with an increased neuron firing rate.

Pharmacologic Effects

The basic pharmacologic effects of the antidepressants are adrenergic, anticholinergic, serotonergic, antihistaminic, and sedative. Antidepressant blockade of neural receptors and uptake sites have been studied *in vivo* and *in vitro*. The studies supporting these impressions include assays of receptor affinity by the binding of radiolabeled compounds to $alpha_1$ (post-synaptic), $alpha_2$ (partly pre-synaptic), and beta-noradrenergic, D_1 and D_2 dopaminergic, H_1 and H_2 histaminergic, $5-HT_1$ and $5-HT_2$ serotonergic and muscarinic acetylcholine receptors, or of their uptake into specific nerve terminals.[14,15,16] As yet there are insufficient correlations between clinical potency and these neuronal receptor data to make them clinically useful.

Clinical Effects

The acute clinical effects of the tricyclic antidepressants are similar to the low-potency phenothiazines in causing sleepiness, postural hypotension, light-headedness, and anticholinergic effects, such as dry mouth and blurred vision. While sedative, adrenergic, and anticholinergic effects are typically reported by patients, acute extrapyramidal effects generally are lacking. With repeated dosing, tolerance to some effects develops but cognitive and affective impairment may persist.[17] Clinically apparent mood elevation typically occurs 2 to 3 weeks after therapy is started although 4 to 6 weeks is needed before an adequate trial is completed. Despite some claims to the contrary, all of the agents have this latency period before a clinical antidepressant effect occurs.

Autonomic nervous system effects include (1) adrenergic agonist effects; (2) variable muscarinic cholinergic blocking effects; (3) cardiovascular effects such as lowered blood pressure, especially postural hypotension, based on uncertain mechanisms that may include alpha-1-adrenergic blockade. Inverted or flattened T waves and prolonged conduction times in the electrocardiogram sometimes are observed, especially on overdosage. A quinidine-like myocardial depression, which may be beneficially antiarrhythmic in some cases, has been found to produce dangerous arrhythmias or heart block if there are pre-existing conduction defects such as bundle branch block. Table 4.1 lists the relative effects of the major tricyclic antidepressants in terms of anticholinergic, sedation, seizure threshold-lowering potential, orthostatic hypotension, and cardiac depressant potential.

Target Symptoms

Neurovegetative symptoms of depression are classified as:

1. Physical, such as loss of energy and libido, somatic complaints, disturbances of sleep and appetite, and poor hygiene
2. Cognitive, such as loss of concentration, reduced IQ performance on WAIS, and indecisiveness
3. Emotional, such as sad, dysphoric mood, anhedonia, suicidal ideation and attempts, feelings of worthlessness, guilt and shame.

These symptoms may be accompanied by psychotic features including delusions and hallucinations. The clinical response to antidepressants is measured as a decrease in neurovegetative symptoms and to a lesser extent to psychotic symptoms, and typically occurs relatively early in treatment. Target responses to psychotherapy are measured in terms of increased productivity in work and other interests, decreased suicidal ideation, and improved mood, although the drug probably contributes to ongoing improvement.

To rule out drug-induced depression, a review of the patient's complete drug regimen is needed. Examples of drugs that have been reported in association with depression are found in the following classes:

Antihypertensive/cardiovascular
    methyldopa, propranolol, reserpine, digitalis glycosides
Sedative and hypnotic
    alcohol, barbiturates, benzodiazepines
Miscellaneous
    antipsychotics, opiates, stimulant overuse or withdrawal,
    indomethacin

Efficacy Studies

Tricyclic Antidepressants.   In a review of 93 double-blind, randomized, controlled clinical trials,[18] 66% of the studies reported greater improvement with a tricyclic antidepressant (usually imipramine or amitriptyline) compared with placebo treatment. Amitriptyline (70% of its trials) and imipramine (60% of its trials) were consistently superior to placebo, although placebo rates can be as high as 20 to 40% (especially in lesser depressions) within 4 to 6 weeks. In 18 similarly designed studies, the efficacy of nortriptyline, desipramine, and protriptyline, compared with placebo, is supported. The efficacy of doxepin is less dramatic at lower (<150 mg per day) dosages but supported at higher dosages. While there is general clinical consensus that the tricyclic antidepressants are effective in the treatment of major depression, these summaries of data across studies do not apply to all patients in the same way. There are significant differences in outcome for subgroups of patients (patient by treatment interactions) that account for the unsuccessful results that occur in 20 to 30% of patients treated in clinical practice.

A large NIMH collaborative study[19] involved 555 hospitalized depressed patients in 10 settings and compared imipramine, chlorpromazine, and placebo. The study findings do not permit an unequivocal statement of the efficacy of the antidepressant. The lack of a strong response attributable to imipramine or a clear difference between imipramine and chlorpromazine is believed to be due to drug-diagnostic subgroup-symptom pattern interaction as well as differential outcomes due to inconsistencies in the measurement of response. Imipramine was predicted to be superior for endogenous, psychotic depression but not better than placebo for exogenous, neurotic depression, although these conclusions were not verified by the study. These drug-placebo differences may better be explained by symptom severity differences between the two groups. Age, sex, and drug interaction effects have been reported for amitriptyline[20] with older, severely depressed women more effectively treated with amitriptyline than men or younger women. In general, a confounding factor in evaluating studies of depression is the occurrence of spontaneous remissions in 20 to 30% of depressions within 4 to 6 weeks which increases to more than 70% after several months. The addition of a placebo increases the nonactive drug-treated response rate to 30 to 50% by the end of two months.[20]

Overall, the efficacy of the tricyclic antidepressants is most clearly and consistently supported for the treatment of severe depressions (variously termed endogenous, manic depressive, retarded, involutional, agitated or psychotic depression) especially regarding physical symptoms, such as anorexia, insomnia, loss of energy, and libido. Nevertheless, issues of concern include the fact that agitated/psychotic depression may require combination therapy with an antipsychotic or may require ECT.

Lesser depressions (variously termed dysthymic, minor, reactive, neurotic, situational, and anxious depression) tend to remit spontaneously, respond to psychotherapy and to nonspecific drug treatments (such as anxiolytics and placebo) about as well as to the tricyclic antidepressants.[21] Issues of concern among lesser depressions include the fact that some minor illness may represent lesser severity of "real" depression that may respond to a tricyclic or MAO inhibitor on the one hand, or become chronic on the other. The focus of clinical research in the past decade has been on identifying the specific subtypes of clinical depression based on differential response to drug therapy. For example, Quitkin et al.[22] consider neurotic or atypical depression to be a heterogeneous syndrome, and expect subgroups to be responsive to specific antidepressant drug regimens. Recent studies by Liebowitz et al.[23] on the treatment of outpatients with atypical depression as defined by the target symptoms of low reactivity, hyperphagia, and hypersomnia demonstrated superiority of phenelzine over imipramine.

Clomipramine for Depression and Obsessive-Compulsive Disorder.
Clomipramine is the 3-chloro derivative of imipramine, a tertiary amine

type of antidepressant that has been widely used for more than 30 years. As such, its pharmacology is similar to imipramine with major adrenergic, serotonergic, and anticholinergic effects. Compared with imipramine, clomipramine has a tenfold greater inhibition of serotonin (5-hydroxytryptamine) re-uptake and twice the re-uptake of inhibition of norepinephrine.[24] Clomipramine has anticholinergic activity equivalent to imipramine;[25] this represents half that of amitriptyline, which is the most potent tricyclic as measured by the affinity for muscarinic receptors in the rat brain. There are additional neurotransmitter effects involving the blockade of dopamine (D_2), histamine (H_1), and α-1-adrenergic receptors.

The relative affinity for these receptors suggests that side effects and long-term risks related to dopamine-blockade, anticholinergic and hypotensive effects as well as problems associated with serotonergic excess should be monitored for effective use of this agent. In addition, the relative activity among these basic pharmacologic effects, despite the relatively greater serotonergic re-uptake blocking effect, makes the serotonin hypothesis a necessary but insufficient basis to explain the effectiveness of this and other agents such as fluoxetine for Obsessive-Compulsive Disorder (OCD).[26]

The serotonin hypothesis controversy: In a detailed review of serotonin re-uptake inhibitors, Boyer and Feighner[26] list the following problems with the serotonin hypothesis:

1. The lack of specificity of abnormal serotonergic functioning. Decreased function has been reported with many psychiatric disorders such as panic disorder, eating disorders, alcoholism, premenstrual syndrome and schizophrenia, as well as Parkinsonism, Alzheimer's Disease and other dementias. Low 5-HIAA levels in the cerebrospinal fluid were reported in idiopathic pain, Tourette's syndrome, multiple sclerosis and myoclonic epilepsy.

2. The interrelationship of the serotonergic system with other neurotransmitter systems (e.g., dopaminergic and noradrenergic). Consequently, changes in the serotonergic system may be producing changes in secondary systems which are etiologically responsible for the clinical effect that is attributed to the serotonergic system.

3. The lack of association between serotonin markers and response to treatment. In addition to the tricyclic antidepressants (TCAs),

bromocriptine, trazodone, and ECT alter serotonin activity in different ways but all are clinically effective treatments.

4. Inconsistent relationship between 5-HIAA levels and suicide. While low levels were found in suicide attempters, high levels were found in successful suicides if the plasma sample was obtained within 10 hours of death.

5. Inability to replicate the finding of an association between low levels of serotonin in plasma or platelets and depression in a significant number of well-designed studies.

6. Assumptions of the correlation between CSF and brain levels of serotonin must be validated.

This conflict does not invalidate the use of serotonergic agents like clomipramine for OCD. Rather, it should make clear that the basis for drug selection is not a drug-receptor specificity but the greater *clinical* efficacy demonstrated in specific study populations for agents with pronounced serotonergic effect such as clomipramine and fluoxetine. The same argument has been made before in regard to the lack of specificity of tricyclic and other antidepressants for the treatment of depression. Baldessarini[17] emphasized the growing doubt that the inhibition of serotonin or norepinephrine per se are necessary and sufficient reasons to explain the antidepressant effect of these drugs.

Despite the lack of biochemical specificity, these agents have more support for their clinical effectiveness in OCD than previous agents. Thus, the clinical data support a relationship between drug use and symptom control in selected diagnostic groups such as OCD and depression, without implying unique, mutually exclusive neurotransmitter effects.

Clinical pharmacology: The elimination half-life of clomipramine (CLO) was reported to average 20 ± 6 hours and 37 ± 13 hours for its metabolite, Desmethylclomipramine (DCMI) in a single dose study with healthy volunteers.[27] Prolonged elimination was reported in depressed patients (mean values for CLO = 34–36 hours and DCMI = 50 hours).[28] However, the increased time to metabolize the drug after repeated administration is more likely to be explained as a pharmacodynamic and pharmacokinetic effect than as a diagnostic effect. In view of these data, clinical monitoring should include a 2 to 3 week period to achieve steady state initially and then 2 to 3 week intervals between subsequent dose changes. Longer time intervals between dose increments should be allowed for the elderly or the patient with liver impairment. Plasma levels for therapeutic usage have not been established due to the relatively small sample of patients studied[29] and wide inter-individual variation.

Efficacy in adults: Drug therapy alone: In 3 double-blind studies[30,31,32] ranging from 4 to 16 weeks' duration, clomipramine was significantly more effective than a placebo as measured by symptom improvement from baseline scores. A multicenter collaborative study[30] was developed by Ciba-Geigy to meet the FDA standard for a Phase 3 clinical trial. The resulting 2 studies assessed more than 500 adult outpatients with OCD as a primary diagnosis (excluding those with other major psychosis on Axis I) and with dosage in the range of 150 to 250 mg per day. At the end of 10 weeks, study 1 and study 2 had, respectively, 38% and 44% of the clomipramine-treated patients improved compared with 3% and 5% of the placebo-treated patients.

A number of adult comparative studies[33,34,35] evaluated clomipramine in relation to other antidepressants. For example, clomipramine in doses of 75 to 300 mg per day was comparable in response to amitriptyline;[34] at similar doses, clomipramine was more effective than clorgyline[35] and slightly more effective than nortriptyline at doses of 50 to 150 mg per day.[33] Volavka et al.[36] evaluated the relative efficacy of clomipramine and imipramine in 23 adult outpatients with OCD symptoms and reported that among the two-thirds of patients completing 12 weeks of treatment, there were modest reductions in OCD symptoms and an antidepressant effect when measures were compared against baseline in both treatment groups.

Combined drug and psychotherapeutic interventions: During the 1970s, behavioral training known as systematic live exposure therapy was introduced for the treatment of OCD and studied by means of controlled clinical trials. The behavioral technique was found to be effective in reducing obsessive-compulsive rituals and the effect persisted for periods up to 2 to 3 years.[37,38] In addition, a double-blind comparison of clomipramine and placebo (mean dose of 164 mg per day) was made in 40 patients receiving either 15 or 30 hours of therapist-accompanied live exposure plus self-exposure homework or 3 weeks of relaxation followed by 3 weeks of exposure. The clomipramine group improved more than the placebo group during weeks 4 to 18, but this drug effect began to wane by week 36, the point at which medication was tapered.

In a two-year follow-up of the two-factor study, gains had been maintained and previous clomipramine treatment conferred no advantage in ritual reduction.[39] At 6 years, 85% of the group was reassessed. The group as a whole remained significantly improved on obsessive-compulsive symptoms, work, social adjustment, and depression; however, general anxiety returned to pretreatment levels (slight to moderate). Drug therapy appeared to have no effect on outcome because the clomipramine-treated patients were no more improved than those who were not taking antidepressants. Better long-term outcome correlated with more exposure therapy (6 weeks vs. 3 weeks) and with better compliance with the exposure therapy homework.[40] These findings are unique in terms of the length of follow-up and suggest that behavioral training should play a significant role in treatment programs for the OCD patient; they are consistent with the limited effectiveness of short-term drug treatment per se to control this often severely disabling disorder.

Efficacy for unlabeled indications: At the present time, no randomized double-blind controlled clinical trials have been reported on the efficacy of clomipramine in panic disorder with and without agoraphobia. One pertinent study is that of Waxman[41] who reported on 58 patients with mixed phobic and obsessional disorders and after randomized double-blind assignment to clomipramine (N = 14) versus diazepam (N = 27) showed significantly greater improvement (global assessment) for clomipramine-treated patients between weeks 4 and 6. The utility of clomipramine as an antidepressant is evidenced by its widespread use in Europe,[42] although differences from standard tricyclics are unremarkable in terms of clinical experience.

Clomipramine target populations and contraindications: Safety in cardiac patients: There was a relatively benign profile in terms of the ratio of pre-ejection period to left ventricular ejection time when compared to baseline measures in a group of 26 depressed adults receiving clomipramine at daily doses of 2 mg per Kg.[43] Compared with previous studies of imipramine,[44,45] clomipramine appeared more benign although a study bias was detected. Specifically, the clomipramine sample had fewer baseline cardiac disturbances suggesting a patient sample with less severe cardiovascular disease.

Contraindication in pregnancy: Two cases of neonatal convulsions and elevated clomipramine levels[46] were reported to be due to withdrawal from maternal clomipramine and corroborated an earlier case report.[47] To avoid such risks, women in the child-bearing years should be informed of the risks and benefits of drug treatment during pregnancy. Clinical notes should document the advantages over nondrug interventions; informed consent for such decisions is emphasized. Clomipramine is found in the milk of lactating women; therefore nursing should be avoided if drug therapy is undertaken.

Atypical Antidepressants

Fluoxetine.   Efficacy studies of fluoxetine include a 540 outpatient trial conducted in 6 centers in a double-blind controlled 3-group randomized design.[48] In group one, fluoxetine, initially up to 60 mg per day, was used in doses of 80 mg per day for 62% of the group. Group two consisted of imipramine-treated patients initially dosed at 125 mg per day, and raised to doses at or above 150 mg per day in 85% of the group. Both groups were significantly improved compared with the placebo-treated group in a study period up to 6 weeks. Fluoxetine was comparable to imipramine in clinical response but *less* effective that imipramine on the sleep disturbance ratings. Anorexia, nausea, anxiety, restlessness, and sexual dysfunction were reported by the fluoxetine-treated patients significantly more often than by imipramine-treated patients who more often reported anticholinergic side effects. Fluoxetine, as with most of the second generation of antidepressants, has not yet been sufficiently evaluated in severe inpatient depression. Dosing is an important question with this drug since Wernicke et al.[49] found no significant difference in the response rates among 3 groups who were treated with fixed doses of 20, 40, and 60 mg per day. Comparable efficacy data for these doses along with the increased adverse event rate at higher doses is the basis for the recommendation that 20 mg daily dosage be used in most patients. Feighner et al.[50] evaluated elderly outpatients with depression in a 6-week, double-blind, parallel group study. Improvement with fluoxetine was comparable to that of doxepin. Nervousness, anxiety, and insomnia were the chief side effects reported by fluoxetine-treated patients whereas anticholinergic effects were reported by doxepine-treated patients.

Bupropion.   In May 1989, bupropion was marketed for the treatment of depression after several years of delay. During the early 1980s, bupropion clinical trials in bulimic patients were halted after reports of grand mal seizures suggested a 5.4% prevalence (i.e., a

10- to 50-fold greater frequency than with standard tricyclics, 0.1–0.3%).[51,52] After reviewing the seizure-related experience of bupropion, several changes were made. For example, there is now a revised protocol with greater time between dose adjustments and a lower maximum dose as well as better identification of the suitable target population. Following these changes, bupropion was approved for marketing by the FDA.

Bupropion is an atypical antidepressant, specifically an aminoketone in the phenethylamine class and is similar in structure to the sympathomimetic stimulant, diethylpropion, a drug used to treat obesity. The mechanism of antidepressant action is essentially unknown but is hypothesized to be related to the drug's receptor action which is weak pre-synaptic dopamine re-uptake blockade (dopamine agonist).[53] Bupropion was reported to induce a marked inhibition of prolactin which suggests that it increases dopaminergic function[54] although this finding was not replicated when 10 patients were given low (12.5–100 mg) *single* doses of bupropion.[55] The reported absence of significant effects on receptors regulating norepinephrine, serotonin, acetylcholine, and histamine is the basis for the expectation that the drug would be useful to the depressed patient who is intolerant of tricyclic antidepressant (TCA) side effects or those with inadequate response to previously marketed antidepressants of tricyclic and atypical types.

Bupropion is rapidly absorbed with peak plasma levels after 2 hours and undergoes extensive first-pass liver metabolism.[56] The kinetics appear to follow a linear (first-order) elimination process and several metabolites having weak antidepressant activity are produced. The parent compound is stored in tissue at 25 times the concentration in plasma.[57] Bupropion is approximately 80% bound to plasma proteins and has an estimated elimination half-life ($t_{1/2}$) of 14 hours. This time interval suggests that dosing twice a day is feasible if each dose is below 150 mg.

The relationship of plasma monitoring to outcome warrants further study but preliminary findings are intriguing. In one study, 12-hour (trough) steady state bupropion plasma levels among 50 patients with a diagnosis of major depressive disorder from a 6-week double-blind comparison to amitriptyline were examined.[58] A curvilinear relationship between antidepressant effectiveness and trough plasma level of bupropion was observed with maximum response in the range of 75 to 100 ng/mL and none below 25 ng/mL. Thus, levels *above* 100 ng/mL were associated with *poor* response and, if validated in larger patient samples, would suggest dose *lowering* when poor response occurs at relatively high doses.

Similar findings were reported by Golden et al.[59] for 11 patients receiving bupropion (225 to 500 mg per day). They evaluated steady state plasma concentrations of hydroxybupropion (HB), threohydroxybupropion, and erythrohydrobupropion which predominated over the parent compound. Higher plasma concentrations were associated with poor clinical outcome. More specifically, HB levels exceeded 1250 ng/mL in the 5 nonresponders and less than 1200 ng/mL in the 7 responders. Fixed dose studies in a larger patient population will help to validate these findings. In the meantime, cautious incremental increases of 50 to 75 mg every 3 to 6 days would minimize the chance of passing through the "therapeutic window" and producing a lack of effectiveness as well as risking toxicity.

The effectiveness of bupropion is based on the findings of double-blind studies in several hundred patients and is summarized by Zung.[60] In the multicenter, randomized, double-blind, placebo-controlled, parallel group clinical trial at 5 sites there were 400 patients with DSM-II diagnoses of bipolar or unipolar depression. The depressive episode ranged from 3 to 24 months in duration and the treatment was evaluated for 4 to 6 weeks. Approximately 20% of the patients were dropped because of (1) intolerable side effects, (2) refusing to continue treatment, or (3) clinical decompensation. Dropouts rose to 35% in the high dose group that was medicated at mean doses of 687 mg per day and the trial was stopped because so many patients were intolerant of higher doses of bupropion.

At the end of 4 weeks, bupropion mean daily doses ranged from 331 to 735 mg per day. The primary efficacy analyses compared measurements made with the Hamilton Depression, Anxiety, and Clinical Global improvement and severity scales at weekly intervals up to 4 weeks from baseline. In 3 of the 5 reports (2 public and 1 private psychiatric hospital) bupropion-treated patients had statistically significant increases in improvement from baseline on depression, anxiety and overall improvement compared with placebo-treated patients. The remaining 2 sites (an outpatient and a VA inpatient setting) showed *no* significant differences on the same outcome measures.

The modest findings of placebo-controlled studies were followed by results from comparative trials with standard antidepressants, such as amitriptyline[55,61] and doxepin.[62] In a 2- to 4-week double-blind comparative trial, 40 depressed inpatients from a state mental hospital were randomized to bupropion (450–750 mg per day) or amitriptyline (75–225 mg per day). Benzodiazepines were used to control severe agitation during the first 7 days and chloral hydrate was used for sleep throughout the trial. High doses of bupropion relative to amitriptyline (respectively, 700 mg and 167 mg at 4 weeks) were administered. No significant differences between the 2 groups were observed on the Hamilton Depression and Anxiety scales and Clinical Global rating scale scores at day 21 and 28. The side effect profiles indicated that bupropion-treated patients reported more agitation and hallucinations (23%) while amitriptyline-treated patients reported more mania, depersonalization, and insomnia (27%). Tremor was 3 times more frequent in bupropion-treated patients and the occurrence of autonomic side effects appeared remarkably similar in bupropion- and amitriptyline-treated patients (dry mouth 64% versus 89%, constipation 41% versus 39%, sweating 18% versus 22%) except for blurred vision which was twice as frequent among amitriptyline-treated patients.

In a large double-blind comparative trial involving bipolar and unipolar outpatients (up to 13 weeks) as well as inpatients (up to 6 weeks)[54] similar findings of equivalent effectiveness were reported for bupropion and amitriptyline. As in the previously mentioned inpatient study,[61] mean daily doses of inpatients receiving bupropion reached 619 mg per day while amitriptyline mean doses were 171 mg per day on average. The outpatients received mean bupropion doses of 374 mg compared with 119 mg of amitriptyline. There were 3 times more outpatient dropouts in the bupropion group than the amitriptyline-treated group, with an overall 20% dropout rate for the study. Additional medication (e.g., neuroleptics) and more than 7 days of benzodiazepine treatment, was required in 66% (N = 31) of bupropion patients and 62% (N = 26) of amitriptyline patients and 4 of these were subsequently excluded from the data analysis. Early dropouts among bupropion patients occurred significantly more often than amitriptyline patients (20% versus 8% p < .05). Together with the previous study, these results were sufficient to support marketing of bupropion but they lack relevance to the current situation because many study patients were medicated with doses of 500 to 900 mg per day and these exceed the current recommended dosage of 300 to 450 mg per day.

More relevant findings for the current dosage guidelines are provided by Feighner et al.[62] This double-blind outpatient trial was designed in a similar fashion to the previous studies but compared bupropion to doxepin. The authors concluded that bupropion in doses of 300 to 400 mg per day was no different in effectiveness than doxepin at doses of 150 to 200 mg per day. Doxepin favored bupropion at weeks 2 and 3 ($p < .05$) and particularly with respect to cognitive disturbance and anxiety somatization factors at weeks 3 and 10 ($p < .05$). Dry mouth, tiredness, sleepiness, increased appetite, and constipation were 2 to 3 times more frequently reported by doxepin patients (statistically significant) while insomnia, headache, and nausea were more frequent in bupropion patients (nonsignificant). Understandably, data on the long-term effectiveness of bupropion is lacking at this time. One exception concerns a 6-month double-blind comparative effectiveness study which reported no difference in the effectiveness of bupropion compared with amitriptyline.[63]

Several studies on the efficacy and safety of bupropion in elderly depressed patients have been reported. For example, depressed outpatients aged 55 to 77 years with mean bupropion doses of 150 mg per day (low) or 323 mg per day (high) were compared with imipramine-treated patients (mean dose = 146 mg per day) for 4 weeks of double-blind treatment. Bupropion was reported to have antidepressant activity and to be tolerated in this population.[64] A similar study at another site[65] found the high-dose bupropion group had significantly greater anxiolytic effect than low-dose bupropion or imipramine. Cognitive improvement was attributed to a practice effect since all treatment groups improved to the same extent. The authors concluded that bupropion would benefit the elderly because they would avoid the anticholinergic and cardiovascular effects of currently marketed antidepressants, although additional empirical support is needed.

Cardiovascular effects of bupropion in depressed patients with pre-existing left ventricular impairment ($N = 15$), ventricular arrhythmias ($N = 15$), and/or conduction disease ($N = 21$) were evaluated by Roose et al.[66] Patients received a mean dose of 442 mg per day of bupropion for 3 weeks. The drug was discontinued in 5 (14%) patients because of adverse effects, including exacerbation of baseline hypertension in 2 patients. Bupropion caused an increase in supine blood pressure but no significant problems in conduction, ventricular arrhythmias, orthostatic hypotension, or pulse rate. These preliminary findings were viewed as hopeful that the generally uneventful use of bupropion in short-term usage will also occur with longer duration of treatment and in larger samples of patients with pre-existing cardiac disease.

Bupropion was found to be ineffective in treating panic disorders.[67]

Bupropion is indicated for the treatment of depression in individuals who have failed to improve on standard antidepressants and do not have any of the following risk factors: history of seizure, head trauma, psychotic symptoms, history of bulimia, or anorexia nervosa and need for concurrent medications that are known to lower the seizure-threshold (e.g., neuroleptics, tricyclic antidepressants, and lithium).[68]

Bupropion appears to be a suitable second-line antidepressant for the mild-moderate nonpsychotically depressed patient in whom standard antidepressants are ineffective or intolerable due to side effects or the presence of pre-disposing risk factors for adverse events.

Atypical antidepressants, particularly those recently marketed such as fluoxetine and bupropion, are enjoying widespread usage. Nevertheless, their benefit-to-risk assessment vis à vis tricyclics in areas such as efficacy for severe depression, side effect profiles, and cost-effectiveness demand additional pharmacoepidemiologic study and clinical experience.

Drug Selection

The tricyclic antidepressants are drugs of first choice for severe depression which consists of typical neurovegetative symptoms unless the risk of suicide or psychosis suggests that electroconvulsive therapy is a better alternative. For the estimated one-third of patients who fail to respond to tricyclic antidepressants, the monoamine oxidase inhibitors are drugs of second choice. Because of their comparable efficacy, the selection of a specific tricyclic agent is based on the patient's past experience or on the side effect profile. If greater sedation is desired for psychomotor agitation, amitriptyline, doxepin, or trazodone may be appropriate, while target symptoms of psychomotor retardation suggest that a less sedating agent (e.g., imipramine or a secondary amine compound) might be selected. Patients sensitive to the strong anticholinergic effect of amitriptyline may better tolerate weaker anticholinergic agents such as desipramine without an expected loss of effectiveness. Patients at risk for cardiotoxic effects include elderly congestive heart failure patients and those with presenting cardiac problems such as bundle branch disease and other A-V conduction blocks. Glassman and Bigger[69] suggest caution in using tricyclic agents such as amitriptyline and imipramine in patients with pre-existing left ventricular dysfunction because of the severe orthostatic hypotension requiring discontinuation of the drug that was observed in 50% of the patients they studied. The decision to treat these patients with low doses of nortriptyline, amoxapine, or trazodone should be made on an individual basis with careful monitoring for orthostatic hypotension and with the collaboration of an experienced cardiologist.

If pre-existing seizure disorder or risk of seizure is a concern, amoxapine, maprotiline, and bupropion should be avoided. Less pronounced sedative effects have been observed with secondary amine tricyclic compounds. The effect of antidepressants on REM sleep has been investigated as a possible predictor of drug responsiveness.[70] Specifically, amitriptyline increased latency time of rapid eye movement (REM) sleep, in effect reducing REM activity in the sleep pattern of depressed patients.

As with the other classes of psychotropics, a patient's past experience with medications is important. In reviewing the patient's current medications for drug-drug interactions, consideration should be given to all drugs that pass the blood-brain barrier, whether for medical or psychiatric purposes, because they may alter the existing balance among the adrenergic, cholinergic, and dopaminergic systems. Many of the drugs that are used to treat heart disease, hypertension, and parkinsonism are in this group.

Patient Factors

A preliminary assessment should be made to establish baseline cardiovascular (recent myocardial infarction, conduction defects, severe perfusion deficits), cerebrovascular, gastrointestinal (e.g., adynamic ileus, esophageal reflux and hiatal hernia may preclude the safe use of any drug which produces an anticholinergic effect), urinary (particularly prostatic hypertrophy), and ophthalmic [specifically, narrow (closed) angle glaucoma] risk factors, especially in the elderly patient. Consultation with experienced medical specialists may be needed to resolve drug selection when such factors are present.

Adequate liver and kidney function are needed to avoid drug intoxication. Elderly patients and those with concomitant physical disorders affecting liver function should be evaluated at baseline and, with appropriate specialty consultation, monitored if abnormal values occur.

Prediction Tests

Several challenge tests have been developed that are designed to assist in the diagnosis of depressive subgroups and selection of medications.[71] Among these is the amphetamine challenge test that involves a behavioral or cardiovascular activation in response to 20 to 30 mg of d-amphetamine administered in one day as a predictor of a favorable response to tricyclics or ECT. The test is a weak and unreliable predictor and negative test responses do not rule out positive drug responses. Thyrotropin-releasing hormone test is a neuroendocrine challenge test in which the response to a 500 μg infusion of TRH was blunted in 25 to 56% of patients with major depression. The test's sensitivity and specificity is very weak. In the metabolic marker group, the presence of normal or high urinary metabolites of norepinephrine (MHPG) are hypothesized to predict serotonergic depression and a positive amitriptyline response while low levels predicted noradrenergic depression and a positive imipramine response, although these drug-specific findings have not been upheld. Overall, these findings are *not* sufficient to support their clinical application.

The dexamethasone suppression test is related to the concept of abnormal secretion of neurotransmitters in depressed patients. Norepinephrine inhibits secretion of corticotrophin releasing factor (CRF) and ACTH secretion with an increase in adrenal cortisol production. In the depressed patient, reduced levels of norepinephrine and other unknown factors may alter control of CRF and produce abnormal steroid levels. To test the individual's response to exogenous steroid, 1 mg of dexamethasone p.o. is administered at 11 PM and blood samples for measuring serum cortisol are drawn at 4 PM and 11 PM the following day. Serum cortisol greater than 5 μg/Dl is considered a positive test for depression and differs from the nondepressed individual's response of suppressed serum cortisol levels.

The low sensitivity of the test is suggested by the false negative results that have been reported in more than 40% of patients with major depression[71] as well as by false positive results in conditions other than depression including panic disorder, mania, dementia, diabetes, and others. Numerous factors can produce artifactual results. For example, false positive tests may be caused by interfering drugs such as phenytoin, barbiturates, carbamazepine, and alcohol while false negative tests may occur with high-dose benzodiazepine therapy and on retesting when the patient is still clinically depressed. The response to tricyclic antidepressants also is not well predicted by the test.

Despite the great clinical need for useful predictors of response to treatment, none of these tests has achieved adequate sensitivity and specificity in sufficiently large populations to recommend their routine clinical use.

Dosing Considerations

Estimated Equivalent Dosage

The tertiary amines, amitriptyline and imipramine, are equipotent (range 50–300 mg per day) while their secondary amine metabolites, nortriptyline and desipramine, are somewhat more potent (range 50–150 and 75–200 mg per day, respectively). Nevertheless, on a mg-equivalent basis the tertiary and secondary amines are about equally effective. Protriptyline is the most potent tricyclic and doses of 15 to 60 mg per day are used to achieve responses comparable to those of the other agents. Overall, the tricyclics and their N-desmethylated (nor) metabolites are approximately equally effective.

Pharmacokinetic Factors

The tricyclic antidepressants resemble the phenothiazines in their pharmacokinetic and metabolism profile. The drugs are well absorbed (peak levels occur within 2–8 hours with extremes of 12 hours) after undergoing variable but generally extensive "first pass" hepatic metabolism. They are relatively lipophilic and have significant plasma and tissue binding resulting in a high volume of distribution (10–20 L/kg). The drugs are metabolized in the liver and undergo dealkylation and oxidation by the cytochrome P-450 enzyme system followed by urinary excretion after oxidation and glucuronidation. Numerous active metabolites of imipramine and amitriptyline in varying ratios to the parent drug exist but plasma levels are usually reported only as that of parent and demethylated product; potentially cardiotoxic hydroxy-tricyclic antidepressant metabolites are rarely assayed even though they may be present in similar amounts as parent and nor-metabolite.

Plasma elimination half-lives of the tricyclic agents range from approximately 16 hours for amitriptyline and imipramine to 30 hours for nortriptyline and desipramine, and secondary amines generally have longer half-lives than tertiary amines. Usually, steady state serum levels are achievable in 4 to 7 days or 4 to 5 times the half-life. Side effect monitoring is appropriate from the start of treatment but clinical monitoring takes a longer period since the clinical antidepressant response cannot be evaluated before 3 to 4 weeks of therapy. Protriptyline is notable for its long half-life of 80 or more hours which makes less frequent dosing possible but which may present added risks in acute organic brain syndrome. Fluoxetine and its active nor-metabolite have very long half-lives, on the order of 90 and 190 hours, respectively, and this fact necessitates cautious use particularly when *adding* this drug to "on board" drugs that rely on liver metabolizing enzymes, such as antipsychotics or benzodiazepines. Trazodone is at the other extreme with a half-life of 5 hours which makes multiple dosing necessary.

Plasma Level Monitoring

Analytical and clinical aspects of plasma level monitoring of the antidepressants have been reviewed by Cooper et al.[72,73] There is significant interindividual variation in the plasma level-dose-response relationships of the tricyclic antidepressants. This variation may be explained partly by genetic differences among individuals. In addition, the ratio of parent to demethylated metabolite varies as much as 50-fold within individuals.[74] There is also additional intra-individual variation, and the reliability of assays performed by commercial laboratories sometimes is uncertain or poor.

To help resolve the problems of variation in dose/plasma level, Cooper and Simpson.[75] among other groups developed a prediction test based on the level observed 24 hours after administration of a single small, safe dose. Their approach makes possible the prediction of an approximately adequate and safe level at steady state with fewer adjustments during the first week of therapy. Table 4.2 provides

TABLE 4.2. Suggested dosage regimen based on 24-hour blood levels after ingestion of 50 mg of nortriptyline.

Blood Level (ng/ml)	Suggested Dosage Regimen
< 12	50 mg three times a day
13–19	50 mg twice a day
20–24	25 mg three times a day
25–34	25 mg twice a day
35–40*	10 mg three times a day
> 41	10 mg twice a day

* Extrapolated from the regression line after graphing the plasma level versus dose for patients who were given a 50 mg oral test dose. For each dose, the 24-hour plasma levels were recorded.[75]

predicted plasma levels after a single 50 mg dose of nortriptyline based on their work. Other studies lead to similar results and have shown the method to be cost-effective and to reduce days in hospital and out of work. As yet, the method is rarely used in clinical practice and needs more systematic evaluation before it can be recommended for routine clinical practice.

The general clinical utility of plasma levels in dosing is the subject of ongoing debate. A major obstacle involves the 10- to 20-fold or greater interindividual variation in levels at a given dose of the same drug that has been observed. To resolve the dilemma, the APA Task Force on Laboratory Tests[76] reviewed the validity and reliability data available in 1985 and found that plasma assays of only 3 tricyclic antidepressant drugs had sufficient support to recommend their use in certain clinical situations. These situations include nonresponsive patients, noncompliant patients, suspected drug toxicity in the elderly and in individuals on drug combinations.

The 3 drugs recommended are nortriptyline, imipramine, and desipramine. In the case of imipramine and desipramine, there are consistent demonstrations of a monophasic plasma level response curve, with maximum benefit usually formed at total tricyclic antidepressant levels at or above 200 ng/ml. Nortriptyline produces a biphasic curvilinear relationship.[77] This inverted U-shaped curve yields what is described as a "therapeutic window" with poor response to nortriptyline expected outside both the upper and lower concentration ranges. Nortriptyline doses that produce levels between 50 and 150 ng/ml may produce maximum therapeutic effect without excessive risk of toxicity. To achieve these levels, doses as high as 100 to 150 mg per day may be required.

The use of plasma drug assay methods often can be helpful when problems arise. For example: (1) to manage a patient with high risk of toxicity due to age or cardiac disease; (2) to interpret toxicity at unusually low levels or lack of effect at high dosages; (3) when concomitant drugs which are hepatic enzyme inducers produce unreliable, reduced antidepressant levels. The use of EKG is an additional monitoring procedure to consider in high risk patients when high dosages are used to achieve a clinical effect while levels remain low.

Dosing Guidelines

Severe Depression: Acute Phase.   Tricyclic antidepressants should be introduced gradually at 50 to 75 mg per day in the healthy adult with increases every 2 to 3 days up to 100 to 150 mg per day of imipramine or its equivalent. Initial inpatient dosages of 100 to 150 mg per day may be increased rapidly to 150 to 250 mg per day. Doses above 200 to 250 mg per day of imipramine or its equivalent, along with adequate plasma levels, increase the risk of toxicity without the likelihood of increased efficacy. This situation may suggest the need for hospitalization to monitor increasing dosages above 250 mg per day especially in those without closely supervised side effect monitoring. In the elderly, debilitated or multi-drug regimen patient 10 to 25 mg per day may be a safer starting dose. Table 4.1 lists usual and extreme dose ranges. The extreme lower dose is a guide for the infirm or elderly (above 65 years) while the upper extreme is suggested during weeks 4 to 6 after an initial period of 3 to 4 weeks in the usual dose range is unsuccessful in healthy adults. Wherever possible, plasma level values and EKG monitoring should be incorporated into dosage decision-making with such patients.

Injectable forms are available for imipramine and amitriptyline and permit the patient who is unmanageable with oral products to receive adequate dosage more easily. Despite faster peak plasma levels and greater bioavailability, there is no therapeutic advantage of injectables over oral products since both forms have similar clinical onset of 2 to 3 weeks and comparable efficacy.

If mood, appetite, sleep, work, and social interactions do not improve after several weeks at dosages up to 300 mg per day of imipramine or its equivalent, the usual course is to switch to a second-choice agent such as a monoamine oxidase inhibitor, an atypical antidepressant or ECT. Prominent authors urge a 7- to 10-day washout period of tricyclic before adding an MAO inhibitor[21] (p. 207) to avoid the potentially life-threatening interaction of an MAO inhibitor and a tricyclic agent although the published clinical reports only document these events when the tricyclic followed the MAO inhibitor. Because there is very limited clinical experience of a safe transition from tricyclic to MAO inhibitor without a washout,[78] it is not recommended until safety has been demonstrated in larger groups and multiple settings.

Severe Depression: Maintenance Phase.   The prescription of maintenance antidepressants was the subject of an NIMH Consensus Development Conference and was endorsed in the following specific situations.[79] Maintenance antidepressants in doses of 75 to 150 mg per day are usually prescribed to reduce the risk of relapse in individuals with recurrent mood disorders.[80] Maintenance drug therapy is more likely to be used when patients have had severe incapacity in the acute episode, or have chronic medical conditions, chronic and psychotic depressive symptoms, older age, and family history of affective disorders.

The efficacy studies for maintenance treatment compare relapse rates in drug- and placebo-treated groups. Summarizing across 7 studies of major depressive patients who were followed for 3 to 8 months after an acute episode, 52% of placebo-treated patients relapsed compared with 21% of imipramine- or amitriptyline-treated patients.[81] Data from 4 longer term studies were reviewed by Baldessarini and Tohen.[82] In these studies, patients were treated with imipramine or placebo and there was 77% relapse on placebo and 54% on antidepressant suggesting that the protective effect is much stronger in the few months following an acute episode. Overall, these data support the short-term (up to 1 year) maintenance treatment following an acute depression.

Additional relapse studies involve a comparison between lithium, antidepressant, the combination, and placebo. In a 1-year follow-up, the relapse rates for these treatments were: placebo (60%), antidepressants (41%), lithium (27%), and combination (29%). At 2- and 3-year follow-up, the protective effect of active drugs in preventing recurrent depression was considerably reduced.[82, 83] For example, at 3 years the relapse rate for placebo was 82%, but for antidepressants (70%), lithium (62%) and the combination (64%), the figures are not remarkably lower. Although lithium and tricyclic combined appears to have an additive effect in clinical trials of unipolar depression, the use of long-term tricyclic agents in bipolar patients may induce mania or psychotic reactions even if lithium is used concomitantly. Moreover, by 3 years of treatment, relapse was likely to have occurred in nearly three-quarters of the cases irrespective of treatment.

Psychotic Depression

When major depression is complicated by psychotic features such as hallucinations and delusions, and when agitation is present, the use of an antipsychotic agent in combination with the antidepressant may be useful. Nevertheless, it is important to remember that a worsening of agitation in the misdiagnosed bipolar or mixed disorders patient may be due to the tricyclic antidepressant. There are a few controlled studies to establish the efficacy of antipsychotic-antidepressant combinations and there is supportive clinical experience. The combined regimen should be optimal when the lowest effective dose of antipsychotic with aggressive antidepressant dosing is used and when monitoring to avoid the toxicity that may follow the additive anticholinergic effect of the combination. Single drug dose changes of no more than 25% at no less than 3 to 5 day intervals provide the opportunity for steady state dosing to be achieved and behavioral response to be assessed. Long-term combination therapy adds the risk of tardive dyskinesia, especially if the association between mood disorder diagnosis and increased risk of tardive dyskinesia is further corroborated.[84]

Clomipramine Dosing for Obsessive-Compulsive Disorder (OCD)

According to the package insert[85] clomipramine should be initiated slowly with low doses (e.g., 25 mg per day and increased in 25 mg per day increments up to 75 mg after one week, 100 mg in the second week, 150 mg in the third, and 200 mg in the fourth). However, after titration to an initial moderate dose to control symptoms, 2 to 3 week intervals between dose increments are consistent with the expected time to achieve steady state pharmacokinetic conditions. The maximum recommended dosage is 250 mg per day. Initially, divided doses with meals may reduce gastrointestinal disturbance but, once stabilized, single bedtime dosing is appropriate. Single bedtime doses have been shown to be equivalent to 3 times a day dosing.

Bupropion Dosing

Bupropion is usually used in adults at 300 mg per day but can be used up to 450 mg per day. Literature from early reports citing doses above this maximum should be disregarded because of the increased risk of seizures. At maximum daily doses of 450 mg, 3 times a day dosing is suggested. The recommendation to use bupropion for insomnia associated with depression in the elderly[86] is inconsistent with the literature that cites the drug's activating properties; avoidance of bedtime dosing is recommended.

Drug Discontinuation and Withdrawal Effects

Abrupt cessation of tricyclic antidepressants has been reported to produce nightmares, insomnia, epigastric distress, anxiety, irritability, and mania. The symptoms are postulated to be the result of noradrenergic hyperactivity (rebound effect) due to increased norepinephrine turnover in the presence of decreased α-2 adrenergic receptor sensitivity.[87] To avoid these withdrawal effects, gradual reduction of antidepressants at about 25% every 3 to 5 days at higher doses and 50% at lower doses is suggested. For example, extreme dosages of 300 mg per day may be reduced in 50 mg decrements every three days over a 2.5 week period. Even more gradual withdrawal of up to 1 month may be required in some cases. Fluoxetine, with its average half-life of 90 hours, may require many weeks to leave the body regardless of the rapidity of discontinuation. The difficulty of distinguishing between drug withdrawal and depressive relapse has been recognized[88] and requires consideration of the timing of symptoms. If symptoms occur within 2 to 14 days after drug withdrawal, then depressive relapse is a less likely explanation. The cumulative probability of depressive relapse increases with time,[21] up to 85% in major unipolar depression by three years on placebo (about 50–60% at one year).[82] This principle implies that the greater the time period between drug discontinuation and recurrence of symptoms, the less likely that the symptoms are drug withdrawal effects.

As with other tricyclic antidepressants, withdrawal effects are expected upon abrupt withdrawal of clomipramine. When a trial of clomipramine is being terminated, a gradual taper over at least 4 weeks should be considered unless toxic conditions or extremely low dosage suggest otherwise. Like other tricyclic antidepressants, several groups of withdrawal symptoms may be found: (1) physiological symptoms such as sweating and elevated temperature; (2) mood and sleep changes such as irritability, difficulty sleeping, increased dreaming; and (3) psychopathological symptoms such as increased aggression, depression, and suicidal ideation. It is important to recognize that new behavioral symptoms following drug withdrawal may not be part of the underlying disorder but merely a transient effect of drug withdrawal.

Both a rigorously designed, double-blind, placebo-controlled withdrawal of clomipramine[89] and anecdotal reports[90] support a clomipramine withdrawal syndrome. For example, a 4-day withdrawal of clomipramine was followed by placebo treatment for 7 weeks and blind ratings were used to assess the outcome of drug withdrawal.[89] The study group consisted of 18 adult patients with OCD treated with doses of 100 to 300 mg per day for a period of 5 to 27 months. Sixteen patients had a substantial recurrence of obsessive-compulsive symptoms by the end of 7 weeks and 11 had an increase in depressive symptoms.

Additional Pharmacodynamic and Clinical Principles

Precautions in the Suicidal Patient. Special attention to the risk of suicide is needed early in tricyclic antidepressant treatment because of the delayed effect of the antidepressants. In addition, the drugs commonly are involved in self-poisoning either deliberately by the patients in acute suicidal overdoses or accidentally by children and adult family members who gain access to the drugs.

The prescription of quantities in excess of a few days supply (less than 1250 mg of imipramine or its equivalent in other agents, which is approximately 25 doses of 50 mg or 1250 mg) may be avoided by involving family members in managing the treatment of outpatients. Another approach involves multiple refills of a 1 week supply provided the total is not more than approximately 1000 mg imipramine-equivalent (much less for higher potency tricyclics).

Age as a Dosing Factor. The selection and dosing of antidepressants in children and adolescents is discussed in Chapter 7.

Geriatric dosing of the antidepressants is a subject of special clinical attention, in part, because of the greater sensitivity of the elderly person's nervous and cardiovascular systems to toxic effects of the drugs. A second factor is the reduced rate of drug metabolism in the elderly (see p. 23). Third, central anticholinergic or other neurotoxic effects can produce an organic mental syndrome with delirium, mental confusion, and agitation. Fourth, cardiovascular problems, especially orthostatic hypotension in those with pre-existing cardiac conduction disease, stroke, hip fractures secondary to falling episodes, and glaucoma are also common complicating problems in the elderly. Fifth, falling episodes which can have serious orthopedic consequences in the elderly patient have been shown to occur more frequently and to be a dose-dependent effect in those exposed to psychotropic drugs[91] especially doxepin, amitriptyline, chlorpromazine, and thioridazine. For these reasons, reduced dosages of nortriptyline or desipramine in the range of 10 to 75 mg per day in divided daily doses with gradual increases over weeks are suggested. Drugs with relatively less anticholinergic activity, such as nortriptyline, desipramine, fluoxetine, and trazodone may be suitable choices. Ami-triptyline, doxepin, and imipramine are less suitable choices in the elderly and in cardiac and CNS disorder patients.

Safety during Pregnancy and Lactation. The safety of the antidepressants to the fetus or newborn during pregnancy and lactation is not established but neither is there evidence of teratogenicity. The drugs cross the placental barrier and are found in breast milk in low levels. Neonatal distress including muscle spasms, congestive heart failure and respiratory distress, has been reported in rare instances.[92] Avoiding the drugs wherever possible is the safest course; electroconvulsive therapy may be a suitable alternative for severe depression in the pregnant and postpartum patient. If medication is unavoidable, low dosage of nortriptyline or desipramine may be considered.

Medication Administration Factors

Smoking.   Laboratory studies support the general notion that smoking enhances drug metabolism by inducing liver enzymes and reducing the plasma level for a given dose of drug. However, early studies of the effect of smoking on antidepressant plasma levels had inconsistent findings. In a more recent study, Perry[93] reported significantly decreased mean total nortriptyline levels but no significant difference in mean free (active) drug levels. The application of these preliminary findings to clinical practice is limited. To be applicable, studies must demonstrate reductions in free drug plasma levels over time for a given dose of antidepressant in large numbers of smokers who receive antidepressants.

Dosing Schedules and Costs.   Total daily doses at or below 150 mg per day may be conveniently administered in once-a-day dosing after dosage is stabilized. Clinical experience with single bedtime doses up to 300 mg has been reported.[80] When given an hour or so before bedtime the drugs may serve to promote sleep as well. The pamoate ester of imipramine is a special, long-acting product formulation that is marketed for this purpose. However, because of its relatively long half-life, imipramine hydrochloride will serve this purpose as well as the special pamoate salt and at a lower price. Table 4.3 lists the price of the frequently prescribed antidepressants. Imipramine pamoate is nonformulary and is listed only for comparison purposes. Newer agents are substantially more expensive than older comparison products. For example, bupropion (300 mg per day) is *40* times more expensive than imipramine HCl (150 mg per day). Similarly, fluoxetine and clomipramine are substantially more expensive than older comparison products.

Noncompliance.   Noncompliance with the antidepressants is a frequently encountered problem. Noncompliance with antidepressant medications was reported for 25% or 43% of a cohort of depressed

TABLE 4.3. Price comparison for frequently prescribed antidepressants.

Agent	Brand Name	Typical Dosage (mg/day)	Price[a] (Dollars)	Relative Cost[b]
Tertiary Amines				
Imipramine HCl	Tofranil[d]	100–300	0.08	1
Imipramine Pamoate[c]	Tofranil-pm	100–300	1.58	20
Amitriptyline	Elavil[d]	100–300	0.07	1
Doxepin	Sinequan[d]	100–300	0.19	2
Trimipramine	Surmontil	100–300	2.23	28
Clomipramine	Anafranil	50–250	2.62	33
Secondary Amines				
Desipramine	Norpramin[d]	100–250	0.36	5
Nortriptyline	Pamelor[d]	75–150	1.89	24
Protriptyline[c]	Vivactil	10–60	1.50	19
Amoxapine	Ascendin	100–400	1.18	15
Maprotiline[c]	Ludiomil	100–300	1.06	13
Atypical Agents				
Trazodone	Desyrel	100–400	0.26	3
Bupropion[c]	Wellbutrin	300–450	1.77	22
SSRIs				
Fluoxetine	Prozac	20–40	1.76	22
Paroxetine	Paxil	20–50	1.53	19
Sertraline	Zoloft	50–200	1.55	19
MAO Inhibitors				
Isocarboxazid	Marplan	30	1.41	1.6
Phenelzine	Nardil	45–75	0.90	1
Tranylcypromine	Parnate	30–60	1.02	1.1

[a] New York State Office of Mental Health contract or direct prices (updated February 1993) for a 150 mg daily dose of amitriptyline or its equivalent based on published approximate equivalencies.

[b] Relative cost based on the comparable dose of the least expensive agent in a class; for example, compared with a bioequivalent generic form of imipramine hydrochloride dosed at 200 mg per day for the tricyclic and atypical compounds. MAO inhibitors are compared with phenelzine in daily doses of 60 mg.

[c] Nonformulary status: not recommended because of lack of rationale (pamoate product), insufficiently demonstrated benefit for the reported risks (maprotiline) insufficient benefit to justify the cost in most patients (trimipramine and protriptyline), and limited evaluation in inpatient settings as well as relatively weak benefit to risk profile (bupropion).

[d] Additional brand names or generic products are available.

outpatients depending on the detection method employed.[94] Noncompliance is a factor contributing to the treatment failure that occurs in 20 to 30% of patients treated with antidepressants. Developing methods for patient participation in side effect monitoring and switching to a drug with a different relative side effect profile may reduce the risk of patient noncompliance. For the long-term maintenance of outpatients with low incomes and those without reimbursement for prescription charges, the cost of antidepressant medication may be a factor in their compliance.

Generic versus Brand Name Products.   For many widely used psychotropic drugs, patent expiration leads to the availability of multiple, equivalent generic products. In recent years, government and third-party reimbursement policies have fostered the substitution of generic products and as this trend has grown, the need for standards increased. To meet the need for an assessment of the quality of generic products, the FDA publishes a list of product ratings ("The Orange Book").[95]

In the FDA rating, the generic product is compared to the product marketed by the company that holds the original patent and the generic is required to be: (1) chemically or pharmaceutically equivalent (i.e., to have identical pharmacologically active ingredients) and (2) bioequivalent (i.e., to have similar bioavailability when administered in identical dosage regimens to the same individuals). The term bioavailability refers to both the rate and extent of drug absorption.

Drugs that are chemically and biologically equivalent are assumed to be therapeutically equivalent, that is, essentially the same in regard to efficacy and toxic effects at equivalent doses. Bioequivalence testing of generic oral products involves healthy subjects who are given a single oral dose of both generic and reference products in a randomized crossover study with washout. Serial blood samples are collected and then assayed for the drug content. Pharmacokinetic parameters (e.g., AUC, C_{max}, and T_{max}) are then compared and are equivalent if they do not differ by more than 20% with 90% confidence and the power of the test at 80%.[96] The NYS Office of Mental Health follows the Orange Book recommendations in its purchasing of generic products.

Despite anecdotal clinical concern, reports documenting clinical problems due to the inequivalence of generic and brand name products are rare.[97] The reported cases usually involve a drug classified as having a narrow therapeutic range (e.g., phenytoin[98] and carbamazepine[99] for seizure control). The extent to which the narrow therapeutic range of carbamazepine for seizure control applies to the use of carbamazepine for psychiatric symptoms of mania and behavioral control is unknown.

Ostroff and Docherty[100] reported differences in amitriptyline blood levels between generic and brand name for a single patient. However, this finding was not supported by a later report from the same authors.[101] The authors found no significant difference among 5 different amitriptyline products in steady state plasma concentrations or clinical effects in 10 chronically depressed patients taking the products in random sequence. A more compelling incident concerns Dubovsky's[97] report of serious nortriptyline intoxication (which might easily have been mistaken for a worsening of the depression) when a patient was switched from generic product to brand name.

Experts agree that a general avoidance of generic products is unwarranted. In rare instances, such as when control of seizures is difficult or incomplete, one might want to avoid any risk of altered bioequivalence. But, in most cases, a general policy of careful change from one manufacturer's product to another is feasible. Unnecessary switching of manufacturers should be avoided and patients should be educated that if a switch is necessitated, weekly plasma level monitoring during the first month is advisable. Monitoring for drug intoxication or return of previously controlled symptoms should allow the generic product's clinical comparability to the previous product to be safely evaluated.

In 1990, the FDA reviewed 24 narrow therapeutic range drugs and found their generic products within acceptable limits of bioequivalence. Nevertheless, there is a general consensus among clinical experts in medical, neurologic, and psychiatric specialties that switching from generic to brand name products or vice versa for narrow therapeutic range drugs requires attention to minimize problems in an individual patient.

Electroconvulsive Therapy

If ECT is begun, antidepressants should not be administered during the treatment. ECT protocols vary depending on the policy of the particular provider. Protocols restricting ECT to 10 to 14 days following withdrawal of antidepressants are generally observed for the MAO inhibitors although there is a single report of successful ECT in a small number of patients who were receiving the drugs.[102] The use of pre-ECT anticholinergic treatment to reduce or dry secretions should be decided after consultation with the anesthesiologist.

Side Effect Monitoring

Side effects of the tricyclic antidepressants may be categorized into the following groups according to their basic pharmacologic actions.

Anticholinergic

Dry mouth, urinary retention, reduced gastrointestinal motility, constipation, and blurred vision are commonly reported. At usual doses these effects are endured by most patients despite frequent reports of discomfort. The notion that pharmacologic tolerance develops with long-term use was challenged in a study in which the frequency of patient-reported side effects of amitriptyline was not significantly different in short-term and long-term users.[103] At higher doses and in acute overdose, severe antivagal effects can produce paralytic ileus and urinary retention, especially in prostatic hypertrophy.

Central Effects

Sedative effects may produce sleepiness and fatigue. Central body temperature regulation may be altered producing hyperthermia. Low-grade confusion can be misdiagnosed as part of depression, or as "dementia," especially in the elderly. Manic switching in bipolar patients should be considered when hyperactivity, agitation and insomnia emerge following the introduction of an antidepressant agent. There is also the risk of inducing or precipitating psychosis or mania in vulnerable individuals[21] as well as manic switching from mixed states.

Cardiovascular Effects

At therapeutic doses in persons with normal heart function, the tricyclic agents exert a quinidine-like effect on the heart muscle. This side effect has been observed to be beneficially anti-arrhythmic in patients with premature ventricular contractions (PVCs).[69] However, at toxic dosages, the drugs produce severe depression of myocardial conduction and contractility as well as potentially dangerous arrhythmias along with palpitations and tachycardia. The lengthening of the PR, QRS, and QTc duration is observed in the electrocardiogram (EKG) pattern. Severe cardiac conduction delays that may produce bundle branch block and atrio-ventricular block, and ventricular tachyarrhythmias are common in acute toxic overdosage. Other cardiovascular effects include syncope due to postural hypotension. Intensive care unit and heart monitoring can be discontinued if the patient is awake and the EKG is totally clear for 24 or more hours after the tricyclic antidepressant overdose.[104]

Neurologic Effects

Dizziness, insomnia, restlessness, and fine and gross resting tremors have been reported. In acute toxic overdosage, epileptic seizures can occur. Amoxapine has been associated with neuroleptic-like extrapyramidal effects, withdrawal dyskinesias and rarely, tardive dyskinesia. Antidepressant-related akathisia has been the subject of recent investigation and underscores the need to distinguish between earlier reports of adverse behavioral effects consisting of restlessness, agitation and hyperactivity from motor restlessness associated with the lower extremities and accompanied by dysphoria.[105] Psychotic patients receiving antipsychotic agents may experience a worsening of psychosis and agitation when a tricyclic agent is added to the regimen. The seizure-threshold lowering of the secondary amines may be greater than that of the tertiary compounds and is a frequent problem among the newer agents such as amoxapine and maprotiline[8] but also occurs with imipramine, other tertiary amines and with bupropion.[68]

Miscellaneous Effects

Skin reactions, allergic obstructive jaundice, purpura and rarely, agranulocytosis have been reported. Weight gain is routine except with fluoxetine and bupropion and is a significant factor in reducing compliance. Increased sweating is also reported.

Acute Intoxication: Symptoms and Management

Acute tricyclic intoxication[106] has the symptoms and signs of anticholinergic toxicity. Centrally-mediated effects that the patient may experience include anxiety, agitation, restlessness, overactivity, delirium, disorientation, impaired memory, hallucinations, and seizures. Autonomic effects include tachycardia, arrhythmias, dilated and unreactive pupils, warm, dry, flushed skin, and increased body temperature. The usefulness and safety of a cholinergic agonist to reverse the anticholinergic blockade is controversial. In this procedure, 1 to 2 mg of physostigmine salicylate (eserine) is administered IM or by *slow* IV injection and repeated in 15 to 30 minute intervals if needed. The technique may be useful when mild intoxication occurs and the vital signs are stabilized. Maintaining the patient's airway, blood pressure, and proceeding to ICU monitoring, if severe, is the general approach. Due to the high morbidity and mortality, acute intoxication is a medical emergency requiring an intensive care unit with constant cardiac monitoring.

Drug-Specific Side Effects

Clomipramine.   Pre-marketing trials involving more than 3000 patients resulted in the manufacturer's report of drug discontinuation in approximately 20%. Reasons for discontinuation involving CNS symptoms, such as abnormal thinking and vertigo, were frequent ($\geq 1/100$) while motor and gait problems and dyskinesias were infrequently reported (1/1000–1/100). Psychiatric symptoms such as delusions, hallucinations, hostility, mania, and suicidal ideation were infrequently reported as side effects of the medication.

The major side effects of clomipramine include CNS effects, anticholinergic effects, and cardiac effects. Anticholinergic effects typically include blurred vision, dry mouth, constipation, and urinary retention. Cardiac effects include conduction changes and orthostatic hypotension. A significant drop in systolic blood pressure was attributed to clomipramine at 150 mg per day during a 5 week study of 17 depressed patients.[107] The effect was judged to be comparable to earlier results with imipramine and amitriptyline. Other effects such as weight gain and sexual dysfunction have been reported. Sleep disturbances described as nocturnal "cataclysms" of frightening illusions of head burning and myoclonus was reported in a woman receiving 200 mg per day. The unusual effects remitted upon discontinuation and recurred upon reinstitution.[108] In addition, the effects of serotonergic excess such as nausea and tremor have been noted. Seizures have been reported to occur in 0.7% of the U.S. clinical trials representing 3000 patients. Serum transaminase levels have been reversibly increased. Elevated plasma prolactin levels with accompanying galactorrhea have been observed and were attributed to both dopaminergic and serotonergic effects.[109]

Spontaneous yawning in 4 individuals accompanied by sexual orgasm in 3 of them was reported to occur within 2 weeks of initiating moderate doses of 50 to 100 mg per day in depressed outpatients. The problems resolved upon discontinuation of the medication.[110]

Aside from monitoring for the typical side effects of imipramine and its congeners, clomipramine's side effects and toxicity may be related to its serotonergic effects. For example, nervousness, headache, nausea may occur as well as dopaminergic effects (e.g., galactorrhea, amenorrhea, dyskinesias) and appropriate monitoring should be undertaken.

Fluoxetine. Nausea, nervousness and insomnia are reported more frequently than with tricyclic antidepressants.[111] Anxiety, nervousness, insomnia, and tremor were reported with significantly greater frequency than with comparison antidepressants (e.g., imipramine and doxepin). These side effects are particularly noteworthy because of the ease with which they might be misinterpreted as worsening depression or psychosis.

Bupropion. The general side effect profile emerging from the clinical trials of bupropion suggests a relatively safe drug with fewer of the troublesome side effects reported at higher doses of tricyclics (e.g., anticholinergic effects, orthostatic hypotension, and sedation). However, the data in these studies reflect the experience of patients who *completed* the trials. Further, by design, the studies tended to exclude patients with major predisposing risk factors for seizures (e.g., history of seizures) and concomitant medication with the potential to lower the seizure-threshold.

Bupropion and seizures: A review of the relationship between bupropion and seizures as reported to the manufacturer is provided by Davidson.[68] In an analysis of all clinical trial patients (N = 4262), there were 37 seizure reports for a crude incidence of 0.80%. If the 19 patients receiving doses above 450 mg are estimated separately then the incidence is 2.2% and those below 450 mg per day yield an estimated incidence of 0.4% which is the same order of magnitude as the seizure risk for previously marketed antidepressants. Thus, the revised product information has a maximum dose of 450 mg per day. In examining the time at risk for seizures, the author found that the median time on dose at which seizures occurred was 8 days and 11 cases had seizures within 2 days of the dosage they were receiving at the time. Although a consistent relationship was not apparent, a majority of cases had a proximate escalation of dose which was thought to play a role in provoking seizures. Therefore, the revised product information suggests that dosage adjustments should be made no sooner than 3 days after the initial daily dose.

Bupropion and psychosis: Among patients discontinued from bupropion treatment during clinical trials, a substantial number had intolerable side effects of a psychotic nature.[112] Auditory and visual hallucinations, severe agitation, and disorientation to time were reported by an adult with no prior history of psychosis and in 2 adults (1 elderly) with a prior history of psychotic depression. In 2 of these 3 cases, the occurrence of psychosis appeared to be related to the dose (dose-dependent). In an earlier report, subjective perceptual changes were reported in 6 patients at mean bupropion doses of 560 mg per day.[113] Unlike the newer report of more severe reactions, the earlier report interpreted effects such as vivid dreaming and altered time perception as possibly beneficial activating effects of the antidepressant. Those engaged in debating the significance of these effects are grappling with an increasingly common psychiatric problem related to the behavioral toxicity of psychotropic agents. It would be useful to undertake intensive post-marketing surveillance to determine if an etiologic relationship can be substantiated.[114]

Monitoring for treatment-emergent psychosis in nonpsychotic depressed patients would consist of regular ratings of symptoms from Hamilton Depression, Hamilton Anxiety and Symptom Checklist-90 (or other scale appropriate for treatment-emergent events). Increased or newly emergent psychotic behaviors would suggest the need for dosage lowering or discontinuation of the drug if the symptoms do not resolve with a dose reduction. If psychotic behavior resolved after discontinuation, the evidence for an association would be strengthened.

Drug-Drug Interactions

A detailed discussion of the following interactions and suggested clinical actions are provided in the books by Hansten and Horn[115] and Baldessarini.[27]

Medical Drug Interactions

Centrally-acting substances and drugs primarily produce additive depressant effects in combination with tricyclic antidepressants.

Examples include alcohol, narcotic analgesics, such as meperidine and morphine, and sedating antihistamines.

The barbiturates may diminish the antidepressant effect by decreasing the plasma level of tricyclic agents. This effect is hypothesized to be due to increased drug metabolism by means of enzyme induction and is supported by the reported increase of levels of hydroxylated metabolites. Avoiding barbiturate use should improve the response to the tricyclic agent.

The antiepileptic agents may decrease the effectiveness of the tricyclics. In the past, the combined use of carbamazepine and the tricyclics was avoided because of their structural similarities. Recent use of carbamazepine in treatment-resistant affective disorder patients and for other unlabeled indications has produced anecdotal reports of a change in the effectiveness of other psychotropics. In part, this may be attributed to reduced plasma levels of the other psychotropics due to increased metabolism. The enzyme-induction effect of carbamazepine supports these drug interaction findings.[116]

Cardiovascular Agents. Alpha-adrenergic agonists such as norepinephrine and phenylephrine may potentiate tricyclics by blocking their neuronal uptake.

Beta-adrenergic agonists such as epinephrine may be potentiated by tricyclics.

Alpha-methyldopa, a centrally-acting hypotensive agent, may reduce the effectiveness of a tricyclic.

Clonidine, a hypotensive which may act by stimulating central alpha-2-adrenergic receptors and inhibit vasomotor function, may be diminished by tricyclics. Moreover, the reports of hypertensive crisis[117] or loss of blood pressure control[118] when a tricyclic was added to a clonidine-stabilized hypertensive patient and the possibility of alternative control of blood pressure with beta-blockers and diuretics led to the recommendation that tricyclics and clonidine be avoided.

Additional cardiac agents that may interact with tricyclics are quinidine and digitalis glycosides. Since tricyclics have a quinidine-like effect they can generally substitute for quinidine. This approach avoids potentiating effects (e.g., intraventricular (H-V) prolongation).[69] Consultation with a cardiologist to monitor gradual switching of the medication is recommended. If digoxin for congestive heart failure is used with a tricyclic agent, there should be monitoring for increased cardiac depression and irritability.

Gastrointestinal Agents.   Cimetidine may impair the hepatic metabolism of tricyclic agents and increase plasma levels of the tricyclic agent.

Gel type antacids containing aluminum, magnesium and calcium salts may directly bind the tricyclics in the gut and can reduce their absorption. To avoid this effect, the antacid may be administered 1 hour before or 2 hours after the tricyclic.

Psychotropic Drug Interactions

Central and autonomic effects of drugs used for psychiatric treatment may interfere with tricyclic agents.

Centrally-Acting Depressants.   Agents such as glutethimide (nonformulary, not recommended) for insomnia produce additive depressant effects with the tricyclic agents. Additive effects due to central anticholinergic activity occur with antihistamines, antipsychotics and antiparkinson drugs. While benzodiazepines have been widely used with tricyclics, the addition of diazepam to amitriptyline increased the plasma level of the latter. Monitoring for additive CNS depressant effects should be undertaken.

Central Stimulants.   These agents may enhance the clinical effect of the tricyclics but are avoided on the theoretical grounds that the combination will produce serious hypertension. There is a recent clinical report of a small number of treatment-resistant patients who gave written consent and were successfully treated with the combination of a tricyclic agent and methylphenidate.[119] Nevertheless, the combination requires study before its efficacy and safety are established.

Monoamine Oxidase Inhibitors.   These agents have produced severe fatal cerebrotoxic crisis along with seizures and hyperpyrexia when used with the tricyclic agents.[120,121] Since hypertension is not always present, the mechanism may not be a tyramine-type effect.

Bupropion.   Dopamine agonists are not routinely prescribed with antipsychotics because of the likelihood of physiological antagonism, ineffectiveness, and the difficulty of managing any behavioral toxicity that the combination may produce. Consequently, the effectiveness of the weak dopamine agonist, bupropion in combination with antipsychotics, which are dopamine antagonists, is controversial. Bupropion clinical trials generally did not include patients with psychotic depression and little is known about the effectiveness of bupropion and antipsychotics. There are 3 open studies[122, 123, 124] with small numbers of patients with schizoaffective disorder who were treated with combined low dose antipsychotic and bupropion. In one study, thiothixene and placebo patients did better than thiothixene and bupropion patients at 4 weeks.[122] The second study had few completers in the "bupropion only" group so that the finding is equivocal.[123] The third study reported on an unselected group of treatment-responsive patients who were successfully managed with low doses of bupropion and either antipsychotic or benzodiazepines. The manufacturer does *not* recommend the combination of antipsychotics with bupropion in clinical practice settings until efficacy is established by randomized, double-blind trial findings.

In addition, bupropion and antipsychotic combinations are not recommended on the basis of the seizure-threshold lowering potential of the antipsychotics. Bupropion and antipsychotics or other antidepressants is a Severity 2 interaction. If it is used, there should be close monitoring to document effectiveness, safety, and lack of behavioral toxicity in each specific case. Combination with other dopamine agonists increases the likelihood of hallucinations and other psychotic symptoms; the combination has been reported to be ineffective for Parkinsonian patients. Combination with levodopa or amantadine, dopamine agonists with known psychotogenic potential, is not recommended. The addition of bupropion to a regimen of haloperidol, amantadine (for parkinsonism), and benztropine in an elderly parkinsonian patient with depression after completing a course of ECT led to delirium and resolved upon discontinuation of bupropion.[125] The combination led the authors to speculate on "dopaminergic overdrive" caused by the dopaminergic activity of bupropion, amantadine, and benztropine, while others have suggested this dopaminergic excess may also be caused by ECT.[126]

Fluoxetine. Fluoxetine has been reported to produce adverse clinical effects and toxicity when added to various psychotropics. The interaction is postulated to be due to fluoxetine interference with the metabolism of the other psychotropics. These interaction reports concern haloperidol,[127] tricyclics,[128] L-tryptophan,[129] buspirone,[130] carbamazepine,[131] lithium,[132] and benzodiazepines.[133,134]

Goff et al.[135] reported relatively modest elevations of haloperidol levels (20% $p < .05$) in 7 of 8 psychotic patients after 7 to 10 days of the addition of 20 mg per day of fluoxetine. Patients received relatively low stable haloperidol doses (average = 14 mg per day). Unfortunately, fluoxetine could not have achieved steady state in most subjects and the relatively low dosing does not preclude the possibility of more severe interactions at higher doses and after steady state of fluoxetine.

Clomipramine.   Clomipramine may compete with drugs that are highly protein bound (e.g., digoxin and warfarin). If clomipramine is added to a regimen of such agents, changes in the dosage of the primary drug may be necessary. Although there is limited experience with low doses of a tricyclic antidepressant in combination with an MAO inhibitor, clomipramine as well as imipramine are considered definitely contraindicated with an MAO inhibitor. Three deaths, and possibly a fourth, were attributed to the addition of clomipramine to patients receiving an MAO inhibitor.

Other drug-drug interactions for clomipramine should follow the general guidelines for tricyclic antidepressants, particularly, imipramine.[136]

These previously reported interactions include interference with hypotensive agents (e.g., clonidine leading to loss of blood pressure control; competitive inhibition of the hypotensive effect of guanethidine, debrisoquine, and bretylium). In Britain, since 1964, there have been 12 reports of serious adverse events related to dental procedures involving the use of local anesthetics containing norepinephrine in patients medicated with TCAs. Headaches led to loss of consciousness in all and death in one patient. Similarly, potentiation of the pressor effect of phenylephrine and epinephrine with imipramine has been reported. The adverse behavioral effects of amphetamines were observed to increase upon addition of tricyclic antidepressants. Methylphenidate was reported to interfere with the metabolism of imipramine and produce increased plasma levels of the antidepressant. High-dose estrogen was reported to interfere with the metabolism of imipramine although whether this interaction extends to patients receiving oral birth control pills is a controversial question.

MONOAMINE OXIDASE INHIBITORS

Shortly before the introduction of the tricyclics in the late 1950s, the antidepressant properties of iproniazid were attributed to the inhibition of monoamine oxidase, the enzyme responsible for the oxidative deamination of norepinephrine, serotonin, and dopamine. In addition to iproniazid, other agents of the hydrazine type such as phenelzine and isocarboxazid as well as nonhydrazine type agents such as tranylcypromine, clorgyline, and deprenyl were developed. However, the popularity of the original agents declined because of several problems. Among these were hypertensive fatalities, liver toxicity, supposedly limited efficacy, and difficulties related to dietary restrictions. Some of these problems have been put into perspective and their current status is second-choice agents after tricyclic agents fail to control severe depression.

In retrospect, clinical experience suggests that underdosage may have contributed to the lack of efficacy, and recent studies at adequate doses support efficacy similar to that of the tricyclic agents. Recent research suggests that platelet MAO (MAO B) should be inhibited by at least 85% before clinical improvement is expected, provided that the patient can tolerate the high doses that are often required, especially for phenelzine.

After oral dosing, the MAO inhibitors exert their enzyme-inhibiting effect within days, although 4 to 6 weeks is needed before the antidepressant effect emerges. Upon withdrawal of MAO inhibitors, MAO activity returns when new MAO enzyme molecules are created in 7 to 14 days, so that a waiting period of at least 2 weeks is recommended to avoid subsequent interactions.

Drug Selection

The 3 currently available MAO inhibitors in U.S. practice are listed in Table 4.1. Phenelzine and isocarboxazid are hydrazine-derived and irreversibly bind MAO while tranylcypromine is nonhydrazine-derived and reversibly but very tenaciously binds MAO. Tranylcypromine is an amphetamine analog with stimulating properties. More selective irreversible type agents that are of current experimental interest are clorgyline, a type A MAO inhibitor and (-) deprenyl, a type B MAO inhibitor. MAO-A inhibition seems more likely to produce antidepressant effects. Experimental, short-acting MAO-A inhibitors are currently under study.

Efficacy

In reviewing 17 published studies Baldessarini,[21] summarizing Davis[80] and Morris and Beck,[18] concluded that phenelzine (doses up to 90 mg per day) and isocarboxazid were inferior to a standard tricyclic agent in 44% and 40% of the trials, respectively. Tranylcypromine was similar to the tricyclic agent in 3 studies. Overall, the MAO inhibitors had inferior efficacy when compared with tricyclics and ECT, but more recent results with doses of phenelzine at or above 45 mg per day showed efficacy as good as the tricyclic agents.

Target Patient Population

Monoamine oxidase inhibitors are indicated for a severely depressed patient who fails to respond to an adequate trial of a tricyclic agent, is not acutely suicidal (or has a protective, hospital environment) and can cooperate with the restrictions imposed by a low-tyramine diet. In addition, the drug regimen should not include interacting sympathomimetic drugs. Besides severe depression, the MAO inhibitors have been used in chronic dysthymia, chronic anxiety, phobic and panic disorders; their usefulness in the long-term prophylaxis of major depression is not yet proven but is reasonable, as with TCAs, for periods of 6 to 12 months after recovery from an acute episode of depression. Because of the possible occurrence of severe hepatocellular toxic reactions with MAO inhibitors, patients being introduced to these drugs should be assessed at baseline and during the initial weeks of treatment for bilirubin and transaminase functions. Chronic liver disease patients should not be treated with these agents.

Dosage Considerations

Phenelzine: To achieve adequate platelet MAO inhibition phenelzine doses between 45 and 90 mg per day[137] may be required. One 15 mg tablet per day on days 1 and 2 may be followed by gradual increases to 3 to 4 per day (45–60 mg) over a two-week period.

Other agents: The utility of platelet MAO measurements is not established for the dosing of the other agents. Clinical response is the best guide to dosage. Tranylcypromine may produce a more rapid response than the other MAO inhibitors.

MAO Inhibitor Withdrawal

If the MAO inhibitor is followed by a trial of a tricyclic, a 10- to 14-day period is needed to allow replenishment of MAO molecules. Failure to do so has produced reports of rare but severe and sometimes fatal MAOI-TCA interactions involving seizures, delirium and hyperyrexia, usually with hypertensive crisis. Despite the serious risks of combination therapy, for the most severe treatment-resistant cases, there is some limited experience with the *low-dose* combination of an MAO inhibitor and a tricyclic agent.[138] In cases warranting this risk, the MAO inhibitor would be added to the TCA. The justification for such trials is based on the severity of the depression, failure of adequate trials of more established treatments, and should be done with written consent, cautious dosing, close monitoring and the avoidance of injectable forms of the drugs and large doses of either agent. Further evidence of the safety of this combination is needed.

Dietary Restrictions

The MAO inhibitors prevent the metabolism in the gut and liver of tyramine contained in foods, allowing more tyramine to enter sympathetically innervated tissue and causing the release of norepinephrine

TABLE 4.4. Dietary restrictions for the patient receiving monoamine oxidase inhibitors.[139]

Foods which must be avoided

    Chianti and other wines and beer
    Cheese (except cottage and cream cheese)
    Smoked or pickled fish (herring)
    Beef or chicken liver
    Summer (dry) sausage
    Fava or broad bean pods (Italian green beans)
    Yeast vitamin supplements (Brewer's Yeast)

Foods which are questionable—unlikely to cause problems unless consumed in large quantities

    Other alcoholic beverages
    Ripe avocados
    Ripe fresh banana
    Sour cream
    Soy sauce (? individual sensitivity to MSG)
    Yogurt

Foods which may be used—insufficient evidence to support exclusion

    Chocolate
    Figs
    Meat tenderizers
    Raisins
    Yeast breads
    Coffee, tea and caffeine-containing beverages

from adrenergic nerve endings. Table 4.4 lists common foods and their relative tyramine content.[139] The current theory holds that intra-neuronal accumulation of excessive norepinephrine may be a crucial aspect of the high blood pressure effect of tyramine.

Drug Discontinuation

Dosage reductions are required to achieve the lowest effective mainte-nance dose and should be done gradually over several weeks. The same process should be used when discontinuing the medication to avoid the possibility of rebound depression effects, a common behavioral with-drawal symptom.

Side Effect Monitoring

Postural hypotension, weight gain, sexual dysfunction (specifically, retarded ejaculation and anorgasmia), daytime sedation, and edema are frequently reported side effects, especially with high doses of phenelzine.

Anticholinergic effects of dry mouth, constipation, and urinary retention are less severe than with the tricyclic antidepressants but dysautonomic changes occur probably through altered adrenergic function.

Acute psychosis has been reported after acute intoxication of MAO inhibitors. Restlessness, agitation, insomnia, and manic switching in bipolar patients have been reported.

Hydrazine-type MAO inhibitors such as phenelzine and isocarbox-azid in rare instances have induced severe, life-threatening hepatocel-lular liver toxicity.

Drug-Drug Interactions

More detailed discussion of drug-drug interactions of the MAO in-hibitors is found in the textbooks by Hansten and Horn[115] and Baldessarini.[21]

Medical Drug Interactions

Analgesics.   Meperidine and probably its congener, alfaprodine, should **NEVER** be used with an MAO inhibitor (for example, to treat "headache" which may be secondary to increased blood pressure) be-cause it has produced severe, immediate crises including excitation, rigidity, hypertension, circulatory collapse, and death. The morphine-related compounds have not been associated with the severe, fatal reaction of meperidine and MAO inhibitors but their safety is relatively uncertain. There is some experience with codeine that has been suggested as an alternative.[140]

Hypoglycemic Agents. Hypoglycemic agents such as insulin and the sulfonylureas may be potentiated by MAO inhibitors and result in hypoglycemic shock.

Anesthetics may cause moderate to severe hypotension and CNS depression when administered with MAO inhibitors. Freese[102] reviewed reports of 42 surgical patients who were receiving MAO inhibitors and were successfully anesthetized during surgery.

Levodopa, Alpha-Methyldopa and L-Tryptophan. Levodopa or alpha-methyldopa may have a potentiated, toxic effect with MAO inhibitors because they are precursors of the neurotransmitters dopamine and norepinephrine, respectively. Analogously, L-tryptophan and especially 5-hydroxytryptophan, may have a potentiated, toxic effect through stimulation of the serotonergic system.

In 1989, the Center for Disease Control received reports of 30 cases of eosinophilia[141] and severe generalized myalgia in association with L-tryptophan. The drug was marketed as a dietary supplement without a prescription and improper formulation was thought to cause the allergic reaction. Patients should be advised to avoid self-medication of psychological and behavioral problems especially when they are supplementing prescribed psychotropic medication.

Antihypertensives. Antihypertensive agents such as guanethidine (rarely used at present), reserpine, and methyldopa may produce hypertensive reactions in a gradual rather than immediate onset due to the release of accumulated catecholamines.

Sympathomimetics. Sympathomimetics, such as phenylpropanolamine and ephedrine, frequently are contained in nonprescription cold or "sinus" products and weight-reducing products. They will augment sympathomimetic activity and can induce severe hypertension with MAO inhibitors. Appropriate education of the patient is needed to insure their avoidance.

Psychotropic Drug Interactions

As previously discussed, tricyclic antidepressants and MAO inhibitors are regarded as a combination to be avoided because hypertensive crises have produced hyperpyrexia, seizures and death in humans. However, some cautious use of reduced dosage combinations has been reported as safe and feasible. If used at all, the combined use of a tricyclic antidepressant and MAO inhibitor must be used with extreme caution, in reduced doses, and carefully justified by the treatment-specific situation. Moreover, there is still no evidence that the combination is more effective than aggressive use of a single agent or ECT.

Centrally-acting sympathomimetics such as amphetamine may produce a hypertensive crisis and stroke (especially hemorrhagic).

Centrally-acting drugs such as opiates, barbiturates, anesthetics, and alcohol may have their central depressant effects potentiated by MAO inhibitors.

ANTIDEPRESSANTS IN OTHER DRUG CLASSES

A discussion of the use of the benzodiazepine, alprazolam, as an antidepressant will be found in Chapter 5.

POLYPHARMACY

There is no rationale for prescribing more than one antidepressant, although occasional cases of combinations may be justified. Combinations within or between classes of antidepressants are not supported by randomized controlled clinical trials and present problems in terms of dosage adjustments and attribution of side effects. Alternatively, lithium has been added to the TCA when the response to the TCA is insufficient.

Combinations of antipsychotics, antidepressants, and anticholinergic agents are a difficult management problem in terms of assessing the additive anticholinergic exposure. The combined anticholinergic effects of the 3 drug classes may produce adverse somatic symptoms as well as cognitive and mood changes in themselves (i.e., behavioral toxicity). Despite growing multi-drug usage, distinguishing drug-induced behavioral symptoms from those that are illness-based is a clinical and research task that has received little systematic attention. In order to produce clearer dose-plasma level-clinical response-side effect relationships among the psychotropics, drug regimens should be as uncomplicated as possible.

REFERENCES

1. Hirschfeld, RMA, Shea MT: Mood disorders: psychosocial treatments, in Comprehensive Textbook of Psychiatry/V, Vol 1, 5th ed. Edited by Kaplan HI, Sadock BJ. Baltimore, Williams and Wilkins, 1989, pp. 933–934; 942–944

2. DiMascio A, Weissman MM, Prusoff BA, Neu C, Zwilling M, Klerman GL: Differential symptom reduction by drugs and psychotherapy in acute depression. Arch Gen Psychiatry 1979; 36:1450–1456

3. Elkin I, Parloff MB, Hadley SW, Autry JH: NIMH treatment of depression collaborative research program. Arch Gen Psychiatry 1985; 42:305–316

4. Elkins I, Shea MT, Watkins JT, Imber SD, Sotsky SM, Collins JF, Glass DR, Pilkonis PA, Leber WR, Docherty JP, et al: NIMH treatment of depression colloborative research program. General effectiveness of treatments. Arch Gen Psychiatry 1989; 46:971–981

5. Kline NS: Present status of psychopharmacological research. Hearings before the subcommittee of the Committee on Appropriations. U.S. Senate, 85th Congress, First Session HR 6287. Washington, DC: U.S. Government Printing Office, May 1957

6. Nelson RC, Baum C: Maprotiline and seizures: An analysis of FDA's adverse reaction system. Abstracts of the 1985 American Public Health Association Meeting, and Nelson RC, unpublished data

7. Bryant SG, Brown CS: Current concepts in clinical therapeutics: major affective disorders, part I. Clin Pharmacy 1986; 5:304–318

8. Prien RF, Blaine JD, Levine J: Antidepressant drug therapy: The role of the new antidepressants. Hosp and Community Psychiatry 1985; 36:513–516

9. Schildkraut JJ: The catecholamine hypothesis of affective disorders: A review of supporting evidence. Am J Psychiatry 1965; 122:509–522.

10. Van Praag HM: Amine hypotheses of affective disorders, in Handbook of Psychopharmacology, Vol 13. Edited by Iversen LL, Iversen SD, Snyder SH. New York, Plenum Press, 1978

11. Axelrod J, Whitby LG, Hertting G: Effect of psychotropic drugs on the uptake of H_3-norepinephrine by tissues. Science 1961; 133:383–384

12. Charney DS, Menkes DB, Heninger GR: Receptor sensitivity and the mechanism of action of antidepressant treatment. Arch Gen Psychiatry 1981; 38:1160–1180

13. Siever LJ, Davis KL: Overview: Toward a dysregulation hypothesis of depression. Am J Psychiatry 1985; 142:1017–1031

14. Richelson E: Antimuscarinic and other receptor-blocking properties of antidepressants. Mayo Clinic Proceedings 1983; 58:40–46

15. Baldessarini RJ: Biomedical Aspects of Depression and Its Treatment. Washington, DC, APA Press, 1983

16. Lipinski JF, Jr., Cohen BM, Zubenko GS, Waternaux CM: Adrenoceptors and the pharmacology of affective illness: A unifying theory. Life Sciences 1987; 40:1947–1963

17. Baldessarini RJ: Drugs and the treatment of psychiatric disorders, in Goodman and Gilman's Pharmacological Basis of Therapeutics. 8th ed. Edited by Gilman AG, Rall TW, Nies AS, Taylor P. New York, Pergamon Press, 1990

18. Morris JB, Beck AT: The efficacy of antidepressant drugs. A review of research (1958–1972). Arch Gen Psychiatry 1974; 30:667–674

19. Raskin A, Schulterbrandt JG, Reatig N, McKeon JJ: Differential response to chlorpromazine, imipramine, and placebo. A study of subgroups of hospitalized depressed patients. Arch Gen Psychiatry 1970; 23:164–173

20. Hodern A, Holt NF, Burt CG, Gordon, WF: Amitriptyline in depressive states. Brit J Psychiatry 1963; 109:815–825

21. Baldessarini RJ: Antidepressants, in Chemotherapy in Psychiatry: Principles and Practice. 2nd ed. Cambridge, Harvard University Press, 1985

22. Quitkin F, Rifkin A, Klein DF: Monoamine oxidase inhibitors. A review of antidepressant effectiveness. Arch Gen Psychiatry 1979; 36:749–760

23. Liebowitz MR, Quitkin FM, Stewart JW, McGrath PJ, Harrison WM, Markowitz JS, Rabkin JC, Tricamo E, Goetz DM, Klein DF: Antidepressant specificity in atypical depression. Arch Gen Psychiatry 1988; 45:129–137

24. Hall H, Ogren SO: Effects of antidepressant drugs on different receptors in the brain. European J Pharmacology 1981; 70:393–407

25. Lindbom LO, Malatray J, Hall H, Ogren SO: Cardiovascular and anticholinergic effects of zimelidine. Progress in Neuro-Psychopharmacology and Biological Psychiatry 1982; 6:403–406

26. Boyer WF, Feighner JP: The serotonin hypothesis: necessary but not sufficient, in Selective Serotonin Re-uptake Inhibitors. Edited by Feighner JP, Boyer WF. Chichester, John Wiley & Sons, 1991 pp. 71–80

27. Evans LE, Bett JH, Cox JR, Dubois JP, Van Hees T: The bioavailability of oral and parenteral chlorimipramine (Anafranil). Progress in Neuro-Psychopharmacology and Biological Psychiatry 1980; 4:293–302

28. Nagy A, Johansson R: The demethylation of imipramine and clomipramine as apparent from their plasma kinetics. Psychopharmacology 1977; 54:125–131

29. McTavish D, Benfield P: Clomipramine. An overview of its pharmacological properties and a review of its therapeutic use in obsessive compulsive disorder and panic disorder. Drugs 1990; 39:136–153

30. Anonymous: Clomipramine in the treatment of patients with obsessive compulsive disorder. The Clomipramine Collaborative Study Group. Arch Gen Psychiatry 1991; 48:730–738

31. Mavissakalian M, Turner SM, Michelson L, Jacob R: Tricyclic antidepressants in obsessive-compulsive disorder: antiobsessional or antidepressant agents? II. Am J Psychiatry 1985; 142:572–576

32. Montgomery SA: Clomipramine in obsessional neurosis: a placebo-controlled trial. Pharmaceut Medicine 1980; 1:189–192

33. Thorén P, Asberg M: Clomipramine treatment of obsessive-compulsive disorder. I. A controlled clinical trial. Arch Gen Psychiatry 1980 37: 1281–1285

34. Ananth J, Pecknold JC, van den Steen N, Engelsmann F: Double-blind comparative study of clomipramine and amitriptyline in obsessive neurosis. Progress in Neuro-Psychopharmacology and Biological Psychiatry 1981; 5:257–262

35. Insel TR, Murphy DL, Cohen RM, Alterman I, Kilts C, Linnoila M: Obsessive-compulsive disorder. A double-blind trial of clomipramine and clorgyline. Arch Gen Psychiatry 1983; 40:605–612

36. Volavka J, Neziroglu F, Yaryura-Tobias JA: Clomipramine and imipramine in obsessive-compulsive disorder. Psychiatry Research 1985; 14: 85–93

37. Marks IM, Hodgson R, Rachman S: Treatment of chronic obsessive-compulsive neurosis by in-vivo exposure. A two year follow-up and issues in treatment. Brit J Psychiatry 1975; 127:349–364

38. Foa EB, Goldstein A: Continuous exposure and complete response prevention of obsessive-compulsive neurosis. Behavior Therapy 1978; 9:821–829

39. Kasvikis Y, Marks IM: Clomipramine, self-exposure, and therapy accompanied exposure in obsessive-compulsive ritualizers, two year follow-up. J Anxiety Disorders 1988; 2:291–298

40. O'Sullivan G, Noshirvani H, Marks I, Monteiro W, Lelliott P: Six-year follow-up after exposure and clomipramine therapy for obsessive-compulsive disorder. J Clin Psychiatry 1991; 52:150–155

41. Waxman D: A clinical trial of clomipramine and diazepam in the treatment of phobic and obsessional illness. J Intl Medical Research 1977; 5 Suppl 5:99–110

42. Trimble MR: Worldwide use of clomipramine. J Clin Psychiatry 1990; 51 Suppl:51–54

43. Faravelli C, Brat A, Marchetti G, Franchi F, Padeletti L, Michelucci A, Pastorino A: Cardiac effects of clomipramine treatment. ECG and left ventricular systolic time intervals. Neuropsychobiology 1983; 9:113–118

44. Burckhardt D, Raeder E, Müller V, Imhof P, Neubauer H: Cardiovascular effects of tricyclic and tetracyclic antidepressants. JAMA 1978; 239:213–216

45. Giardina EG, Bigger JT, Jr., Glassman AH, Perel JM, Kantor SJ: The electrocardiographic and antiarrhythmic effects of imipramine hydrochloride at therapeutic plasma concentrations. Circulation 1979; 60:1045–1052

46. Cowe L, Lloyd DJ, Dawling S: Neonatal convulsions caused by withdrawal from maternal clomipramine. Brit Med J 1982; 284:1837–1838

47. Musa AB, Smith CS: Neonatal effects of maternal clomipramine therapy (letter). Arch of Disease in Childhood 1979; 54:405

48. Stark P, Hardison CD: A review of multicenter controlled studies of fluoxetine vs. imipramine and placebo in outpatients with major depressive disorder. J Clin Psychiatry 1985; 46:3(sec 2) 53–58

49. Wernicke JF, Dunlop SR, Dornseif BE, Zerbe RL: Fixed-dose fluoxetine therapy for depression. Psychopharm Bull 1987; 23:164–168

50. Feighner JP, Cohn JB: Double-blind comparative trials of fluoxetine and doxepin in geriatric patients with major depressive disorder. J Clin Psychiatry 1985; 46:3(sec 2):20–25

51. Trimble MR: Non-monoamine oxidase inhibitor antidepressants and epilepsy: a review. Epilepsia 1978; 19:241–250

52. Jick H, Dinan BJ, Hunter JR, Stergachis A, Ronning A, Perera DR, Madsen S, Nudelman PM: Tricyclic antidepressants and convulsions. J Clin Psychopharmacology 1983; 3:182–185

53. Cooper BR, Hester TJ, Maxwell RA: Behavioral and biochemical effects of the antidepressant bupropion (Wellbutrin): evidence for selective blockade of dopamine uptake in vivo. J Pharmacol Exptl Therapeutics 1980; 215:127–134

54. Chouinard G: Bupropion and amitriptyline in the treatment of depressed patients. J Clin Psychiatry 1983; 44:121–129

55. Whiteman PD, Peck AW, Fowle ASE, Smith PR: Failure of bupropion to affect prolactin or growth hormone in man. J Clin Psychiatry 1983; 44:209–210

56. Lai AA, Schroeder DH: Clinical pharmacokinetics of bupropion: a review. J Clin Psychiatry 1983; 44:82–84

57. Schroeder DH: Metabolism and kinetics of bupropion. J Clin Psychiatry 1983; 44:79–81

58. Preskorn SH: Antidepressant response and plasma concentrations of bupropion. J Clin Psychiatry 1983; 44:137–139

59. Golden RN, DeVane CL, Laizure SC, Rudorfer MV, Sherer MA, Potter WZ: Bupropion in depression II. The role of metabolites in clinical outcome. Arch Gen Psychiatry 1988; 45:145–149

60. Zung WWK: Review of placebo-controlled trials with bupropion. J Clin Psychiatry 1983; 44:104–114

61. Davidson J, Miller R, Van Wyck Fleet J, Strickland R, Manberg P, Allen S, Parrott R: A double-blind comparison of bupropion and amitriptyline in depressed inpatients. J Clin Psychiatry 1983; 44:115–117

62. Feighner JP, Hendrickson G, Miller L, Stern W: Double-blind comparison of doxepin versus bupropion in outpatients with a major depressive disorder. J Clin Psychopharmacology 1986; 6:27–32

63. Othmer E, Othmer SC, Stern WC, Van Wyck Fleet J: Long-term efficacy and safety of bupropion. J Clin Psychiatry 1983; 44:153–156

64. Kane JM, Cole K, Sarantakos S, Howard A, Borenstein M: Safety and efficacy of bupropion in elderly patients: preliminary observations. J Clin Psychiatry 1983; 44:134–136

65. Branconnier RJ, Cole JO, Ghazvinian S, Spera KF, Oxenkrug FG, Bass JL: Clinical pharmacology of bupropion and imipramine in elderly depressives. J Clin Psychiatry 1983; 44:130–133

66. Roose SP, Dalack GW, Glassman AH, Woodring S, Walsh BT, Giardina EG: Cardiovascular effects of bupropion in depressed patients with heart disease. Am J Psychiatry 1991; 148:512–516

67. Sheehan DV, Davidson J, Manschreck T, Van Wyck Fleet J: Lack of efficacy of a new antidepressant (bupropion) in the treatment of panic disorders with phobias. J Clin Psychopharmacology 1983; 3:28–31

68. Davidson J: Seizures and bupropion: a review. J Clin Psychiatry 1989; 50:256–261

69. Glassman AH, Bigger JT, Jr.: Cardiovascular effects of therapeutic doses of antidepressants: a review. Arch Gen Psychiatry 1981; 38:815–820

70. Kupfer DJ, Spiker DG, Coble PA, Neil JF, Ulrich R, Shaw OH: Sleep and treatment prediction in endogenous depression. Am J Psychiatry 1981; 138:429–434

71. Sternberg DE: Biologic tests in psychiatry. Psychiatric Clinics North Am 1984; 7:639–650

72. Cooper TB: Analytical aspects of the pharmacokinetics of psychotropic drugs. Handbook of Neurochem 1983; 2:281–300

73. Cooper TB, Simpson GM, Lee JH: Thymoleptic and neuroleptic drug plasma levels in psychiatry: Current status. Intl Review Neurobiol 1976; 19:269–309

74. Nagy A, Johansson R: Plasma levels of imipramine and desipramine in man after different routes of administration. Nanunyn-Schmiederbergs Archives of Pharmacology 1975; 290:145–160

75. Cooper TB, Simpson GM: Prediction of individual dosage of nortriptyline. Am J Psychiatry 1978; 135:333–335

76. American Psychiatric Association Task Force on the use of laboratory tests in psychiatry: Tricyclic antidepressants—blood level measurements and clinical outcome: An APA Task Force Report. Am J Psychiatry 1985; 141:155–162

77. Asberg M: Treatment of depression with tricyclic drugs—Pharmacokinetics and pharmacodynamic aspects. Pharmakopsych Neuro-Psychopharmakologie 1976; 9:18–26

78. Klein DF: personal communication

79. Anonymous: NIMH/NIH Consensus Development Conference Statement. Mood disorders: pharmacologic prevention of recurrences: Consensus Development Panel. Am J Psychiatry 1985; 142:469–476

80. Davis JM: Overview: maintenance therapy in psychiatry: II. Affective disorders. Am J Psychiatry 1976; 133:1–13

81. Prien RF: Schizophrenia and Affective Disorders: Biological and Drug Treatment. Edited by Rifkin A. Boston, Wright-PSG, 1983

82. Baldessarini RJ, Tohen M: Efficacy of long-term antidepressant and mood-stabilizing treatment in unipolar major depression, in Current Trends in Psychopharmacology. Edited by Christensen AV, Casey DE. Heidelberg, Springer Verlag, 1987

83. Peselow ED, Dunner DL, Fieve RR, Gulbenkian G, Deutsch SI, Kaufmann M: Maintenance treatment of unipolar depression. Psychopharm Bull 1981; 17:53–56

84. Casey DE: Tardive dyskinesia and affective disorders, in Tardive Dyskinesia and Affective Disorders. Edited by Gardos G, Casey DE. Washington DC, American Psychiatric Press, 1984

85. Anonymous, 1990; Anafranil package insert.

86. Prinz PN, Vitiello MV, Raskind MA, Thorpy MJ: Geriatrics: sleep disorders and aging. New Eng J Med 1990; 323:520–526

87. Charney DS, Heninger GR, Sternberg DE, Landis H: Abrupt discontinuance of tricyclic antidepressant drugs: Evidence for noradrenergic hyperactivity. Brit J Psychiatry 1982; 141:377–386

88. Ayd FJ, Jr.: Depressive relapse or tricyclic antidepressant (TCA) withdrawal? Intl Drug Therapy Newsletter 1987; 22:20

89. Pato MT, Zohar-Kadouch R, Zohar J, Murphy DL: Return of symptoms after discontinuation of clomipramine in patients with obsessive-compulsive disorder. Am J Psychiatry 1988; 145:1521–1525

90. Diamond BI, Borison RL, Katz R, DeVeaugh-Geiss J: Rebound withdrawal reactions due to clomipramine. Psychopharm Bull 1989; 25:209–212

91. Ray WA, Griffin MR, Schaffner W, Baugh DK, Melton LJ: Psychotropic drug use and the risk of hip fracture. New Eng J Med 1987; 316:363–369

92. Goldberg HL, DiMascio A: Psychotropic drugs in pregnancy, in Psychopharmacology: A Generation of Progress. Edited by Lipton MA, DiMascio A, Killam KF. New York, Raven Press, 1978

93. Perry PJ, Browne JL, Prince RA, Alexander B, Tsuang MT: Effects of smoking on nortriptyline plasma concentrations in depressed patients. Therapeutic Drug Monitoring 1986; 8:279–284

94. Willcox DRC, Gillan R, Hare EH: Do psychiatric outpatients take their drugs? Brit Med J 1965; ii:790–792

95. Approved Drug Products with Therapeutic Equivalence Evaluations, 11th ed. Rockville, MD: US Dept HHS, PHS, FDA, Center for Drug Evaluation and Research, 1991

96. FDA. Bioequivalence Task Force Report. Rockville, MD, 1988

97. Dubovsky SL: Severe nortriptyline intoxication due to change from a generic to a trade preparation. J Nerv Ment Dis 1987; 175:115–117

98. Bochner F, Hooper WD, Tyrer JH, Eadie MJ: Factors involved in an outbreak of phenytoin intoxication. J Neurol Sci 1972; 16:481–487

99. Sachdeo RC, Belendiuk G: Generic versus branded carbamazepine (letter). Lancet 1987; 1:1432

100. Ostroff RB, Docherty JP: Tricyclics, bioequivalence, and clinical response. Am J Psychiatry 1978; 135:1560–1561

101. Giller EL, Ostroff R, Bialos D, Altshul S, Jatlow P, Patrick W: Steady state bioequivalence and therapeutic equivalence of different amitriptyline compounds with various dissolution rates. J Clin Psychopharmacol 1984; 4:299–300

102. Freese KJ: Can patients safely undergo electroconvulsive therapy while receiving monoamine oxidase inhibitors? Convulsive Therapy 1985; 1:190–194

103. Bryant SG, Fisher S, Kluge RM: Postmarketing surveillance of long-term amitriptyline side effects. Psychopharm Bull 1986; 22:995–998

104. Goldberg RJ, Capone RJ, Hunt JD: Cardiac complications following tricyclic antidepressant overdose. Issues for monitoring policy. JAMA 1985; 254:1772–1775

105. Zubenko GS, Cohen BM, Lipinski JF: Antidepressant-related akathisia. J Clin Psychopharmacol 1987; 7:254–257

106. Frommer DA, Kulig KW, Marx JA, Rumack B: Tricyclic antidepressant overdose: A review. JAMA 1987; 257:521–526

107. Christensen P, Thomsen HY, Pedersen OL, Gram LF, Kragh-Sörensen P: Orthostatic side effects of clomipramine and citalopram during treatment for depression. Psychopharmacology 1985; 86:383–385

108. Myers BA, Klerman GL, Hartmann E: Nocturnal cataclysms with myoclonus: a new side effect of clomipramine (letter). Am J Psychiatry 1986; 143:1490–1491

109. Anand VS: Clomipramine-induced galactorrhea and amenorrhoea. Brit J Psychiatry 1985; 147:87–88

110. McLean JD, Forsythe RG, Kapkin IA: Unusual side effects of clomipramine associated with yawning. Can J Psychiatry 1983; 28:569–570

111. Wernicke JF: The side effect profile and safety of fluoxetine. J Clin Psychiatry 1985; 46:3 (Sec2) 59–67

112. Golden RN, James SP, Sherer MA, Rudorfer MV, Sack DA, Potter WZ: Psychoses associated with bupropion treatment. Am J Psychiatry 1985; 142:1459–1462

113. Becker RE, Dufresne RL: Perceptual changes with bupropion, a novel antidepressant. Am J Psychiatry 1982; 139:1200–1201

114. Johnston JA, Lineberry CG, Freiden CS: Prevalence of psychosis, delusions, and hallucinations in clinical trials with bupropion (letter). Am J Psychiatry 1986; 143:1192–1193

115. Hansten PD, Horn JR: Drug Interactions and Updates. 6th ed. Philadelphia, Lea and Febiger, 1990

116. Morselli PL, Biandrate P, Frigerio A, Garattini S: Pharmacokinetics of carbamazepine in rats and humans. Europ J Clin Invest 1962; 2:297

117. Hui KK: Hypertensive crisis induced by interaction of clonidine with imipramine. J Am Geriatrics Society 1983; 31:164–165

118. Briant RH, Reid JL, Dollery CT: Interaction between clonidine and desipramine in man. Brit Med J 1973; 1:522–523

119. Feighner JP, Herbstein J, Damlouji N: Combined MAOI, TCA and direct stimulant therapy of treatment-resistant depression. J Clin Psychiatry 1985; 46:206–209

120. Brachfeld J, Wirtshafter A, Wolfe S: Imipramine-tranylcypromine incompatibility, near fatal toxic reaction. JAMA 1963; 186:1172

121. Jarechi HG: Combined phenelzine and amitriptyline poisoning. Am J Psychiatry 1963; 120:189

122. Dufresne RL, Kass DJ, Becker RE: Bupropion and thiothixene versus placebo in the treatment of depression in schizophrenia. Drug Dev Res 1988; 12:259–266

123. Goode DJ, Manning AA: Comparison of bupropion alone and with haloperidol in schizoaffective disorder, depressed type. J Clin Psychiatry 1983; 44:253–255

124. Wright G, Galloway L, Kim J, Dalton M, Miller L, Stern W: Bupropion in the long-term management of cyclic mood disorders: Mood stabilizing effects. J Clin Psychiatry 1985; 46:22–25

125. Liberzon I, Dequardo JR, Silk KR: Bupropion and delirium (letter). Am J Psychiatry 1990; 147:1689–1690

126. Rudorfer MV, Manji HK, Potter WZ: Bupropion, ECT, and dopaminergic overdrive (letter). Am J Psychiatry 1991; 148:1101–1102

127. Tate JL: Extrapyramidal symptoms in a patient taking haloperidol and fluoxetine. (letter) Am J Psychiatry 1989; 146:399–400

128. Aranow RB, Hudson JI, Pope HG, Grady TA, Laage TA, Bell IR, Cole JO: Elevated antidepressant plasma levels after addition of fluoxetine. Am J Psychiatry 1989; 146:911–913

129. Steiner W, Fontaine R: Toxic reaction following the combined administration of fluoxetine and L-tryptophan: five case reports. Biol Psychiatry 1986; 21:1067–1071

130. Bodkin JA, Teicher MH: Fluoxetine may antagonize the anxiolytic action of buspirone. (letter) J Clin Psychopharmacol 1989; 9:150

131. Pearson H: Interaction of fluoxetine with carbamazepine. J Clin Psychiatry 1990; 51:126

132. Salama AA, Shafey M: A case of severe lithium toxicity induced by combined fluoxetine and lithium carbonate. Am J Psychiatry 1989; 146:278

133. Moskowitz H, Burns M: The effects on performance of two antidepressants, alone and in combination with diazepam. Prog In Neuropsychopharmacol and Biol Psychiatry 1988; 12:783–792

134. Lemberger L, Rowe H, Bosomworth JC: The effect of fluoxetine on the pharmacokinetics and psychomotor responses of diazepam. Clin Pharmacol Therapeutics 1988; 43:412

135. Goff DC, Midha KK, Brotman AW, Waites M, Baldessarini RJ: Elevation of plasma concentrations of haloperidol after the addition of fluoxetine. Am J Psychiatry 1991; 148:790–792

136. Beaumont G: Drug interactions with clomipramine (Anafranil). J Intl Medical Research 1973; 1:480–484

137. Post RM: Mood disorders: Somatic Treatment, in Comprehensive Textbook of Psychiatry/V Vol 1, 5th ed. Edited by Kaplan HI, Sadock BJ. Baltimore, Williams and Wilkins, 1989, p. 921

138. Blackwell B: Adverse effects of antidepressant drugs I: Monoamine oxidase inhibitors and tricyclics. Drugs 1981; 21:201–219

139. McCabe B, Tsuang MT: Dietary consideration in MAO inhibitor regimens. J Clin Psychiatry 1982; 43:178–181

140. Davidson J, Zung WWK, Walker JI: Practical aspects of MAO inhibitor therapy. J Clin Psychiatry 1984; 45(7, Sec 2):81–84

141. Anon. Eosinophilia-myalgia syndrome associated with ingestion of L-tryptophan. Morbidity and Mortality Weekly Reporter 1989; 38:842–843

CHAPTER 5

Pharmacotherapy of Anxiety and Sleep Disorders

INTRODUCTION

Terms such as anxiolytic, antianxiety agent, minor tranquilizer, and sedative have been used interchangeably to describe the sedative action of a diverse group of chemical agents. Among this group are the benzodiazepines, barbiturates, propanediol carbamates (e.g., Meprobamate), and sedative antihistamines. When used in doses to produce sleep, these compounds are called hypnotics. In this discussion, the terms antianxiety agents and hypnotics will be used.

Historically, the barbiturates and chloral hydrate were the major sedatives and hypnotics until the discovery of the clinical effects of chlordiazepoxide in 1958. By the 1980s, the benzodiazepines had become the most frequently prescribed class of sedative/hypnotics. In 1980, benzodiazepines were estimated to account for more than 500 million patient exposures since they were marketed 20 years earlier.[1] Approximately 80% of the U.S. benzodiazepine prescriptions are written by medical practitioners, as opposed to psychiatrists, suggesting that much of the time anxiety and insomnia are presented to the medical practitioner who responds with a prescription. It also suggests that anxiety and insomnia often accompany medical problems.

Anxiety

Anxiety is a familiar concept but differs in its definition, interpretation, and management according to whether a psychologist, pastoral counselor or psychiatrist is defining it, the degree of symptom severity and functional impairment and according to the attitudes, beliefs, and experience of the anxious individual. As a distinct clinical disorder, DSM-III-R lists the following anxiety disorders: panic disorder (with and without agoraphobia), agoraphobia with a history of panic, social and simple phobias, obsessive-compulsive disorder (OCD), post-traumatic stress disorder, and generalized anxiety. The annual prevalence of anxiety disorders based on recent American household surveys is 4.3/100 which was differentiated into generalized anxiety (2.5/100), phobic disorders (1.4/100), and panic disorders (0.4/100).[2]

Biochemical theories of anxiety in humans have been proposed in the hope of gaining more understanding of the pathophysiology of anxiety, to develop pharmacologic treatments and to identify high-risk populations by the use of challenge tests. Adrenergic agonists such as epinephrine and the α_2 receptor blocker yohimbine (which induces the release of norepinephrine) have been used experimentally to provoke anxiety although each has distinct limitations.[3]

In the late 1960s, lactate infusions were shown to produce similar or identical symptoms of anxiety in anxious patients.[4] Repeat studies corroborated this finding and reported that 80% of patients with panic disorder (compared with less than 20% of normal subjects) experience a panic attack when given lactate.[3] Panic induced by sodium lactate was blocked by imipramine or desipramine[5] an effect that has been used to support the use of antidepressants in the treatment of panic. The use of challenge tests must be further validated in large samples and there must be sufficient sensitivity (predictive accuracy for a positive test result[6]) and specificity (predictive accuracy for a negative test result) before they will have practical clinical meaning.

The diverse physiological and psychological symptoms of acute anxiety may be grouped into 4 types:

1. Motor tension: shakiness, jitteriness, jumpiness, trembling, tension, muscle aches, fatigability, easily startled, and strained face.
2. Autonomic hyperactivity: sweating, cold clammy hands, paresthesias (tingling hands and feet), lump in the throat, palpitations, tachycardia, easy fatigability, difficulty breathing or breathlessness, chest tightness, pain, lightheadedness, and dizziness.
3. Apprehensive expectation: anxiety, worry, fear, irritability, rumination, and anticipation of misfortune to self or others.
4. Vigilance and scanning: hyperattentiveness resulting in distractibility, difficulty in concentrating, insomnia, irritability, and impatience.

In the diagnosis of anxiety, symptoms may occur secondary to or be related to medical disorders, such as angina pectoris, caffeinism, hyperthyroidism, withdrawal from substances such as alcohol and benzodiazepines, complex partial seizures, and mitral valve prolapse. Clinicians' misdiagnosis or underrecognition of drug-induced effects that mimic anxiety has been reported.[7] For example, akathisia, a drug-induced extrapyramidal effect of the antipsychotic agents, may be mistaken for anxiety and treated with an antianxiety agent instead of the preferred decision of a trial dose reduction of the antipsychotic. Similarly, withdrawal from other centrally-acting drugs may produce transient anxiety.

Much of the treatment of anxiety occurs with anxiety as a target symptom of an anxiety disorder such as obsessive-compulsive or phobic disorder. Also, anxiety may be treated in the course of a psychotic disorder such as agitated depression or acute schizophrenia. In the latter instance, complicated treatment regimens composed of antipsychotics, antianxiety agents, and hypnotics are sometimes used in treatment-resistant or violent patients who fail to be managed with simpler regimens. These complex regimens require careful longitudinal monitoring such as suggested by the "N-of-1" study design[8] because of the lack of established effectiveness and safety of the combinations and the dilemma of not recognizing drug-induced behavioral toxicity.

The wide range of target symptoms is matched by the variety of mechanisms of antianxiety effect depending on the drug class selected for treatment. The benefits and risks of these classes will be described next. Decisions to use drug treatment require consideration of nondrug alternative treatments. For example, insight-oriented and supportive individual and group psychotherapy are a standard part of the treatment of anxiety disorders.[9] In addition, there are preliminary studies to support the effectiveness in selected individuals of self-help activities such as biofeedback for cardiac neurosis and chronic situational anxiety.[10] Successful treatment programs also include group therapy for phobias and community-based peer support programs such as Al-Anon for those with severe anxiety associated with alcohol and drug dependence.

A number of nonpharmacologic factors influence the effectiveness and safety of the antianxiety agents. Among these are: (1) patients' attitudes toward their symptoms and treatment, (2) their propensity to misuse or abuse medications with significant potential for dependence, (3) the severity of their symptoms as reflected by the degree of vocational and social impairment, and (4) the degree of motor and cognitive performance required in activities of daily living. The antianxiety agents are recommended for short-term use (4 months is the FDA recommendation) because they are not curative, lack data supporting their long-term effectiveness, and have documented dependence potential.[11]

Insomnia

Insomnia is a subjective state in which patients are unable to fall asleep, may wake frequently and may be unable to resume sleep. This may be associated with early morning wakening. The problem may reflect patients' exalted expectations and consequent dissatisfaction with their sleep pattern.

The treatment of insomnia is complicated by the risk of failing to diagnose the physical or psychological basis for the insomnia. In addition, long-term pharmacologic treatment readily subjects patients to the risks of accidental overdosage, and hypnotic hangover and tolerance, conditions that lead to increasing dosage and possible physiologic dependency.

Insomnia is usually treated for short intervals of 1 to 2 weeks in conjunction with situational medical treatment or surgery, time-limited or acute crises (e.g., deaths, family crises). If symptoms persist, a referral for psychotherapy is indicated. In psychotic patients, short-term insomnia may require treatment during the acute phase of management while antipsychotics are being stabilized. Until the antipsychotic dosing is stabilized, a benzodiazepine hypnotic may be needed. Continuous usage is not recommended.

DRUG SELECTION

Anxiety

The drugs used to treat anxiety and insomnia are virtually identical with lower frequent daily dosing for the treatment of anxiety and larger single nighttime dosing for insomnia. More refined distinctions among the benzodiazepines can be made based upon pharmacokinetic characteristics (e.g., onset of action, extent of distribution, and rate of elimination).[12] Clinical researchers have developed the residual fraction quotient (C_{12}/C_{max}) as a measure of antianxiety versus hypnotic utility.[13] The antianxiety agents vary according to drug class and include the benzodiazepines, carbamates, barbiturates, and miscellaneous agents. The sedating antihistamines are not usually considered to be antianxiety agents although several (e.g., diphenhydramine) are used for insomnia. Also, several beta-blockers (e.g., propranolol) have been used as antianxiety agents. The barbiturates and propanediol carbamates (e.g., meprobamate) enjoyed extensive usage until the 1960s when the benzodiazepines virtually replaced these classes whether comparing dollars spent or the number of patients given prescriptions. Today, there is a general consensus that the risk-to-benefit ratio supports the benzodiazepines as the class of choice for both anxiety and insomnia when a drug is indicated. The benefits of benzodiazepines include less acute toxicity than barbiturates and carbamates, and less severe addiction and withdrawal syndromes.

Table 5.1 lists the 8 benzodiazepines that are indicated for anxiety by chemical class and provides product forms, duration and half-life information, active metabolites and daily dosage guidelines. A relative potency scale[14,15] relates dosage to a standard compound, lorazepam, for ease in switching among these agents. Pro drugs are chemical precursors of active agents. To illustrate, clorazepate is a pro drug which is metabolized to desmethyldiazepam and produces the same antianxiety effect as diazepam, although the rates of absorption, distribution, and metabolism differ.

Insomnia

Table 5.2 lists the major classes of agents for the treatment of sleep disorders along with comparative duration data and daily dosage information. Table 5.3 lists barbiturates for historical and relative dose purposes. Table 5.4 lists nonbenzodiazepine agents that are occasionally used as alternatives when a benzodiazepine is not indicated.

TABLE 5.1. Benzodiazepines commonly indicated for the treatment of anxiety according to the available dosage forms, duration of clinical action, half-life (hours) of key metabolites, and usual and extreme daily dosage (mg).

Generic Name (Brand)	Rel[a] Potency	Form[b]	Duration	$t_{1/2}$	Active Metabolites	Usual Dose/Day	Extreme Dose/Day
3-Hydroxy							
Oxazepam (Serax)	15	O	Short	8 ± 2	None	30–60	30–120
Lorazepam (Ativan)	1	O,I	Short	10 ± 20	None	2–6	1–10
2-Keto							
Diazepam (Valium)	5	O,I	Long	43 ± 13 62 ± 16	ND, OXA	4–40	2–40
Chlordiazepoxide (Librium)	10	O,I	Long	112 ± 31 80 ± 21	DMC,ND,OXA	15–40	10–100
Halazepam (Paxipam)	?	O	Long	2 ± 1 62 ± 16	ND, OXA	60–160	20–160
Prodrugs							
Clorazepate (Tranxene)	7.5	O	Long	80 ± 20	ND,OXA	30	7.5–90
Prazepam (Centrax)	10	O	Long	80	ND,OXA	20–40	10–60
Triazolo							
Alprazolam[c] (Xanax)	0.5	O	Intermed.	11 ± 3	α-HA	0.75–1.5	0.5–4(6)[d]

[a] Approximate dose equivalence cited in Rosenbaum.[14]

[b] Drug products are identified as available in oral(O) or injectable(I) forms.

[c] Approximate dose equivalence cited in Dawson.[15]

[d] Outpatients with panic disorder were treated with doses of 6 mg per day for 8 weeks.[16]

147

TABLE 5.2. Benzodiazepines commonly indicated for the treatment of insomnia according to the available dosage forms, duration of clinical action, half-life (hours) of key metabolites, and usual and extreme daily dosage (mg).

Generic Name (Brand)	Form	Duration	$t_{1/2}$	Active Metabolites	Usual Dose/Day	Extreme Dose/Day
2-Keto						
Flurazepam (Dalmane)	O	Long	74 ± 24	NF, NF, 3-H	15–30	30
3-Hydroxy						
Temazepam (Restoril)	O	Short	13 ± 3	OXA	15–30	30
Triazolo						
Triazolam (Halcion)	O	Ultra-short	2 ± 0.4	α-HT	0.25–0.5	0.125–0.5

TABLE 5.3. Barbiturates previously used for the treatment of insomnia.

Generic Name (Brand)	Form[a]	Class[b]	$t_{1/2}$	Usual Dose/Day	Extreme Dose/Day
Pentobarbital (Nembutal)	O,I	C-III	15 ± 48	100	—
Secobarbital (Seconal)	O,I	C-III		100	200
Amobarbital (Amytal)	O,I	C-III		65	200

[a] Drug products are available in oral (O) or injectable (I) forms.
[b] Federal narcotic classification system.

TABLE 5.4. Miscellaneous agents occasionally used for the treatment of insomnia.

Generic Name (Brand)	Form[a]	Class[b]	$t_{1/2}$	Usual Dose/Day	Extreme Dose/Day
Chloral hydrate (Noctec)	O	C-IV	4 ± 9.5	500	1000
Diphenhydramine	O,I	—	8.5 ± 32	50	150
Hydroxyzine (Vistaril, Atarax)	O,I	—	$2.5 - 3.4$[c]	50	150
Buspirone[d] (Buspar)	O	—	2.4 ± 0.5	15–30	15–60

[a] Drug products are available in Oral (O) or Injectable (I) forms.
[b] Federal narcotic classification system.
[c] Fouda HG, Hobbs DC, Stambaugh, JE, J Pharm Sci 1979; 68:1456–1458.
[d] Nonformulary status.

BENZODIAZEPINES

Mechanism of Action

The brain-type benzodiazepine receptors are the site of action of these drugs and they are most heavily concentrated in the limbic-forebrain and cortical areas. The drugs bind with high affinity to these receptors with a rank-order of affinities, potencies, and *in vitro* binding systems which parallels their rank-order of clinical potencies in animals[17] and humans.[18] Lipophilicity has been suggested as a factor in clinical potency[19] but this remains an open question without further experimental evidence. Activation of the benzodiazepine-receptor complex is postulated to lead to an enhanced inhibitory action of gamma-amino butyric acid (GABA) through increased chloride conduction at the neuronal membrane. From a clinical practice standpoint, the selection factors for the benzodiazepines include receptor affinity to estimate potency, lipophilicity to estimate onset of action and the number and half-life of metabolites to estimate duration.

Clinical Effects

The pharmacologic actions of the benzodiazepines include antianxiety, anticonvulsant, muscle-relaxant, and sleep-inducing (hypnotic) effects. When given in equivalent doses, all of the commercially available benzodiazepines are equally effective for treating anxiety and insomnia.[20]

Psychiatric usage of the benzodiazepines is based on the behavioral pharmacologic effects in animals which is collectively termed disinhibition.[16] Disinhibition includes increased spontaneous and exploratory activity, active and passive avoidance, and attenuation of the sequelae of stress and frustration. Taming effects in animals refer to reduced aggression and hostility, although paradoxical rage, hostility, and violence following benzodiazepine use are known in both animals and humans.

Eight benzodiazepines commonly used as antianxiety agents are listed in Table 5.1 along with pharmacokinetic and dosing data. Table 5.2 lists the three benzodiazepines commonly used to treat insomnia. Triazolam has been reported to have an insufficient hypnotic effect, perhaps due to its very short half-life[21] (p. 241). This problem may explain the recent report[22] of extreme doses as high as

1.0 mg. A discussion of the anticonvulsant usage of clonazepam, lorazepam, and diazepam is located in Chapter 6.

Pharmacokinetics and Pharmacodynamics

While there are no major differences in clinical efficacy, the rationale
for selecting, dosing and comparing benzodiazepines is based on reviewing pharmacokinetic and pharmacodynamic principles.[23] Specifically, the characteristics related to absorption, distribution, and
metabolism of the benzodiazepines should be reviewed to understand
their selection and dosing. Differences in time to onset of action, intensity, and duration of a single dose administered by a particular
route of administration are the factors on which clinical selection is
based.[24] For example, rapid onset and distribution is related to the degree of lipophilicity. The half-life of most benzodiazepines depends
primarily on the rate at which metabolic enzymes convert the drugs to
hydrophilic inactive forms after which they are rapidly excreted.

The rate, extent, and consistency of absorption for the oldest and
best studied agents, chlordiazepoxide and diazepam, is *lower* for intramuscular (IM) than for oral administration. This is explained by
physicochemical factors such as the degree of fat solubility and crys-
tallization at the injection site. Oral administration is more likely to
produce rapid onset of effects than IM injection and serves the typical
situation for the treatment of anxiety and insomnia. Emergency treatment of severe agitation, alcoholic detoxification or the rapid control
of status epilepticus may require IV injectable benzodiazepines. Diazepam by IM injection is better absorbed from the high blood region
of the deltoid muscle area rather than from gluteal or vastus lateralis
sites. Lorazepam is well-absorbed by intramuscular injection.[24]

First-pass liver metabolism, the production of numerous pharmacologically active metabolites and kidney excretion are involved in the
metabolic disposition of the benzodiazepines. Multiple dosing reaches
a steady state pharmacokinetic pattern when the drug no longer accu-
mulates, a process that is controlled by the elimination half-life of the
parent drug and its active metabolites. Steady state implies that a drug
is administered at the same rate at which it is metabolized and excreted, after equilibrium has been reached. To estimate the time to
achieve steady-state for a very long-acting agent such as flurazepam
with its slowly metabolized N-demethyl metabolite, one multiples the
half-life of the longest metabolite by 4 or 5 which is approximately 3

weeks for the normal individual. This would be much longer in those with risk factors for reduced drug metabolic functioning such as the elderly and those with liver disease. To illustrate, the elimination half-life of diazepam is approximately 20 hours in a healthy 20-year-old, but increases to approximately 100 hours in a healthy 70-year-old.[25] Thus, the time to steady state in young healthy persons is approximately 5 days, whereas 3 weeks may be needed for a healthy older adult. Dosing increments that occur more often than the time interval suggested by these numbers present a risk of toxicity and excessive dosing and may help to explain the numerous reports of adverse effects in the elderly.

There has been considerable discussion devoted to determining the most favorable pharmacokinetic profile (i.e., the drug with most rapid onset, fewest active metabolites, and rapid metabolism to minimize hangover and motor and cognitive impairment). However, it appears now that a balancing is needed against the following factors: serious withdrawal incidents reported following abrupt withdrawal of short half-life agents, inadvertent missed doses due to the need for more frequent prescription refills and the importance of successfully accomplishing time-limited treatment episodes. To achieve success, discontinuation of benzodiazepines and the likelihood of rebound anxiety and insomnia must be considered. Benzodiazepines accumulate in plasma, brain, and cerebrospinal fluid as well as liver, adipose tissue and many other organs.[26] Wide interpatient variation in the metabolism of these drugs is reported. For example, the steady state half-life of diazepam was shown to vary 30-fold for a single dose while lorazepam varied 8- to 10-fold.[27] These differences are ascribed to genetic variations in patients' ability to metabolize drugs. In practical clinical terms, dosage titration is made in increments until the symptoms are controlled or side effects emerge. This process should take account of the estimated time to achieve steady state in order to achieve the lowest effective dose and minimize dose-dependent CNS-related adverse effects.

The benzodiazepines may be classified as short, intermediate and long-acting according to the number and average elimination half-life time of the drug and its active metabolites. This time interval is described as the dispositional half-life.[28] As stated earlier, the degree of lipophilicity and rate of absorption also affect their clinical selection. Consequently, consulting a table of half-life of the parent drug does *not* provide sufficient information for selecting and determining the dosing intervals of a benzodiazepine.

Plasma Level Monitoring

Therapeutic plasma level ranges of the benzodiazepines for anxiety and insomnia are not established generally because of the wide inter-patient variation in dose and response. Plasma range data for seizure control are available for diazepam and clonazepam and will be discussed in Chapter 6. Among the possible uses of plasma level data for anxiety and insomnia are to verify compliance (adherence) and to establish "normal" ranges for *individual* patients at steady state for the purpose of explaining new developments at a future time. Although drug-drug interactions often cannot be predicted on the basis of plasma concentrations, one might monitor levels to establish the effect of the addition or deletion of a second drug on the plasma level of the benzodiazepine. Plasma levels may be of some use when drug withdrawal (i.e., discontinuation) follows long-term use and is complicated by rebound effects.

Clinical Use

Efficacy Studies for the Anxiety Disorders

The effectiveness of the benzodiazepines in treating adjustment and stress disorders is widely accepted based on clinical practice. Due to the sudden onset and acute and unpredictable nature of this type of anxiety, it has not been the subject of controlled clinical trials.[29]

The control of symptoms of neurotic anxiety with benzodiazepines in outpatients during 4-week double-blind trials has been demonstrated to be significantly greater than placebo,[30] barbiturates,[31] propanediols,[32] and low-dose antipsychotic drugs.[33] However, in a review of 52 clinical trials comparing benzodiazepines with other anti-anxiety agents, Greenblatt and Shader[34] found only 3 instances of superiority of the benzodiazepines. In 48 studies, a benzodiazepine was comparable to another agent used to treat anxiety such as doxepin (an antidepressant), the tricyclic antidepressants, major and minor tranquilizers or a beta-blocker.

When accompanied by depressive symptoms, antidepressants may be more suitable for the treatment of anxiety. Johnson reviewed 25 double-blind studies comparing the relative efficacy of benzodiazepines and tricyclic antidepressants.[35] Twelve studies showed the tricyclic antidepressant to be superior, 1 showed the benzodiazepine to be superior, and 12 studies showed no statistically significant differences between the 2 drug groups.

No long-term efficacy studies of the benzodiazepines have been done because of the methodologic and logistic problems associated with long-term, "blinded" (i.e., when patient and evaluator are unaware of the status of medication as either active test agent or comparison agent or placebo) drug compliance. One exception is the 6-month evaluation of the use of diazepam in anxious outpatients by Fabre et al.[36] who reported a return to pre-treatment levels of symptoms after drug discontinuation. Numerous studies by Rickels et al.[37] report on clinical effectiveness and safety issues of the benzodiazepines. Questions about long-term efficacy were raised by recent data[37] indicating that 5 weeks after benzodiazepines were abruptly withdrawn from regular outpatient use of at least 1 year's duration, anxiety scores were significantly *lower* than at pre-taper baseline ($p < .01$). Behavioral toxicity (i.e., abnormal behavior due to medication) may explain the higher ratings while they were receiving medication. Alternatively, the finding raises the question of whether initial effectiveness was sustained.

Panic has been identified by Klein as a specific subgroup of the anxiety disorders characterized by severe, sudden, overwhelming anxiety with autonomic effects, such as rapid heart rate, and a feeling of impending death. Klein recommends prophylactic treatment with a tricyclic such as imipramine. Alternatively, clomipramine, the 3-chloro-analog of imipramine which was recently marketed in the United States for Obsessive-Compulsive Disorder (OCD), or an MAO inhibitor,[38] has been suggested, although controlled trials are lacking. The benzodiazepines have the advantage of rapid action for the acute panic attack. The dosing of antidepressants for panic attacks is usually less than half of the dose for major depression.[21] British researchers do not support a differential drug response for panic and they recommend treatment with benzodiazepines.[35] The triazolo benzodiazepine, alprazolam, has been investigated for indications such as panic and obsessive-compulsive disorder (OCD). The compound has been widely promoted for mixed anxiety and depression but the claimed antidepressant effect should not be interpreted as a reflection of either chemical or receptor specificity. At this time, the data support its efficacy based on studies with panic and obsessive-compulsive disorder patients. Such favorable clinical effects are not unique among the benzodiazepines[21]

(p. 253). Rapid escalating dosage and abrupt withdrawal of alprazolam should be avoided to prevent management difficulties. The treatment of OCD with clomipramine and other interventions is discussed in Chapter 4.

Phobic disorders including agoraphobia (restricted activity) and social phobias have been successfully treated with benzodiazepines although drug treatment should be specific to the patient situation and targeted to reduce anticipatory anxiety associated with the phobic stimulus. The timing of the occasional dose of benzodiazepine should be related to the exposure to the phobic stimulus. Behavior modification techniques include systematic desensitization in imagination and *in vivo*, (in practice) as well as flooding in imagination and *in vivo*. At 4-year follow-up, 58% of a study cohort were improved after psychosocial treatment.[39] Benzodiazepines have been shown to be efficacious for circumscribed phobias but less so for agoraphobia.[40] Zitrin et al.[41] found moderate to marked improvement in both imipramine- and placebo-treated patients who were given randomized assignment in this double-blind trial of drug and group exposure therapy. Thus, the behavioral treatment of phobic disorders with the occasional use of medication to reduce anticipatory anxiety is the major treatment approach.[41,42]

In the controlled trial by McNair and Kahn[43] agoraphobia with panic attacks was found to be more effectively treated with imipramine than chlordiazepoxide. The combined use of drug and psychotherapy treatment of agoraphobia has been modelled using path analysis.[42] Similarly, the MAO inhibitors were shown to be more effective than placebo in treating phobic disorders.[44] Alprazolam has been shown to be more effective than placebo in anxiety with panic.[45] Comparisons of alprazolam's effectiveness with antidepressants await further study.

Obsessive-compulsive disorder has been treated with either a benzodiazepine or an antidepressant with relatively poor response in many patients. Alprazolam has been proposed as a drug which may provide the effectiveness of both drug groups. Such hypotheses must be tested in rigorous double-blind studies.[46]

Efficacy Studies in Insomnia

In a discussion of flurazepam, the first benzodiazepine marketed for insomnia, Greenblatt et al.[47] reviewed the clinical studies that evaluated the drug against placebo and other hypnotics. In 17 studies, flurazepam was more effective than placebo. Most of these studies provided short-term efficacy usually of less than 2 weeks' duration. In regard to dosage, 15 mg nightly doses were consistently superior in 3 studies but less effective than 30 mg doses in 2 studies. Among sleep research studies, comparisons between flurazepam and non-benzodiazepine hypnotics such as chloral hydrate, glutethimide, and barbiturates, indicated that flurazepam was superior at 2 weeks[48] and at 1 month.[49]

These studies have focused on the elaborate monitoring of patients that is made possible by studying insomnia in a sleep laboratory environment. Some of these studies suggest that hypnotics lose their effectiveness after 1 or 2 weeks.[50] Despite the large number of clinical drug studies that exist, the methodologic inadequacies of these studies of hypnotics were emphasized by leading sleep researchers.[51] These include: (1) insufficient study of intermediate and long-term effectiveness, (2) neglect of drug interaction effects, and (3) failure to evaluate withdrawal effects. Thus, the generalization of short-term hypnotic efficacy findings to the typical long-stay psychiatric patient is inappropriate.

Efficacy Studies in Alcohol Withdrawal

The withdrawal reaction to alcohol includes hyperacuity of all sensory modalities, hyperreflexia, muscle tension and tremor, overalertness, anxiety, insomnia, and reduction of seizure threshold. Depending on the intensity and duration of prior alcohol exposure, the symptoms of withdrawal may range from mild to life-threatening events including visual hallucinations, seizures and delirium (delirium tremens or DTs). The benzodiazepines are the drugs of first choice in managing alcohol withdrawal. The effectiveness of IV diazepam was compared with rectally administered paraldehyde and found to control severe delirium tremens in half the time and with fewer side effects.[52] The effectiveness of a benzodiazepine was demonstrated against placebo in 3 studies and against phenothiazines and paraldehyde-chloral hydrate in 2 studies.

Efficacy of Benzodiazepine-Antipsychotic Combinations in Psychotic Disorders

Recently, investigators have been evaluating combinations of antipsychotic agents and benzodiazepines such as lorazepam[53] or alprazolam[54,55] in acute and chronic management of patients who fail to be managed by antipsychotics alone. This approach represents a reversal in pharmacotherapy from well-evaluated monotherapy since there is strong evidence from more than a dozen studies that benzodiazepines are *not* effective in reducing the disordered thinking, hallucinations and delusions of psychosis.[30,56,57] Rather, the goal of adding a benzodiazepine for a short period is to reduce the anxiety and agitation that frequently occur in *acute* psychosis or to avoid the negative symptoms that would occur with high-dose antipsychotic.

Interest in reevaluating combination treatment is related primarily to finding better treatment for the 15 to 33% of patients who are relatively treatment-resistant to the antipsychotic regimens that they have been given. Second, there is interest in finding a treatment regimen which will reduce the lifetime antipsychotic drug exposure. There are a number of case reports[58,59,60] of reduced psychotic symptoms in individuals with varying clinical characteristics. Unfortunately, these findings do *not* generalize without additional study. Among controlled studies, Kellner[61] reported that chlordiazepoxide/antipsychotic regimens produced favorable results in some patients but no improvement in others. When Guz[62] compared haloperidol with placebo and haloperidol with lorazepam, the lorazepam group showed greater improvement. However, the study involved various haloperidol doses and diagnoses. Chou[63] reviewed studies evaluating the role of benzodiazepines along with other nonstandard pharmacologic agents being suggested for acute mania.

There are too few rigorous studies from which conclusions can be drawn; additional studies are currently underway.[63] Among negative findings, Ruskin et al.[64] found no benefit from adding diazepam in daily doses of 40 to 80 mg to a fixed antipsychotic dosage in stabilized schizophrenic patients. Similarly, Karson et al.[65] failed to observe improvement when clonazepam was added to the antipsychotic regimen of schizophrenic inpatients. In a related study, Jus et al.[66] reported no insomnia upon withdrawal of benzodiazepine hypnotics in schizophrenic inpatients and inferred that hypnotic benzodiazepines were overprescribed.

These preliminary studies support the need for careful protocol development, attention to the total dose of antipsychotic (in CPZ-EQ for various antipsychotics) in relation to the past daily dose that was associated with favorable antipsychotic drug response, behavioral side effect monitoring of the antipsychotic agent alone and in combination, and gradual withdrawal of the benzodiazepine to avoid severe withdrawal symptoms. Last, some drug-specific differences should be emphasized: (a) Most of the work that has been reported involves combining a high-potency rather than a low-potency antipsychotic with benzodiazepine. The combination with low-potency agents is not advocated on theoretical grounds of excessive sedation and central depressant effects. (b) Clozapine is *not* recommended for combined therapy because of the common occurrence of hypersalivation and bronchial secretion which may produce an excess frequency of pneumonia and pulmonary edema in the severely sedated individual[67] and, most important, because of acute, severe respiratory depression that has been reported[68] including deaths.[69]

Efficacy of Alprazolam in Depressive Disorders

Among the more recent evaluations of drugs in other chemical classes for depression is the triazolo-benzodiazepine, alprazolam, which is being used to treat depression and panic attacks as well as anxiety in doses up to 5 mg, or rarely 10 mg, per day. Efficacy comparable to imipramine[70] and to amitriptyline and doxepin[71] has been demonstrated in the treatment of depression. This short-acting benzodiazepine has a half-life range of 6 to 16 hours compared with the longer acting diazepam ($t_{1/2}$ = 15 to 90 hours). While the shorter duration of action is an advantage in reducing hangover effects, it produces problems in relationship to abrupt withdrawal syndromes. Alprazolam's limited usage for milder depression awaits further clinical trial support. The selection of alprazolam must also be balanced against long-term usage problems such as tolerance, dependency, and withdrawal syndrome. There are reports of behavioral problems such as mania following alprazolam for the treatment of depression.

Tapering of alprazolam no faster than 0.5 mg every 3 days is recommended by the manufacturer but this has been found too abrupt in three-fourths of a series of patients undergoing treatment for panic disorder.[72] The abrupt withdrawal of alprazolam and other short-acting benzodiazepines has been reported to produce dramatic withdrawal symptoms including generalized tonic-clonic seizures,[73] psychosis, delirium, and rebound anxiety. In one case, seizures occurred despite the use of a long-acting benzodiazepine because the relative potency of the substituted drug was not factored into its dosage. A rough ratio of 1:10 alprazolam:diazepam is suggested.[74] Adequate control of withdrawal from benzodiazepines requires careful consideration of relative potency.

Nonpharmacologic Factors

Age and Gender Differences

Plasma level differences according to gender and age have been reported for the well-studied benzodiazepines such as diazepam[75] and chlordiazepoxide.[76] In the study of diazepam, Greenblatt et al.[75] found increased total (free and bound) plasma concentration of diazepam with increasing age when comparing normal individuals in 2 age groups (21–37 vs. 61–84 years). Females had higher mean plasma levels compared with males. They concluded that a clinically important interaction effect explained the significantly lower clearance of diazepam in elderly males compared with young males, whereas no age effect was seen in females. In addition to these experimental study findings, clinical studies support the increased sensitivity of the elderly of both genders to benzodiazepine central depressant effects such as sedation.[77]

Smoking

Smoking has been reported to increase the clearance (and thereby decrease the clinical effect) of some liver-metabolized drugs.[78] Benzodiazepines were reported to have reduced clinical effects as measured by clinician-observed drowsiness when the amount of smoking increased from nonsmoking to light and heavy smoking groups.[77] The postulated mechanism of action is hepatic enzyme induction caused by the various constituents of smoke. Nevertheless, wide interpatient variation occurs in the dose response of the benzodiazepines. Genetics, age, and gender are among the chief factors that account for this variation. Thus, the application of the smoking data to clinical practice is mainly heuristic (i.e., as a factor to consider when trying to resolve unusually poor response). Dosage changes in anticipation of altered effects in smokers should *not* be made.

Co-Morbid Medical Conditions

Among the most important co-morbid conditions that affect benzodiazepine metabolism is liver disease.[79] To avoid the problems generated by long half-life metabolites of diazepam, chlordiazepoxide, and related prodrugs, oxazepam is often suggested for individuals with liver dysfunction because it has no metabolites. Oxazepam has been found to undergo normal disposition in patients with acute hepatitis and cirrhosis.[80] Patients with respiratory impairment such as chronic obstructive pulmonary disease may be at risk for increased anxiety due to hypoxia when treated with benzodiazepines. Patients in respiratory failure were reported to experience significant deterioration when treated with a benzodiazepine.[81]

Addiction-Prone Patients

The potential of the benzodiazepines for misuse and abuse has received considerable attention. Certain patients tend to escalate dosage and to exhibit drug-seeking behavior. The potential for abuse is greatest in opiate and polysubstance abusers and relatively low among outpatient alcoholics.[11] In recognition of this problem, New York State began to require triplicate prescription forms for benzodiazepines in January 1989. Treatment of anxiety and insomnia with benzodiazepines in individuals who are likely to abuse them requires a different benefit-to-risk assessment than the patient for whom short-term therapy followed by withdrawal is less problematic. For the patient at risk of abusing benzodiazepines, nondrug alternative treatments such as psychotherapy or behavioral techniques, or other medications may be safer, more fruitful approaches.

Overall, adequate liver and respiratory function, reduced dosage with slow titration to the lowest effective dose, especially in the elderly, and avoidance in the addiction-prone individual are important factors in selecting candidates for benzodiazepine therapy.

BENZODIAZEPINE DOSING CONSIDERATIONS

Anxiety

Dosing of diazepam (or equivalent) for the control of anxiety in healthy adults may be initiated with 2 mg 3 times a day and titrated upward gradually in 3- to 5-day intervals unless severity of symptoms or prior medication history suggests other initial dosing. Increases are made until symptom control is achieved. A list of approximate relative doses of the commonly used agents is provided in Table 5.1. Awareness of relative potency is becoming more important as the need grows for effective management of withdrawal from various short-acting benzodiazepines.[82]

Antianxiety drug usage for more than 4 months of continuous usage is not recommended by the FDA approved guidelines and is stated in the package insert information. Safe, periodic withdrawal is especially important for short-acting agents because of the recent reports of severe withdrawal effects such as tonic-clonic seizures observed with triazolo derivatives such as alprazolam[72] and triazolam.[83] In addition, there is the dilemma of distinguishing behavioral withdrawal symptoms (rebound effects) from recurrence of underlying illness which may be worsening. The challenge of behavioral toxicity is particularly difficult in panic disorder.

Acute, anterograde amnesia was recognized as drug-induced when several neurologists took triazolam to prevent jet lag.[84] The serendipitous finding received rapid attention in the professional literature and high credibility in light of the professional training of the users and the novel usage. By contrast, for chronic psychotic patients receiving multi-drug regimens, the likelihood of attributing acute, anterograde amnesia to one of their medications is much lower.

Insomnia

The ideal hypnotic should induce sleep rapidly, leave no residual hangover effects upon awakening, and no withdrawal effects. Despite less severe physiological dependency and greater safety in acute overdosage, this ideal has no more been realized with the benzodiazepines than with the barbiturates.[85] However, this position is not universally held and it is argued that *if used correctly*, the benzodiazepines induce sleep rapidly, leave no residual hangover effects upon awakening and do not produce withdrawal effects. The growing evidence of the abuse or misuse of benzodiazepines challenges this view.[86, 87] In addition to patients' experience of difficulty withdrawing from benzodiazepines, as mentioned earlier, several characteristics emphasized in the marketing of benzodiazepine hypnotics have been criticized by sleep researchers.[51] Specifically, the significance of sleep stage effects is unknown. Despite the fact that the role of rapid eye movement (REM) sleep and stage-4 sleep in normal sleep is unknown, differential drug effects related to these characteristics are used to promote drug selection.

Alcohol Withdrawal

Alcohol withdrawal management is typically a medical emergency and its drug therapy is too detailed for this review. A summary of specific guidelines and the rationale for the guidelines is provided by Koch-Weser et al.[88]

Combination with Antipsychotics

Treatment-resistant chronic and acute psychotic patients who fail to be managed by single antipsychotic agents, may be evaluated in a systematic protocol (see Part IV for sample longitudinal monitoring protocol) using intermittent lorazepam to control agitation along with a regularly scheduled low dose of a moderate or high-potency antipsychotic agent (less than 1000 chlorpromazine-equivalents per day). The addition of benzodiazepines to high doses of antipsychotics is not supported by rigorous double-blind controlled clinical trials and therefore, is not recommended. Clonazepam is indicated for the treatment of seizure disorder while its use for behavioral control in psychiatry constitutes an unlabeled indication. A protocol for short-term trials (up to 4 months) to evaluate its use in combination with antipsychotics in selected individuals should be used.

BENZODIAZEPINE MONITORING

Typical Side Effects

The benzodiazepines have the same side effects whether used for anxiety or insomnia. The major side effects are the dose-dependent central nervous system depressant effects such as daytime drowsiness, hangover following bedtime dosing for insomnia, confusional states, and ataxia (motor incoordination). Anterograde amnesia (lack of recall of recent events),[89] slurred speech, and nausea are frequently reported.

Motor incoordination is especially difficult for elderly patients where falling episodes may result in costly hospitalizations. In an epidemiologic analysis of elderly Medicaid patients, hip fracture cases currently had been prescribed a long-duration hypnotic/anxiolytic significantly more often than controls.[90]

Cognitive effects such as amnesia and confusion have been reported at all ages but the most pronounced effects have been demonstrated in the elderly.[91] Experimental studies document the numerous adverse effects on cognition and motor performance in the elderly. For example, decrements in memory, motor function, and increased fatigue were observed in elderly volunteer males who were treated with diazepam (12 mg per day) compared with placebo.[92] Relatively greater daytime sleepiness,[93] cognitive and motor performance impairment are associated with long half-life agents such as flurazepam compared with short-acting agents such as oxazepam.

Behavioral toxicity (defined as new behavioral symptoms that are drug-induced) when discussed in relation to the benzodiazepines has been described as a paradoxical reaction and includes gross behavioral disturbances, hostility, aggression, and rage.[94] While these reactions rarely have been reported in general, they may be particularly underrecognized in psychiatric patients due to the difficulty of distinguishing drug-induced from illness-based behaviors. DiMascio suggested that a rage reaction produced by benzodiazepine-induced disinhibition should not be considered paradoxical in those with a history of rage, violence, and poor impulse control.[95] Benzodiazepines may ultimately prove to be ineffective in those with a predisposition to these behaviors.

Depression, suicidal ideation, and suicide have been documented in association with diazepam usage in individuals with no prior history of depression and whose abrupt onset of symptoms coincided with drug therapy.[96] These unexpected responses to benzodiazepine therapy were reviewed by Hall and Zisook.[97] Age and co-morbid conditions such as renal or cardiovascular disease which required treatment with medications such as digoxin, phenytoin, and phenobarbital were additional factors in these cases. The severity of the reactions was associated with daily doses exceeding 40 mg per day of diazepam.

Long-Term Usage

Despite the relatively greater safety of the benzodiazepines compared with the older sedative/hypnotics of the barbiturate class, significant dependence and withdrawal problems are recognized.[37,98,99] As the length of exposure and dosage of the benzodiazepine increases, the likelihood of physiological dependence and withdrawal reactions increases.

The clinical reports of increasing long-term use and the difficulties of withdrawing patients from these regimens prompted the FDA to recommend that the treatment of anxiety and insomnia be limited to 4 month intervals after which trial dosage reductions and discontinuation should be attempted.

Withdrawal Effects

Withdrawal reactions due to abrupt discontinuation of the benzodiazepines has been documented for both long- and short-acting compounds. Hollister[100] noted withdrawal symptoms and signs such as insomnia, agitation, depression, worsening of psychosis, tremor, twitches, seizures, nausea, vomiting, loss of appetite, cyanosis, and sweating, in 10 of 11 hospitalized VA psychiatric patients who were abruptly withdrawn from high daily doses of chlordiazepoxide (300–600 mg per day) after up to 6 months of drug exposure. The abrupt withdrawal occurred when a switch to placebo was made in a single-blind study. By the end of 1 week, chlordiazepoxide plasma levels were 10% of their original plasma level. Seizures were coincident with almost complete disappearance of drug from the plasma.

Since the initial reports from the early 1960s, many authors have reported cases of dramatic withdrawal effects following long-term exposure to high therapeutic doses[101] and high illicit doses.[102] Other reports document withdrawal at moderate doses; for example, 15 to 25 mg per day of diazepam after 6 years of usage.[103] Similarly, paranoid behavior in a nonpsychiatric patient undergoing withdrawal was reported.[104] Following reintroduction of two 5 mg IM doses of diazepam at 8-hour intervals and oral tapering over 4 weeks, diazepam was successfully withdrawn.

By the late 1970s, leading investigators concurred that abrupt withdrawal of benzodiazepines at therapeutic levels is likely to produce an organic psychosis consisting of agitation, disorientation, and confusion similar to that of the long-term alcohol or barbiturate user.[105]

Rebound insomnia is the principal effect following the use of hypnotics. The term refers to a worsening of sleep disturbance greater than was initially experienced.[106] The effect is more dramatic with shorter half-life agents. Rebound insomnia is easily mistaken for the original symptoms requiring the medication and can inadvertently lead to dependence. To avoid long-term dependency problems, gradual tapering, especially for the short half-life agents, is recommended.

Withdrawal Protocol

For ease of administration, the following protocol may be used during a one-month discontinuation, unless very high dosage and ultra-short half-life drugs suggests a slower tapering:

Week 1: give the usual dose on day 1, 3, 5 and 7

Week 2: give the usual dose on day 8, 11 and 14

Week 3: give the usual dose on day 15 and 19

Week 4: give the usual dose on day 25

Week 5: give the usual dose on day 29 and discontinue

Drug Interactions

Among the clinically significant drug interactions involving a benzodiazepine are the following:

- Disulfiram was shown to decrease diazepam and chlordiazepoxide clearance by one-half.[107] Substitution of a benzodiazepine without active metabolites (e.g., oxazepam or lorazepam) is recommended because the clearance of these compounds was shown to be unaffected by disulfiram.

- Cimetidine decreased the clearance of diazepam and chlordiazepoxide by more than one-third resulting in increased sedation.[108] The proposed mechanism is the inhibition of microsomal metabolism of the benzodiazepine by cimetidine.

- Magnesium and aluminum-containing antacids reduce the rate but not the extent of absorption of diazepam and chlordiazepoxide. This common effect of antacids with the psychotropics agents can be avoided by separating antacid dosing from *all* medications by administering them 1 hour before or 2 hours after the other medications.[109]

- Antitubercular agents: isoniazid decreased diazepam clearance while rifampin increased the clearance.[109] When antitubercular agents are initiated or discontinued, concomitantly administered benzodiazepines should be closely monitored for changes in plasma levels.

- The effect of levodopa in parkinsonism was decreased and the effect of digoxin was reported to increase upon addition of a benzodiazepine.[110]

- Oral contraceptives were shown to decrease the clearance of chlordiazepoxide and diazepam.[111] Reduced doses of benzodiazepines may be required when women receiving a benzodiazepine begin oral contraceptive treatment.

- Other psychotropic agents generally produce additive central depressant effects with benzodiazepines. In one report, amitriptyline levels were increased in the presence of diazepam. This effect would be particularly difficult in the elderly patient because of the dangers of anticholinergic toxicity. Although the fixed combination of a benzodiazepine and an antidepressant is marketed for the treatment of mixed anxiety and depression, the combination is *not* recommended because of case reports of delusional thinking, confusion, irritability and disorientation.[112] Further, fixed dose combinations do not allow individualized dosing of each drug in the combination.

- Alcohol and benzodiazepines produce an additive central depressant effect and is a frequent combination in suicides. There is evidence that the amount of benzodiazepine absorbed is significantly increased (nearly doubled) by co-administration of alcohol.[113]

- As discussed earlier, clozapine and benzodiazepines are not recommended (Severity 1) due to reports of severe respiratory depression and deaths.[68, 69]

Safety in Pregnancy

The safety of the benzodiazepines in pregnancy is not established and recent studies suggest the potential for harmful effects. There are reports of fetal abnormalities following benzodiazepine administration to pregnant women during the first trimester.[114] Withdrawal symptoms occur in neonates whose mothers chronically ingested benzodiazepines during pregnancy. This "floppy baby" syndrome includes hypotonia and hypothermia and has been documented in mothers after relatively short periods of benzodiazepine usage.[115] Therefore, antianxiety agents should be avoided during the first trimester. Benzodiazepines for the treatment of insomnia are contraindicated during pregnancy. Women of child-bearing age are at risk of unintended pregnancy and consequently, should be informed before treatment is undertaken. Nursing should be avoided because the benzodiazepines pass into breast milk.

OTHER ANTIANXIETY AND HYPNOTIC AGENTS

Barbiturates and Carbamates

The barbiturates have been virtually replaced by the benzodiazepines for the treatment of anxiety and insomnia. Benzodiazepines are preferred because of their greater margin of safety, lesser dependency potential and lower morbidity and mortality in acute intoxication. Phenobarbital, a long-acting barbiturate continues to have limited usage as an antiepileptic agents and for detoxifying patients from shorter acting barbiturates. However, reports of behavioral symptoms such as hyperactivity in children, and irritability in adults[116] have led to a gradual shift away from barbiturates as drugs of first choice. Another disadvantage of barbiturates is their liver enzyme induction effect which produces clinically significant drug interactions.

In the 1960s, synthetic compounds called propanediol carbamates were marketed and widely used to treat anxiety. Meprobamate is the best known of these agents. Gradually they were found to exhibit significant tolerance and severe withdrawal reactions were reported. There is no advantage to recommend these compounds over a benzodiazepine. Neither barbiturates nor meprobamate and its congeners are recommended for the treatment of anxiety or insomnia.

Chloral Hydrate

In the 1940s, a two-carbon alcohol derivative, chloral hydrate, which is metabolized by the alcohol dehydrogenase enzyme of the liver, was found to have sedative properties. The compound has well-documented clinical trial data to support efficacy and is sometimes used because of minimal respiratory and vasomotor function depression at therapeutic doses. However, acute intoxication results in depression of both respiration and blood pressure. The drug is irritating to the gastric mucosa and abuse has been documented. Chloral hydrate is a suitable alternative to benzodiazepines for patients who may require initial sedation during the titration to adequate clozapine dosages.

Sedative Antihistamines

Sedative antihistamines have been utilized as hypnotics because they lack the dependency potential and withdrawal symptoms of the barbiturates and benzodiazepines. Diphenhydramine in a dose of 50 and 150 mg was found to be comparable to a 60 mg dose of pentobarbital.[117] Similarly, hydroxyzine in 50 and 150 mg doses was comparable to a 60 mg dose of pentobarbital.[118]

Caution in psychiatric patients is necessary because the antihistamines have anticholinergic activity which is additive to the anticholinergic effects of the antipsychotics, antidepressants, and antiparkinsonian agents that these patients may be receiving. Following acute ingestion, the antihistamines are very toxic (coma, convulsions, and cardiac arrest are observed) relative to benzodiazepines and they are involved in many suicides.

Buspirone

Buspirone is a nonformulary alternative for the treatment of anxiety which was recently marketed. The compound is a member of the azapirone chemical class with a pharmacologic profile involving interaction with the 5-HT$_{1A}$ subtype of the high affinity 5-HT (serotonin) receptor[119] that is described as a partial agonist with weak serotonin-like activity. In addition to serotonin-like activity, buspirone has moderate affinity for D$_2$ receptors and exhibits both dopamine agonist and antagonist actions. Noradrenergic actions are also postulated. Efficacy was established in a double-blind comparison with placebo[120] and in a comparative trial with diazepam.[121] A dose-dependent increase in prolactin level has been observed[122] suggesting a weak neuroleptic-like action mediated through blockade of the post-synaptic D$_2$ receptor. The short- and long-term effects of dopamine blockade by this drug have not been established, but preliminary case reports suggest caution. Irreversible oral dyskinesia was reported in an elderly woman with dementia (and minimum neuroleptic treatment but no prior movement disorder) after 3 days of buspirone treatment.[123] The report of high-dose buspirone to treat tardive dyskinesia is subject to the alternative interpretation of a "masking" of severe irreversible movements following previous long-term treatment with lithium and neuroleptics.[124] This interpretation is bolstered by additional cases suggesting antidopaminergic mediated worsening of movements in parkinsonian patients.[125, 126] Patients who are given buspirone should be informed of the issue and close monitoring for abnormal involuntary movements is appropriate. The use of this agent merely to avoid triplicate prescription monitoring is inappropriate.

Agents with Unlabeled Indications

Beta-Blockers

Propranolol, the first of the beta-adrenergic receptor blockers, has labeled indications for the treatment of hypertension, angina and migraine. Serendipitously, it was found to relieve the anxiety that accompanied tachycardia. Following these reports, several small studies provided data to support a limited role for propranolol in treating anxiety. In a study of 15 outpatients with anxiety, 9 were less anxious on active drug than on placebo while 6 were not significantly different.[127] However, while there was global improvement, the symptoms that improved were the *physical* and not the mental symptoms of anxiety. Similar findings of a 1 week evaluation of diazepam and propranolol indicated that propranolol was effective in reducing somatic anxiety but failed to control psychic anxiety.[128]

Propranolol should not be used in asthmatics because it increases airway resistance. Caution is needed in patients with pre-existing heart disease to avoid acute heart failure. Side effect monitoring includes daily blood pressure and pulse measures during early treatment and when dose increases are made. An additional problem which makes the use of propranolol in psychiatric patients more difficult is secondary depression.[129] Until there are efficacy data in large samples of patients to support the effectiveness of propranolol or other beta-blockers for the treatment of anxiety, they are not recommended.

Clonidine

Clonidine is a predominantly presynaptic noradrenergic agonist that stimulates central alpha$_2$ adrenergic receptors causing inhibition of sympathetic vasomotor centers. It has labeled indications for the treatment of hypertension. Clonidine has been suggested for the treatment of anxiety based on a theoretical biochemical model of anxiety involving the noradrenergic system and the locus coeruleus. In evaluating this theory, a modest response to clonidine with frequent side effect complaints (e.g., tension, excitation, sleep disturbance, decreased concentration, and sexual dysfunction) was reported in 23 anxiety disorder patients. They were treated in a double-blind crossover study for 2 weeks with active drug and 2 weeks with placebo.[130] After 4 weeks, half the patients continued treatment but, by the end of 10 weeks, only 4 patients continued treatment. More favorable findings are needed before clonidine can be recommended for treatment-resistant anxiety disorder.

CONCLUSION

Among the agents available for the treatment of anxiety and insomnia, the benzodiazepines are the drugs of choice because of their demonstrated effectiveness and wider margin of safety compared with older agents. While short-term use of benzodiazepines is well-established, long-term treatment should generally include psychotherapeutic and behavioral approaches. They have an abuse potential for the person unaware of the need for ongoing, individualized benefit, risk and cost assessment but serious abuse tends to occur within a particular subgroup of patients and the problems of acute intoxication and withdrawal tend to be less severe than with the barbiturates and carbamates. There are challenges to the correct use of these agents (i.e., the lowest dose for the shortest time periods necessary). Among these challenges is the identification and management of short-term rebound effects so that the benzodiazepine can be withdrawn successfully after time-limited periods of treatment. Continuous, long-term use for patients receiving complex, multi-drug regimens deserves case review for the possibility of drug-induced anxiety or insomnia.

REFERENCES

1. Ayd FJ, Jr.: Social Issues: misuse and abuse. Psychosomatics 1980; 21(Suppl):21–31

2. Weissman MM, Leaf PJ, Holzer CE, Merikangas KR: The epidemiology of anxiety disorders: a highlight of recent evidence. Psychopharm Bull 1985; 21:538–541

3. Lader M, Bruce M: States of anxiety and their induction by drugs. Brit J Clin Pharmacol 1986; 22:251–261

4. Pitts FN, Jr., McClure JN, Jr.: Lactate metabolism in anxiety neurosis. New Eng J Med 1967; 277:1329–1336

5. Rifkin A, Klein DF, Dillon D, Levitt M: Blockade by imipramine or desipramine of panic induced by sodium lactate. Am J Psychiatry 1981; 138:676–677

6. Feinstein AR: Clinical Epidemiology. Philadephia, WB Saunders, 1985

7. Weiden PJ: Clinical nonrecognition of neuroleptic-induced movement disorders: a cautionary study. Am J Psychiatry 1987; 144:1148–1153

8. Guyatt G, Sackett D, Taylor DW, Chong J, Roberts R, Pugsley S: Determining optimal therapy—randomized trials in individual patients. New Eng J Med 1986; 314:889–892

9. Uhde TW, Nemiah JC: Anxiety Disorders, in Comprehensive Textbook of Psychiatry/V. 5th ed, vol 1. Edited by Kaplan HI, Sadock BJ. Baltimore, Williams and Wilkins, 1989

10. Wickramasekera I: Heart rate feedback and the control of cardiac neurosis, in Biofeedback, Behavior Therapy and Hypnosis. Edited by Wickramasekera I. Chicago, Nelson-Hall, 1975

11. Ciraulo DA: Abuse potential of benzodiazepines. Bull NY Acad Med 1985; 61:728–741

12. Abernethy DR, Greenblatt DJ, Shader RI: Benzodiazepine hypnotic metabolism: drug interactions and clinical implications. Acta Psychiatr Scand 1986; 332:32–38

13. Amrein R, Eckert M, Haefeli H, Leishman B: Pharmacokinetic and clinical considerations in the choice of a hypnotic. Brit J Clin Pharmacology 1983; 16:5S–10S

14. Rosenbaum JF: The drug treatment of anxiety. New Eng J Med 1982; 306:401–404

15. Dawson GW, Jue SG, Brogden RN: Alprazolam, a review of its pharmacodynamic properties and efficacy in the treatment of anxiety and depression. Drugs 1984; 27:132–147

16. Uhlenhuth EH, Matuzas W, Glass RM, Easton C: Response of panic disorder to fixed doses of alprazolam or imipramine. J Affective Disorders 1989; 17:261–270

17. Squires RF, Braestrup C: Benzodiazepine receptors in rat brain. Nature 1977; 266:732–34

18. Möhler H, Okada T: Benzodiazepine receptor: demonstration in the central nervous system. Science 1977; 198:849–857

19. Arendt RM, Greenblatt DJ, Liebisch DC, Luu MD, Paul SM: Determinants of benzodiazepine brain uptake: lipophilicity versus binding affinity. Psychopharmacology 1987; 93:72–76

20. Greenblatt DL, Shader RI: Drug therapy: Benzodiazepines Part I. New Eng J Med 1974; 291:1011–1015

21. Baldessarini RJ: Antianxiety Drugs in Chemotherapy in Psychiatry: Principles and Practice. 2nd ed. Cambridge, Harvard University Press, 1985

22. Ananth J: Benzodiazepines: selective administration. J Affective Disorders 1987; 13:99–108

23. Greenblatt DJ, Shader RI, Abernethy DR: Current status of the Benzodiazepines (First of two parts). New Eng J Med 1983; 309:354–358

24. Greenblatt DJ, Shader RI, Franke K, MacLaughlin DS, Harmatz JS, Allen MD, Werner A, Woo E: Pharmacokinetics and bioavailability of IV, IM and oral lorazepam. J Pharmaceut Sci 1979; 68:57–63

25. Usdin E (ed): Clinical Pharmacology in Psychiatry. New York, Elsevier, 1981

26. Marcucci F, Mussini E, Guaitani A, Fanelli R, Garattini S: Anticonvulsant activity and brain levels of diazepam and its metabolites in mice. Eur J Pharmacol 1971; 16:311–314

27. Norman TR, Burrows GD: Plasma levels of benzodiazepine antianxiety drugs and clinical response, in Handbook of Studies on Anxiety. Edited by Burrows GD, Davies B. Elsevier/Holland, Biomed Press, 1980

28. Hollister LE: A look at the issues. Psychosomatics 1980; 21:(10) 4–8

29. Tyrer P: Benzodiazepines in the treatment of anxiety and tension states, in Benzodiazepines Divided. Edited by Trimble MR. Chichester, Wiley and Sons, 1983

30. Rickels K: Use of antianxiety agents in anxious outpatients. Psychopharmacol 1978; 58:1–17

31. Lader MH, Bond AJ, James DC: Clinical comparison of anxiolytic drug therapy. Psychol Med 1974; 4:381–387

32. Rickels K, Lipman RS, Park LC, Covi L, Uhlenhugh EH, Mock JE: Drug, doctor warmth, and clinic setting in the symptomatic response to minor tranquilizers. Psychopharmacologia (Berlin) 1971; 20:128–152

33. Smith ME, Chassan JB: Comparison of diazepam, chlordiazepoxide and trifluoperazine in a double-blind clinical investigation. J Neuropsychiatry 1964; 5:593–600

34. Greenblatt DJ, Shader RI: The treatment of emotional disorders in Benzodiazepines in Clinical Practice. New York, Raven Press, 1974

35. Johnson DAW: Benzodiazepines in depression, in Benzodiazepines Divided. Edited by Trimble MR. Chichester, Wiley and Sons, 1983

36. Fabre LF, McLendon DM, Stephens AG: Comparison of the therapeutic effect, tolerance and safety of ketazolam and diazepam administered for six months to outpatients with chronic anxiety neurosis. J Int Med Research 1981; 9:191–198

37. Rickels K, Schweizer E, Case WG, Greenblatt DJ: Long-term therapeutic use of benzodiazepines. İ. Effects of abrupt discontinuation. Arch Gen Psychiatry 1990; 47:899–907

38. Klein DF: Delineation of two drug-responsive anxiety syndromes. Psychopharmacologia 1964; 5:397–408

39. Marks I: Phobic disorders four years after treatment: a prospective follow-up. Brit J Psychiatry 1971; 118:683–688

40. Gelder MG, Marks IM, Wolff HH: Desensitization and psychotherapy in the treatment of phobic states: a controlled inquiry. Brit J Psychiatry 1967; 113:53–81

41. Zitrin CM, Klein DF, Woerner MG: Treatment of agoraphobia with group exposure *in vivo* and imipramine. Arch Gen Psychiatry 1980; 37:63–72

42. Klein DF, Ross DC, Cohen P: Panic and avoidance in agoraphobia. Application of path analysis to treatment studies. Arch Gen Psychiatry 1987; 44:377–385

43. McNair DM, Kahn RJ: Imipramine compared with a benzodiazepine for agoraphobia, in Anxiety: New Research and Changing Concepts. Edited by Klein DF, Rabkin JC. New York, Raven Press, 1981

44. Tyrer P, Candy J, Kelly D: A study of the clinical effects of phenelzine and placebo in the treatment of phobic anxiety. Psychopharmacologia 1973; 32:237–254

45. Sheehan DV, Ballenger JS, Jacobsen G: Treatment of endogenous anxiety with phobic, hysterical and hypocondriacal symptoms. Arch Gen Psychiatry 1980; 37:51–59

46. Chouinard G, Annable L, Fontaine R, Solyom L: Alprazolam in the treatment of generalized anxiety and panic disorders: a double blind placebo-controlled study. Psychopharmacology 1982; 77:229–233

47. Greenblatt DJ, Shader RI, Koch-Weser J: Flurazepam hydrochloride. Clin Pharmacol and Therapeutics 1975; 17:1–14

48. Kales A, Allen C, Scharf MB, Kales JD: Hypnotic drugs and their effectiveness. All-night EEG studies of insomniac subjects. Arch Gen Psychiatry 1970; 23:226–232

49. Kales A, Kales JD, Leo LA, Bixler EO: Evaluation of the effectiveness of hypnotic drugs under conditions of prolonged use. (Abstract) Sleep Research 1973; 2:157

50. Kales A, Bixler EO, Tan T-L, Scharf MB, Kales JD: Chronic hypnotic-drug use: ineffectiveness, drug-withdrawal, insomnia and dependence. JAMA 1974; 227:513–517

51. Kales A, Kales JD: Shortcomings in the evaluation and promotion of hypnotic drugs. (Editorial) New Eng J Med 1975; 293:826–827

52. Thompson WL, Johnson AD, Maddrey WL, Osler Medical Housestaff: Diazepam and paraldehyde for treatment of severe delirium tremens, a controlled trial. Ann Int Med 1976; 294:757–762

53. Arana GW, Ornsteen ML, Kanter F, Friedman HL, Greenblatt DJ, Shader RI: The use of benzodiazepines for psychotic disorders: a literature review and preliminary clinical findings. Psychopharm Bull 1986; 22:77–87

54. Wolkowitz OM, Pickar D, Doran AR, Breier A, Tarell J, Paul SM: Combination alprazolam-neuroleptic treatment of the positive and negative symptoms of schizophrenia. Am J Psychiatry 1986; 143:85–87

55. Csernansky JG, Lombrozo L, Gulevich GD, Hollister LE: Treatment of negative schizophrenic symptoms with alprazolam: a preliminary open-label study. J Clin Psychopharmacol 1984; 4:349–352

56. Jos CJ, Schneider R, Gannon P: Diazepam in the treatment of hallucinations. (Letter) Am J Psychiatry 1985; 142:1130–1131

57. Kramer JC: Treatment of chronic hallucinations with diazepam and phenothiazines. Dis of the Nervous System 1967; 28:593–594

58. Irvine BM: "Valium" in the treatment of schizophrenia. Med J Australia 1969; 1:1387

59. Ansari JMA: Lorazepam in the control of acute psychotic symptoms and its comparison with flupenthixol, in Phenothiazines and structurally related drugs: Basic and Clinical Studies. Edited by Usdin E, Eckert H, Forrest IS. New York, Elsevier North Holland, 1980

60. Greenberg WM, Triana JP, Karajgi B: Lorazepam in the treatment of psychotic symptoms. (Letter) Am J Psychiatry 1986; 143:932

61. Kellner R, Wilson RM, Muldawer, Pathak D: Anxiety in schizophrenia. The responses to chlordiazepoxide in an intensive design study. Arch Gen Psychiatry 1975; 32:1246–1254

62. Guz I, Moraes R, Sartoretto JN: The therapeutic effects of lorazepam in psychotic patients treated with haloperidol: a double-blind study. Current Therapeutic Research 1972; 14:767–774

63. Chou JC: Recent advances in treatment of acute mania. J Clin Psychopharm 1991; 11:3–21

64. Ruskin P, Averbukh I, Belmaker RH, Dasberg H: Benzodiazepines in chronic schizophrenia. (Letter) Biol Psychiatry 1979; 14:557–558

65. Karson CN, Weinberger DR, Bigelow L, Wyatt RJ: Clonazepam treatment of chronic schizophrenia: negative results in a double-blind, placebo-controlled trial. Am J Psychiatry 1982; 139:1627–1628

66. Jus K, Jus A, Villeneuve A, Pires P, Fontaine P: The utilization of hypnotics in chronic schizophrenics: Some critical remarks. Biol Psychiatry 1979; 14:955–960

67. Bitter I, Rihmer Z: Practical Psychopharmacology, 2nd ed. Budapest, Medicina, 1989 (Hungarian)

68. Sassim N, Grohmann R: Adverse drug reactions with clozapine and simultaneous application of benzodiazepines. Pharmacopsychiatry 1988; 21:306–307

69. Citizens Health Research Interest Group, Washington, DC: Personal communication, 1991; Dear Doctor Letter from Sandoz, November 1992

70. Feighner JP, Aden GC, Fabre LF, Rickels K, Smith, WT: Comparison of alprazolam, imipramine, and placebo in the treatment of depression. JAMA 1983; 249:3057–3064

71. Rickels K, Feighner JP, Smith WT: Alprazolam, amitriptyline, doxepine and placebo in treatment of depression. Arch Gen Psychiatry 1985; 42:134–141

72. Fyer AJ, Liebowitz MR, Gorman JM, Campeas R, Levin A, Davies SO, Goetz D, Klein DF: Discontinuation of alprazolam treatment in panic patients. Am J Psychiatry 1987; 144:303–308

73. Noyes R, Jr., Perry PJ, Crowe RR, Coryell WH, Clancy J, Yamada T, Gabel J: Seizures following the withdrawal of alprazolam. J Nerv Mental Dis 1986; 174:50–52

74. Ayd FJ, Jr.: Alprazolam: a new benzodiazepine anxiolytic. Intl Drug Therapy Newsletter 1981; 16:37–40

75. Greenblatt DJ, Allen MD, Harmatz JS, Shader RI: Diazepam disposition determinants. Clin Pharmacol and Therapeutics 1980; 27:301–312

76. Roberts RK, Desmond PV, Wilkinson GR, Schenker S: Disposition of chlordiazepoxide: sex differences and effects of oral contraceptives. Clin Pharmacol and Therapeutics 1979; 25:826–831

77. Boston Collaborative Drug Surveillance Program: Clinical depression of the central nervous system due to diazepam and chlordiazepoxide in relation to cigarette smoking and age. New Eng J Med 1973; 288:277–280

78. Hart P, Farrell GC, Cooksley WGE, Powell LW: Enhanced drug metabolism in cigarette smokers. Brit Med J 1976; 2:147–149

79. Klotz U, Antonin KH, Brügel H, Bieck PR: Disposition of diazepam and its major metabolite desmethyldiazepam in patients with liver disease. Clin Pharmacol and Therapeutics 1977; 21:430–436

80. Shull HJ, Wilkinson GR, Johnson R, Schenker S: Normal disposition of oxazepam in acute viral hepatitis and cirrhosis. Ann Int Med 1976; 84:420–425

81. Model DG, Berry DJ: Effects of chlordiazepoxide in respiratory failure due to chronic bronchitis. Lancet 1974; 2:869–870

82. Albeck JH: Withdrawal and detoxification from benzodiazepine dependence: a potential role for clonazepam. J Clin Psychiatry 1987; 48:10 (Suppl)43–48

83. Heritch AJ, Capwell R, Roy-Byrne PP: A case of psychosis and delirium following withdrawal from triazolam. J Clin Psychiatry 1987; 48:168–169

84. Morris HH, Estes ML: Traveler's amnesia. Transient global amnesia secondary to triazolam. JAMA 1987; 258:945–946

85. Greenblatt DJ, Shader RI: Sleep, in Benzodiazepines in Clinical Practice. New York, Raven Press, 1974

86. Ashton H: Benzodiazepine withdrawal: an unfinished story. Brit Med J 1984; 288:1135–1140

87. P'etursson H, Lader MH: Dependence on Tranquillizers. Oxford, Oxford University Press, 1984

88. Koch-Weser J, Seller EM, Kalant H: Alcohol intoxication and withdrawal. New Eng J Med 1976; 294:757–762

89. Wolkowitz OM, Weingartner H, Thompson K, Pickar D, Paul SM, Hommer DW: Diazepam-induced amnesia: a neuropharmacological model of an "organic amnestic syndrome." Am J Psychiatry 1987; 144:25–29

90. Ray W, Griffin MR, Schaffner W, Baugh DK, Melton LJ: Psychotropic drug use and the risk of hip fracture. New Eng J Med 1987; 316:363–369

91. Pomara N, Stanley B, Block R, Berchou RC, Stanley M, Greenblatt DJ, Newton RE, Gershon S: Increased sensitivity of the elderly to the central depressant effects of diazepam. J Clin Psychiatry 1985; 46:185–187

92. Salzman C, Shader RI, Harmatz J, Robertson L: Psychopharmacologic investigations in elderly volunteers: effect of diazepam in males. J Am Geriatric Society 1975; 23:451–457

93. Bliwise D, Seidel W, Greenblatt DJ, Dement W: Nighttime and daytime efficacy of flurazepam and oxazepam in chronic insomnia. Am J Psychiatry 1984; 141:191–195

94. Ryan HF, Merrill B, Scott GE, Krebs R, Thompson BL: Increase in suicidal thoughts and tendencies: association with diazepam therapy. JAMA 1968; 203:1137–1139

95. DiMascio A: Behavioral toxicity, in Clinical Handbook of Psychopharmacology. Edited by DiMascio A, Shader RI. New York, Science House, 1970

96. Hall RC, Joffe JR: Aberrant response to diazepam: a new syndrome. Am J Psychiatry 1972; 129:738–742

97. Hall RC, Zisook S: Paradoxical reactions to benzodiazepines. Brit J Clin Pharmacology 1981; 11 Suppl 1:99S–104S

98. Marks J: The Benzodiazepines: Use, Overuse, Misuse, Abuse. Baltimore, University Park Press, 1978

99. Swinson RP, Pecknold JC, Kirby ME: Benzodiazepine dependence. J Affective Disorders 1987; 13:109–118

100. Hollister LE, Motzenbecker FP, Degan RO: Withdrawal reactions from chlordiazepoxide. Psychopharmacologia 1961; 2:63–68

101. Pevnick JS, Jasinski D, Haertzen CA: Abrupt withdrawal from therapeutically administered diazepam. Arch Gen Psychiatry 1978; 35:995–998

102. Winokur A, Rickels K, Greenblatt DJ, Snyder PJ, Schatz NJ: Withdrawal reaction from long-term, low-dosage administration of diazepam. Arch Gen Psychiatry 1980; 37:101–105

103. Dysken MW, Chan CH: Diazepam withdrawal psychosis: a case report. Am J Psychiatry 1977; 134:573

104. Preskorn SH, Denner LJ: Benzodiazepines and withdrawal psychosis. Report of three cases. JAMA 1977; 237:36–38

105. Greenblatt DJ, Shader RI, Abernethy DR: Current status of benzodiazepines (second of two parts). New Eng J Med 1983; 309:410–416

106. Kales A, Soldatos CR, Bixler EO, Kales JD: Rebound insomnia and rebound anxiety: a review. Pharmacology 1983; 26:121–137

107. MacLeod SM, Sellers EM, Giles HG, Billing BJ, Martin PR, Greenblatt DJ, Marshman JA: Interaction of disulfiram with benzodiazepines. Clin Pharmacol Therapeutics 1976; 24:584–589

108. Klotz U, Reimann I: Delayed clearance of diazepam due to cimetidine. New Eng J Med 1980; 302:1012–1014

109. Katcher BS: Anxiety and insomnia, in Applied Therapeutics, The Clinical Use of Drugs. 3rd ed. Edited by Katcher BS, Young LY, Koda-Kimble MA. Spokane, Applied Therapeutics, Inc., 1983

110. Hansten PD, Horn JR: Drug Interactions and Updates. 6th ed. Philadelphia, Lea and Febiger, 1990

111. Abernethy DR, Greenblatt DJ, Divoll M, Arendt R, Ochs HR, Shader RI: Impairment of diazepam metabolism by low-dose estrogen-containing oral-contraceptive steroids. New Eng J Med 1982; 306:791–792

112. Beresford TP, Feinsilver DL, Hall RC: Adverse reactions to benzodiazepine-tricyclic antidepressant compound. J Clin Psychopharmacol 1981; 1: 392–394

113. Hayes SL, Pablo G, Radomski T, Palmer RF: Ethanol and diazepam absorption. New Eng J Med 1977; 296:186–189

114. Laegreid L, Olegärd R, Wahlström, Conradi N: Abnormalities in children exposed to benzodiazepines in utero. (Letter) Lancet 1987; 1:108–109

115. Prescott LF: Safety of the benzodiazepines, in The Benzodiazepines: From Molecular Biology to Clinical Practice. Edited by Costa E. New York, Raven Press, 1983

116. Stotsky B: Use of psychopharmacologic agents for geriatric patients. DiMascio A, Shader RI: Clinical Handbook of Psychopharmacology. New York, Science House, 1970, p. 269 see also p. 285

117. Teutsch G, Mahler DL, Brown CR, Forrest WH, Jr., James KE, Brown BW: Hypnotic efficacy of diphenhydramine, methapyrilene and pentobarbital. Clin Pharmacol Therapeutics 1975; 17:195–201

118. Brown CR, Shroff PF, Forrest WH, Jr.: The oral hypnotic bioassay of hydroxyzine and pentobarbital for nighttime sedation. J Clin Pharmacol 1974; 14:210–214

119. Traber J, Glaser T: 5-HT$_{1A}$ receptor-related anxiolytics. Trends Pharmacol Sci 1987; 8:432–437

120. Goldberg HL, Finnerty R: Comparison of buspirone in two separate studies. J Clin Psychiatry 1982; 43:87–91

121. Rickels K, Weisman K, Norstad N, Singer M, Stoltz D, Brown A, Danton J: Buspirone and diazepam in anxiety: a controlled study. J Clin Psychiatry 1982; 43:81–86

122. Meltzer HY, Fleming R: Effect of buspirone on prolactin and growth hormone secretion in laboratory rodents and man. J Clin Psychiatry 1982; 43:76–79

123. Strauss A: Oral dyskinesia associated with buspirone use in an elderly woman. J Clin Psychiatry 1988; 49:322–323

124. Hammerstad JP, Carter J, Nutt JG, Casten GC, Shrotriya RC, Alms DR, Temple D: Buspirone in Parkinson's disease. Clin Neuropharmacol 1986; 9:556–560

125. Ludwig CL, Weinberger DR, Bruno G, Gillespie M, Bakker K, LeWitt PA, Chase TN: Buspirone, Parkinson's Disease and the locus ceruleus. Clin Neuropharmacol 1986; 9:373–378

126. Neppe VM: High-dose buspirone in case of tardive dyskinesia. (Letter) Lancet, 1989; 2:1458

127. Granville-Grossman KL, Turner P: The effect of propranolol on anxiety. Lancet 1966; 2:788–790

128. Tyrer PJ, Lader MH: Response to propranolol and diazepam in somatic and psychic anxiety. Brit Med J 1974; 2:14–16

129. Parker WA: Propranolol-induced depression and psychosis. Clinical Pharmacy 1985; 4:214–218

130. Hoehn-Saric R, Merchant AF, Keyser ML, Smith VK: Effects of clonidine on anxiety disorders. Arch Gen Psychiatry 1981; 38:1278–1282

CHAPTER 6

Anticonvulsants for Seizure Disorder and Behavioral Disorders Resistant to Standard Psychiatric Treatments

INTRODUCTION

Although this manual is focused on psychotropic agents, a section on anticonvulsant agents was added to this edition because of the prevalence of seizure disorder in the long-term mentally ill population. Another reason to do so is related to studies evaluating the anticonvulsant prescribing practice of New York State Office of Mental Health facilities[1,2,3] that recommended guidelines for up-to-date clinical practice. In addition, since the late 1970s, there has been increasing unlabeled usage of carbamazepine and valproic acid as psychotropic agents in the management of treatment-resistant affective disorder as well as anecdotal usage in other psychiatric disorders. To address the need for current drug information on the commonly used anticonvulsants, the following sections will describe relevant clinical epidemiologic issues, drug selection, dosing strategies, additional non-pharmacologic factors, side effect and toxicity monitoring, and drug interactions.

Historical, Diagnostic and Epidemiologic Issues

Anticonvulsant therapy is an important area of clinical pharmacology since drug therapy is the mainstay of the management of seizure disorder. Modern treatment began with barbiturates, principally phenobarbital, which was augmented in 1938 by the development of phenytoin, a hydantoin compound that is structurally related to phenobarbital. Although many barbiturates exhibit anticonvulsant activity, only those with sufficient anticonvulsant activity below the hypnotic dose are useful. Since 1965, additional agents have come into use including carbamazepine, an iminostilbene, benzodiazepines such as diazepam and clonazepam and, since 1978, valproic acid. Absence seizures have been successfully treated with ethosuximide.

The prevalence of seizure disorder is generally considered to be between 0.3 and 0.6% of the general population.[4] Of these epileptic patients, the prevalence of severe psychiatric disorders as measured by random surveys in the community is low while specialty referral clinics report a prevalence of 25 to 50% with the upper range reported for indigent populations.[5]

Although important for diagnostic purposes, the categorization of seizure disorders according to etiology, (e.g., that the primary idiopathic type is differentiated from secondary seizures due to trauma, neoplasm, infection, and developmental abnormalities) is generally not relevant to drug selection. After ruling out correction of any underlying cause of seizures, it is the type of seizure and the epileptic syndrome that is the deciding factor in the selection of an anticonvulsant.

The currently recognized terminology for the description of seizure types utilizes the International League Against Epilepsy classification system.[6] Seizures are broadly divided into two groups: (1) partial (focal, local seizures), which may be either simple (without impairment of consciousness) or complex (with impaired consciousness), each of which may lead to secondary generalized tonic-clonic seizures; and (2) generalized (convulsive or nonconvulsive seizures), which are further classified into absence, myoclonic, clonic, tonic, tonic-clonic (grand mal), and atonic seizures. Once the seizure types are classified, the drug selection is based on effectiveness for the type of seizures and the patient's response to anticonvulsant agents. Additional epidemiologic factors concern the type of epileptic syndrome, the frequency of the seizures and the social and environmental setting in which they occur. For example, a first unprovoked tonic-clonic seizure with normal neurologic examination (EEG and CT scan) has less than a 30% chance of recurrence[7] and long-term treatment for such patients is based on an individualized benefit-to-risk assessment. Table 6.1[8] lists the frequently used anticonvulsants according to the seizure types for which they are usually effective.

Basic and Clinical Pharmacology

Seizures are the result of excess electrical discharge in the brain and the anticonvulsants suppress that activity through various mechanisms. According to Eadie,[9] the mechanism of action of the anticonvulsants can be

TABLE 6.1. Anticonvulsants (generic and brand names) and the seizure types for which they are generally effective.

Generic Name	Brand Name	Seizure Type	Primary or Secondary Choice
Carbamazepine	Tegretol	Gen'd tonic-clonic	Primary
		Simple partial	Primary
		Complex partial	Primary
Clonazepam	Klonopin	Simple partial	Primary
		Complex partial	Secondary
		Myoclonic	Primary
		Absence	Secondary
Ethosuximide	Zarontin	Absence	Primary
Phenobarbital	Luminal	Gen'd tonic-clonic	Secondary
Phenytoin	Dilantin	Gen'd tonic-clonic	Primary
		Simple partial	Primary
		Complex partial	Primary
Primidone	Mysoline	Gen'd tonic-clonic	Secondary
		Simple partial	Secondary
		Complex partial	Primary
Valproic Acid	Depakene	Absence	Primary
	Depakote	Gen'd tonic-clonic	Secondary
		Myoclonic	Secondary

Source: Adapted from *The Epilepsy Handbook,* RJ Gumnit. Raven Press, New York 1983.

described at four levels. Specifically, these are the molecular, neurophysiologic, intact animal and human levels. First, at the molecular level the current theories include: (a) alterations in sodium and potassium ion concentration gradients are postulated to be responsible for hyperpolarization of neuronal cell membranes and these are implicated in phenytoin, phenobarbital and valproic acid drug effects; (b) central neurotransmitter levels of serotonin in rats are increased by phenytoin, phenobarbital, and clonazepam; (c) increased brain concentrations of the inhibitory neurotransmitter gamma-aminobutyric acid (GABA) and a consequent reduced neural excitability have been reported for phenytoin, phenobarbital, ethosuximide, valproic acid, and the benzodiazepines. Second, at the neurophysiologic level there are effects on individual and grouped cells. For example, phenytoin reduces postsynaptic excitatory potentials while valproic acid and benzodiazepines are reported to decrease spontaneous firing rate of neurons. In groups of cells, phenytoin appears to impair the propagation (post-tetanic propagation) rather than the initiation of epileptic activity from experimentally induced epileptic foci. Similarly, phenobarbital, carbamazepine, and clonazepam appear to inhibit the spread of epileptic activity. However, ethosuximide, diazepam, and valproic acid appear to have some effect at epileptic foci. Third, there are animal models with experimentally induced generalized epilepsy using electroshock and chemicals such as pentylenetetrazole, and partial seizures obtained by local electrically kindled seizures and by chemical application. Finally, there are effects in humans with epilepsy that form the basis for clinical trials and the clinical practice that derives from the trial findings. Despite the considerable body of work in this area, the essential biochemical mechanism of antiepileptic action is not known for any of the commonly used anticonvulsants.

Clinical pharmacology of the frequently used anticonvulsants generally lacks data that is based on rigorously designed double-blind controlled studies because drug development preceded newer standards of drug efficacy. In a review of 120 clinical trials conducted between 1920 and 1969, only 3 had any type of controlled design. Most lacking are trials of more than a few weeks or months for a disorder that is usually treated for years.[10] Thus, empirical data of variable validity are the basis for the principles of clinical practice. This situation supports the need for systematic longitudinal monitoring in individual patients in order to determine effectiveness and safety on a patient-by-patient basis. Relevant findings from generally accepted basic and clinical studies are reflected in the drugs of choice for each type of seizure listed in Table 6.1.

Seizures are rarely cured and thus drug therapy typically involves the suppression of recurrent seizures in a long-term situation. For about half the patients treated with medication, seizures are completely controlled, for one-quarter, drugs improve their control, and for the remainder, drug therapy inadequately controls seizures.[11] Thus, the current search for optimal control of intractable seizures involves a systematic approach based on known pharmacodynamic and pharmacokinetic principles and on response measured in the individual patient. The quantitative measures required for this approach involve daily counts of seizure frequency and regularly assessed side effects. The optimal drug regimen is defined as the simplest regimen (fewest drugs) which gives the best control of seizures with the best tolerated side effects. Information from the following sections on the selection, dosing, plasma level, and side effect monitoring of these agents will aid in making systematic drug and dose decisions.

DRUG SELECTION

The most frequently used anticonvulsants are listed alphabetically by generic name in Table 6.2 along with their chemical class, major metabolites, and dosage range in adults. Dosing based on mg per kilogram per day estimates is most useful when initiating therapy after which the relationship of plasma level and seizure frequency to side effects in the individual patient should be the basis for drug or dose changes. The selection of anticonvulsants is also related to the pharmacodynamic and pharmacokinetic characteristics of these agents. Whenever possible, no more than one drug change should be made at a time so that logical attribution of the drug and dose changes in relation to seizure control and side effects can be made.

TABLE 6.2. Frequently used anticonvulsants and their chemical class, major metabolites and dosing information.

Generic Name	Chemical Class	Major Metabolites (Active)	Usual Oral Dose Range: Adult day (mg/kg/day)
Carbamazepine	iminostilbene	cbz-10,11-epoxide	200 bid initially, 600–1200/day[a] (15)
Clonazepam	benzodiazepine	—	0.5 bid initially, 1–20 mg/day[a]
Diazepam[b]	benzodiazepine	N-desmethyl-diazepam	
Ethosuximide	succinimide	—	750–2000[a]
Phenytoin	hydantoin	—	200–400[a] (4–6)
Phenobarital	barbiturate	—	90–240 (1–3)
Primidone	barbiturate	Phenobarbital PEMA	125 bid initially, 750–1500/day[a]
Valproic Acid	carboxylic acid	2-en-VPA 3-hydroxy VPA 3-keto VPA	750–2000[a] (15–30)

[a] Divided dosage is recommended especially as the total dosage increases. Adult dosage is provided for general toxicity information followed by the generally accepted mg/kg/day range in parenthesis. Dosing should be regulated through the relationship between plasma level, seizure frequency and side effects in the individual patient.
[b] Diazepam is *not* recommended for oral usage; it is the drug of choice for the rapid control of status epilepticus by IV administration.

Pharmacodynamic Factors

Oral dosing is the commonly used route of administration of the anticonvulsants. Absorption from the gut tends to be relatively slow with peak plasma concentrations requiring 4 to 12 hours.[9] Significant differences in oral bioavailability of phenytoin and phenobarbital have been reported.[12] As a result of the bioavailability studies on phenytoin, Dilantin Kapseals, a brand of phenytoin sodium, is now labeled an *extended* dosage form (35% dissolution per 30 minutes) while the generic phenytoin sodium products are labeled *prompt* (85+% dissolution per 30 minutes). Extended phenytoin is now available as a generic product, although some neurologists prefer the original product. The loss of seizure control following changes in brands has been reported for primidone[13] and recently the recall of generic carbamazepine was reported. These reports suggest that patients should be maintained on the same product unless a change is necessitated. Any anticonvulsant that is dispensed from OMH facilities is listed by the FDA as therapeutically equivalent to the brand name product.[14] However, when a switch from one manufacturer to another occurs, close observation is warranted and any change in seizure control should be investigated in regard to possible differences in therapeutic equivalency. A more detailed discussion of generic and brand name equivalence is found in Chapter 4.

The distribution of the anticonvulsants is measured in terms of the apparent volume of distribution and ranges from the lowest value for valproic acid, which is essentially found in the extracellular water, to phenytoin, carbamazepine, ethosuximide, and the barbiturates, which are found throughout body water. Distribution is highest for the benzodiazepines as they are reported to be concentrated in lipophilic tissues such as the nervous system. From a theoretical standpoint, highly lipophilic anticonvulsants would be expected to add to the intracellular drug load of highly lipophilic agents. Many such agents are commonly found among the psychotropic agents for treating chronic mental disorders.

The following is the approximate rank order from high to low of the protein binding capacity of the major anticonvulsants:[9]

> diazepam>phenytoin>valproic acid>carbamazepine>
> clonazepam>phenobarbital>primidone>ethosuximide.

Patients who will receive highly protein bound acidic compounds such as phenytoin and valproic acid should be closely monitored when added to other acidic drugs (e.g., warfarin), which may be competitively replaced from their binding sites and induce problems (e.g., acute bleeding). Alterations in binding can also occur due to clinical states which release bilirubin and from compounds produced by renal failure.[15] These compounds will cause displacement of drug from binding sites. The clinical situation may be difficult to recognize because routine plasma levels are misleading—only total levels are reported and these remain unchanged whereas the ratio of free (increased active drug) to bound (decreased inactive drug) has been altered and can lead to drug toxicity. Such special situations can be monitored by requesting "free" rather than total drug plasma levels.

The metabolism of the anticonvulsants requires the hepatic microsomal enzyme system. Phenytoin, phenobarbital, clonazepam, and ethosuximide have essentially no active metabolites, a situation which strengthens the validity of plasma monitoring for these drugs. Primidone, a congener of phenobarbital, is metabolized to PEMA plus phenobarbital; carbamazepine and valproic acid also produce active metabolites. Among the benzodiazepines, diazepam has an active metabolite of long duration while clonazepam has none.

Pharmacokinetic Factors

Most anticonvulsants are presumed to follow first-order (linear) kinetics defined as having a linear relationship between dose and plasma level. The concept implies that doubling the dose doubles the plasma level and that the half-life time of elimination is independent of the dose. By contrast, for the dose-dependent elimination kinetics of phenytoin (a one-compartment open model with zero-order input and Michaelis-Menten elimination) only dosages below 10 micrograms per milliliter have been shown to follow first-order kinetics. Higher doses result in dose-dependent kinetics and the half-life increases nonlinearly with increasing dosage. Thus, the apparent half-life of the drug changes with dose and serum level. Theoretical explanations of this effect include the possibility that the hydroxylation step is saturated or that it is inhibited by the presence of metabolites.[16]

Clinically, drugs with nonlinear kinetics produce considerable difficulty in optimizing dosage especially in the patient with incompletely controlled seizures. Since the half-life depends on the dose as well as individual patient characteristics, accumulation may be occurring for up to 30 days rather than the expected 5 to 7 days based on the average half-life of 24 hours. This theory is supported by clinical study.[17] The greater the dosing rate, the longer the time to reach steady state. Rapid escalation of dosages preceding steady state will result in drug toxicity; this leads clinicians to lower dosage in order to lower plasma levels. This in turn may provoke withdrawal seizures which forces a dosage increase. Thus, a see-saw of plunging and soaring levels can occur which is bewildering unless one recognizes that steady-state dynamics are not operating.[18]

When nonlinear kinetics are operating and there is a narrow dose range within which adequate seizure control to side effect balance occurs, the clinician may find that even slight increases above the optimal range will produce disproportionately large increases in plasma level with resultant drug toxicity. Likewise, interchange of phenytoin products with differing bioavailability may affect the difficult-to-control seizure patient when relatively small changes in available drug cause fluctuations in the seizure control-toxicity balance.

DOSING STRATEGIES

Dosing strategies can be divided into the following areas: (1) status epilepticus, (2) initiation of maintenance therapy with monotherapy, (3) plasma level monitoring, (4) long-term monitoring of stable patients, (5) intractable seizures and polytherapy, (6) trial drug discontinuation in long-term prophylaxis, and (7) anticonvulsants in psychiatric disorders.

Status Epilepticus

Because status epilepticus is a medical emergency, its drug management is beyond the scope of this manual. Intravenous diazepam in conjunction with or followed by phenytoin loading (20 mg/kg) are drugs of choice for control of continuous seizures, with 63 to 83% of patients achieving control of seizures.[19, 20] For a full discussion see the review of Leppik et al.[20]

Initiation of Maintenance Therapy

New Patients

Initiating anticonvulsants in new patients with recurrent seizures should be carefully considered because of the growing awareness of the relative difficulty of discontinuing these medications once they are started.[20] Single seizures are generally not considered an indication for maintenance therapy and the decision to treat recurrent seizures is based on the risk of further attacks. Drug selection is based on the seizure type(s). Table 6.1 indicates the primary and secondary drugs according to the major seizure types. Beyond these generally agreed upon guidelines, there are clinical differences among these agents that may affect drug selection. Some of these distinctions will be considered next.

Benzodiazepines.   The benzodiazepines are among the more recent additions to anticonvulsant treatment. They are effective antiepileptics in animal models and for short-term usage such as in status epilepticus. However, they are generally regarded as less effective for chronic maintenance due to the development of tolerance and increased side effects as doses are raised to offset tolerance.[21,22] Clinical studies show that for oral dosing there is relatively little efficacy data to support the use of long half-life benzodiazepines such as diazepam.[19] In chronic hospitalized mental patients with epilepsy, for example, Chien and Keegan[23] found significantly more severe seizures of the generalized tonic-clonic type and more behavioral problems in those randomly allocated to oral diazepam (10 mg tid) during a 6-month evaluation compared with those on standard treatment (phenytoin or phenobarbital). Another study reported only slight advantage for diazepam compared with pheneturide. Such findings account for the fact that oral diazepam is not useful for seizure disorder[11] (p. 467) and has never found wide acceptance.

Of the numerous oral benzodiazepines on the market, only clonazepam and clorazepate (a carboxylated form of N-desmethyl-diazepam) have FDA-approved indications for seizure disorder. Clonazepam usage has been well-reviewed and has achieved the most acceptance of all the benzodiazepines for orally administered drug treatment. It is indicated for typical and atypical absence, infantile myoclonic, myoclonic and akinetic seizures. It was found to be as effective as ethosuximide and superior to placebo and diazepam[24] for the management of absence seizures[25] and for the management of myoclonic seizures.[26] The efficacy data of clonazepam for generalized tonic-clonic seizures is insufficient to support its use for this type of seizure.

In a study of clorazepate, clorazepate-phenytoin combinations were preferred by patients who were switched from the standard treatment of phenytoin-phenobarbital.[27] No differences in seizure control were observed but less subjectively and objectively measured toxicity was reported for the clorazepate group.

In addition to the relative lack of efficacy based on clinical trials for the orally administered benzodiazepines there is a growing awareness of the problem of tolerance. Tolerance leads to dosage increases and ultimately to switching medications since higher doses are eventually limited by the development of drug toxicity or complete ineffectiveness. Tolerance to the anticonvulsant effect of clonazepam has been noted.[28] There is limited evidence from animal studies to support less tolerance of the desmethyl metabolite of the European product clobazam,[29] but such findings require documentation in large clinical populations before they can be generalized.

Carbamazepine.   Carbamazepine now competes with phenytoin as the drug of first choice for the treatment of tonic-clonic, simple, and complex partial seizures.[30] Its efficacy[31] was equivalent to phenytoin and superior to phenobarbital and primidone in a large double-blind, randomized multicenter trial of 3 years' duration. The choice between these drugs is related to other factors, namely, the potential for decreased cognitive functions such as memory and alertness (described as subacute encephalopathy) and psychomotor performance[32] and dysmorphic effects (e.g., gum hypertrophy, acne, hirsutism, and thickening of the subcutaneous tissues of face and scalp) that are associated with long-term phenytoin use.[33] The structural relationship between carbamazepine and the tricyclic antidepressants has led some clinicians to suggest that the improved mood and behavior of patients who are switched from phenytoin[32] or phenobarbital[33,34] is due to an intrinsic antidepressant effect. However, the effect may simply be due to the loss of adverse effects due to the phenytoin or phenobarbital.[33,34]

The decision to use carbamazepine requires hematologic monitoring early in treatment to determine the effects on bone marrow suppression. Among these effects the risk of aplastic anemia is estimated to be less than 1 in 50,000[35] and appears to be patient-specific and unrelated to the more common fall in white cell count that occurs at the start of treatment. Biweekly monitoring of white cells particularly neutrophils (absolute neutrophil count must remain above 1000) for 3 to 6 months is necessary at the initiation of therapy to insure the ability of the body to fight infection and stress. White cell counts below 3500 to 4000 cells/mm[36] should be referred for neurological consultation to decide the benefits and risks of continuing treatment.

If the count continues to drop the drug must be discontinued. Reticulocyte counts should be maintained above 20,000/mm.[3]

   Valproic Acid.   Valproic acid has been available in the United States
since 1978 with an FDA-approved indication for absence seizures. Preliminary reports of its use in a very small number of treatment-resistant
affective disorder patients have been published.[37,38] Additional study of
its effectiveness for these psychiatric indications is needed before the
drug is recommended.

   There are reports of fatal hepatotoxicity, mainly among infants and
young patients[39] and even more frequent cases of drug-induced pancreatitis, including fatalities.[40] European data is accumulating on these effects in adults and in patients receiving only monotherapy.[41] For example, of 16 fatalities in southern Germany, only 12% were under the age
of 3. In another sample, 15% of those who died were on monotherapy.
In one case, the hepatotoxicity occurred late in treatment.[42] As a result
of these events, standard procedure includes liver function test at baseline, and at one month, and then every 6 to 8 weeks for the first 6
months of treatment.[43] In addition, plasma level monitoring should be
undertaken with the goal of maintaining levels between 50 and 100 ng/
ml, although this range requires further validation.

Chronic Patients

For the chronic seizure patient, drug therapy begins with a review of
the seizure history and the previous response to anticonvulsant therapy. Drug selection should be aimed at selecting the single agent most
likely to control the specific type of seizure(s) given the patient's past
experience of anticonvulsant effectiveness and side effects. A single
agent that is a primary drug for the seizure type(s) under treatment
should be started at the recommended mg/kg/day dose and plasma
levels should be evaluated at steady state (estimate should be based on
5 times the usual elimination half-life) in conjunction with seizure
frequency and toxicity measures. Toxicity is discussed in the side effect section next. Table 6.3 lists the frequently prescribed anticonvulsants according to their duration of action.

   The initial drug is monitored for seizure frequency and toxicity.
Dosage should be increased in gradual intervals based on the estimated time to steady state (Table 6.3, column 6) to the maximum suggested plasma level to achieve seizure control. If seizure control is not
complete, the use of a second drug may be considered although the

TABLE 6.3. Suggested guidelines for anticonvulsant drug dosing based on pharmacokinetic characteristics.[a,b]

Anticonvulsant	Plasma Level Range (mcg/ml)[c]	$t_{1/2}$	Time[d]	Steady State Time[e]	Dose Change Interval
Short-acting					
Carbamazepine					
alone	8–12	12 ± 6	1 day	5 days	Weekly
multi-drug regimen	4–8				
Primidone	5–12	12 ± 6	1 day	5 days	Weekly
Valproic Acid	50–100[f]	12 ± 6	1 day	5 days	Weekly
Intermediate-acting					
Phenytoin	10–20	24 ± 12	2 days	10 days	Biweekly
Ethosuximide	40–150	30 ± 6	2 days	10 days	Biweekly
Clonazepam	40–60[f]	27 ± 5	1½ days	7½ days	Biweekly
Long-acting					
Phenobarbital	20–40	96 ± 12	5 days	25 days	Monthly

[a] To determine if a drug is in the usually effective range, draw a trough level (12 hours after the last dose) at intervals not more frequent than the time interval suggested in column 6 for a dose that is being initiated or is undergoing a change.

[b] Under nonemergency situations, dosage changes (increases or decreases) should not exceed 25 percent of the total daily dose. Changes should not occur more frequently than the suggested dosage change interval (column 6) unless a serious clinical consideration warrants a more drastic change. For example, for an idiosyncratic allergic reaction or when significant drug toxicity occurs, the drug should be discontinued immediately.

[c] These ranges are suggested by Gumnit (1983).

[d] The time period is estimated as the half-life plus twice the standard deviation.

[e] The time to steady state is estimated as the product of 5 times the half-life plus twice the standard deviation.

[f] Not yet reliably established.

decision to switch to an alternative drug is suggested as a more useful strategy.[28,43] This approach is based on the poor efficacy data that emerges from studies in which a second anticonvulsant agent was added. For example, Shorvon et al.[44] found no further improvement with a second drug in trials of phenytoin and carbamazepine although the findings are not conclusive. In a retrospective study of this problem, the same group[45] found only a third of patients improved upon the addition of a second drug. Better results were achieved when the first drug was titrated to within the optimum plasma range than by adding a second drug. In summary, this approach uses one drug unless more than one seizure type is involved. Three and 4 drug regimens are not supported at all because of the great difficulty in making systematic changes and logical decisions.

Plasma Level Monitoring

Anticonvulsants have a relatively narrow range of effective plasma concentrations, narrower in fact, than the antibiotics. The usually effective plasma ranges cited in Table 6.3 are recommended by Gumnit[8] and are consistent with New York State OMH recommended laboratory values.[46] Plasma level monitoring is now established as a standard method for longitudinal monitoring of the anticonvulsants.[20] The principles underlying plasma monitoring of these drugs are: (1) the wide interindividual variation for a given dosage suggests within-patient comparisons (changes in level produced by dosage changes in an individual patient) as the method for using plasma levels in a clinically meaningful way; (2) good correlations between brain and plasma levels have been demonstrated for phenytoin, phenobarbital, primidone, and carbamazepine; and (3) clinical data support level-response effects in some of these agents, principally phenytoin, and some limited data suggest level-adverse effect (toxicity) correlations. The strongest findings exist for phenytoin.[47,48]

In general, the upper limit of a suggested plasma level range should be regarded as the dose above which there may be no further antiepileptic effect and for which there is increasing likelihood of acute toxicity. In some cases, the upper range is unclear. For example, the upper range of phenobarbital is quite variable depending on an individual's tolerance to the soporific effects. Carbamazepine is typically suggested in a range of 4 to 8 ng/ml if used in a multi-drug regimen and 8 to 12 ng/ml if used alone. Despite this generally held rule, a recent study reported seizure control among 86% of a cohort of chronic patients treated with carbamazepine alone at levels between 4 and 8 ng/ml.[28] Thus, additional prospective studies are needed to determine the optimal plasma level range of carbamazepine. Appropriate levels for the management of treatment-resistant affective disorder with carbamazepine lack sufficient data at this time and therefore follow the experience of its use in epileptic patients which suggests that levels above 12 in most patients would be likely to produce intolerable side effects. Valproate has data to support the lower limit of the range but the upper range is not yet established. The usefulness of establishing a clonazepam plasma level range is limited by the tendency for tolerance to the antiepileptic effect to occur.

It should be emphasized that plasma level monitoring is a tool for more effective management of the individual patient. Level-response effects are partly a function of the severity of the underlying seizure process so that one-quarter of patients will fail to be controlled despite optimal use of plasma levels to assist decision-making. This relatively small pool of patients, with an estimated prevalence of 15 to 25%, constitute true drug failures. As a tool for enhancing drug therapy, plasma levels should only be altered in response to clinical need—either seizures or side effects—*never because a level is below the so-called established "therapeutic" range.*[49] The therapeutic range for an individual patient is defined as the range in which maximum seizure control and minimum side effect toxicity occurs. This range may be above or below the established range, although in statistical terms, on average in a population it is likely to be within the range. Recent emphasis on the cost effectiveness of laboratory and plasma level monitoring has led to a reminder[50] that rare drug-specific fatal reactions usually are not preceded by abnormal lab values. On the other hand, routine plasma level monitoring *is* useful for dose-dependent drug toxicity.

To use plasma level monitoring effectively, one must consider the estimated length of time to achieve steady state pharmacokinetics. Levels which are not at steady state will underestimate the eventual plasma level because the drug is still undergoing accumulation in body sites. Only after accumulation is complete, does the plasma level reflect the drug effect for the current seizure frequency/side effect level and the replacement dose represents the drug added to make up for that which is lost to elimination. The suggested time intervals between dose changes (upward or downward) are listed in Table 6.3.

A number of authors have described an increase in seizure frequency in association with high plasma levels of phenytoin,[51,52,53] phenobarbital, primidone, and carbamazepine.[54] For example, carbamazepine was reported to increase seizures in 2 cases of acute overdosage.[55] Of greater clinical significance are the reports in some patients with specific types of epilepsy having increased seizures or new seizure types following *therapeutic levels* of drugs like carbamazepine,[54] valproic acid and clonazepam.[55] For example, carbamazepine was reported to exacerbate myoclonic minor motor seizures in 2 series of pediatric patients with generalized tonic-clonic,[56] mixed seizure types,[57] and Lennox-Gastaut syndrome, most of whom were receiving other anticonvulsants. Edwards[58] reported increased or *de novo* tonic-clonic seizure frequency in a subgroup of adult patients following the addition of clonazepam to other anticonvulsants.

The dilemma of increasing seizure frequency at higher doses or with combinations of agents is a challenge to optimal dosing that can be helped by making dose changes in slow, single drug fashion. As time progresses, the plasma levels, coupled with quantitative measures of seizures and side effects, will help to establish a longitudinal pattern of single drug changes. From this record, the change in seizures with dosing changes can be deduced. A method of graphing cumulative seizure frequency versus time has been developed[59] to decide, based on statistically significant differences, whether seizure frequency has changed enough to warrant a change in drug therapy and might be useful in cases of particular difficulty.

Long-Term Monitoring of Stable Patients

Once stabilized, regular review of drug therapy is mandated by OMH policy[3] to occur not less than monthly. This review should consider whether the seizures, recorded daily on a seizure monitoring form, are acceptably controlled and if the regularly monitored side effects have increased to the point of requiring a change from either the patient's or clinician's perspective. Any change in therapy requires plasma level monitoring to determine the level/dose/side effect relationship. Level/dose relationships are especially useful to rule out noncompliance, the commonest problem in chronic anticonvulsant failure.[60]

At the time of the annual physical examination, the clinical interrelationship of seizure frequency, plasma level/dose, and side effects for the previous year should be reviewed. In the stable well-controlled patient, annual plasma levels are required although, as previously discussed, no change in therapy should be made because of a subtherapeutic level unless the clinical picture supports it. Patients receiving phenytoin should be carefully assessed for Vitamin B_{12} level changes and the condition of the teeth and gums should be assessed to determine the need for dental hygiene to treat gingival hypertrophy secondary to phenytoin use. Consultation with the annual reviewing neurologist should occur by request if the treating psychiatrist finds the current regimen does not adequately control seizures without intolerable side effects. In addition, the annual physical review provides an opportunity for long-term neurological review. To facilitate this process, the annual physical examination report should specify the drug and dosage of all current psychotropic and anticonvulsant medications, side effects monitored, a summary of the patient's seizure history, and laboratory and plasma level test results.

Intractable Seizures and Polypharmacy

Although polypharmacy of the psychotropic agents is not sanctioned for routine clinical practice, the occurrence of polypharmacy in seizure management has been the rule rather than the exception because of the prevalence of inadequately controlled seizures with single anticonvulsants. In recent years, the effectiveness of multi-drug regimens has been seriously challenged by several developments: (1) an awareness of the lack of rigorous studies to support greater efficacy for combinations and (2) studies in which there has been an improvement of seizure control following the withdrawal of an anticonvulsant from polydrug regimens;[61,62,63] (3) In animals, the combined use of phenytoin and carbamazepine failed to show greater efficacy than either alone.[64] The findings from these clinical studies suggest that single agent therapy should be seriously and carefully monitored by the use of plasma levels to rule out noncompliance before adding a second agent. Because of the difficulty of successfully managing anticonvulsant drug withdrawal (seizures often increase upon withdrawal and this may be a temporary phenomenon) strict dosing protocols should be followed in upward and downward titration of these medications. Before adding a second agent, consideration should be given to *switching* agents, especially in the patient who is relatively new to pharmacologic treatment and not yet receiving polytherapy.

Fixed drug combinations such as phenytoin and phenobarbital are nonformulary in NYS OMH facilities.[2] They are *not* recommended because of numerous drawbacks and have fallen into disuse in general clinical practice. These drawbacks have been described for fixed combinations in general[65] but they are particularly important for the anticonvulsants because of their narrow therapeutic index. The drawbacks include: (1) inability to establish the need for the second drug if introduced in fixed combination; (2) inability to alter the amount of one agent without changing the other—this poses difficulties in correct attribution since logical drug therapy changes are deduced from single agent changes; (3) the use of more than one agent increases the risk of adverse effects; (4) the complexity of seizure/side effect monitoring in the patient who is difficult to stabilize is not likely to be resolved by fixed dose combinations.

Trial Drug Discontinuation in Long-Term Prophylaxis

For the fully controlled seizure disorder patient drug therapy is often maintained for 3 to 5 years.[9] A recent study documented the usefulness of attempting withdrawal after 2 years in which the patient remains free of seizures.[66] Patients with generalized seizures or complex or simple seizures without secondary generalization who were withdrawn from monotherapy had lower relapse rates than those with complex partial seizures with secondary generalization.

Discontinuation poses problems in itself because of the growing awareness of transient withdrawal seizures. Gradual reductions of not more than 25% of upper range doses should be made over *several months* so that both biological and behavioral adjustment to the reduced dose can occur. Increased seizures that are transient in nature may require reinstituting the dose and more gradual reductions at a later time. The clinical literature[62] has begun to document the difficulty of withdrawing multiple anticonvulsants once they are "on board" in the chronic seizure disorder patient. Nevertheless, the advantages of freedom from long-term drug toxicity as well as the economic and psychological gains make the process worthwhile. This is particularly true for the psychiatric patient who may be receiving 2 or more concurrent psychotropic agents in addition to the anticonvulsants.

Anticonvulsants in Psychiatric Disorders

It is of historical interest to note that phenytoin was once touted to be beneficial for psychological symptoms and at one point it was popularized as an antidepressant based on the personal experience of a millionaire businessman.[67] Since the 1970s, carbamazepine has been used successfully in treatment-resistant bipolar affective disorder. The literature to date is a collection of open studies with small patient samples, a wide range of diagnoses including manic, schizoaffective and depressed patients, with differing lengths of treatment and widely divergent outcome measures.[68] In the only double-blind, placebo-controlled study reported thus far, 4 of 6 manic patients had marked or moderate therapeutic response and 2 did not respond.[69] Plasma levels followed the general guidelines for seizure disorder and patients were maintained between 6 and 12 mcg/ml. Level-response correlations were not found. A comparative 4-week trial of lithium and carbamazepine in a randomized double-blind design failed to demonstrate significant differences in improvement between the two drugs.[70] The authors concluded that the beneficial effects of carbamazepine occurred in a subgroup (3/14) of patients and that larger samples are needed to determine the clinical characteristics of this subgroup of responders.

ADDITIONAL FACTORS

Co-Morbid Medical Conditions

Successful long-term drug therapy of seizure disorder requires recognition of conditions that may alter drug response. Among these conditions are: (1) fever: reported to produce seizures due to increased drug clearance,[71] (2) pregnancy: the risk of fetal abnormalities in women should be taken only when the severity of seizures warrants it;[72] in addition, pregnancy produces changes in clearance not only during the pregnancy, but also at parturition and after birth and these changes can lead to drug toxicity; (3) decreased levels of metabolic compounds such as glucose and sodium that can lower the seizure threshold.

Co-Morbid Psychiatric Disorders

Historically, temporal lobe epilepsy and abnormal behavior have been clinically associated[73] while an inverse relationship between schizophrenia and seizure disorder was an accepted clinical belief. More recently, researchers report a 2-5:1 predominance of temporal lobe epilepsy compared with generalized epilepsy among patients diagnosed with epilepsy and either schizophrenia or paranoid hallucinatory psychosis, although these data may simply reflect the coincidence of psychosis with adult intractable epilepsy that is found in specialty clinics.[5] These relationships pose many difficult etiologic questions. From the standpoint of drug therapy, they suggest that there is a considerable pool of patients who are likely to receive both anticonvulsant and psychotropic agents. Strong evidence of a lowering of the seizure threshold for the antidepressants[74] is based partly on the prominence of seizures in toxic overdosage. However, there is epidemiologic evidence of an association at usual doses of the phenothiazines, butyrophenones, and other antipsychotics.[75,76,77] The atypical antipsychotic, clozapine has a 10-fold greater risk of seizure disorder compared with older agents and the risk increases with doses above 600 mg/day.[78] The use of antipsychotics or antidepressants in seizure patients receiving anticonvulsants should be managed with attention to the potential for a worsening of seizures by the psychotropic agents.

Compliance

Regular use of anticonvulsants requires the patient's cooperation with treatment. As with other chronic disorders that require long-term treatment, noncompliance is a frequent problem. The psychosocial aspects of epilepsy play a part in determining whether an individual acknowledges and accepts the need for regular medication and whether remaining seizure-free is actually a goal for the patient.[8] Withdrawal seizures due to poor compliance should first be considered whenever an increase in seizure frequency or loss of seizure control occurs. If the increased seizure frequency is caused by irregular compliance patterns, the problem can often be detected by observing changes in the plasma level pattern in relationship to dose. For drugs with good plasma level-dose correlations such as phenytoin and carbamazepine[79] a suggested protocol (to be performed without the patient's advance knowledge of the specific occasions of the checking) is to draw 3 plasma drug levels measured at the same time of day and if the variation among them is greater than 20%, the question of poor compliance should be considered.

Dosing on a once or twice a day schedule aids compliance and needs to be exceeded only if side effects require it. Education, supportive therapy, group social support, and self-report of symptoms and side effects are used in various programs to increase a patient's role in forging a therapeutic alliance with the clinician. Increased compliance (adherence) often results from participation in these approaches. Economic factors may also play a part in an individual's reluctance to take medication on a long-term basis.

SIDE EFFECT MONITORING

General Side Effect Monitoring

Routine side effect monitoring of phenytoin, the barbiturates, and carbamazepine typically consists of an assessment of the degree of lethargy (CNS depressant effect), motor incoordination (ataxia), mental confusion (delirium), and double or blurred vision. The benefits of increasing the dose to try to achieve greater control of seizure frequency must be balanced against the risk of increasing drug toxicity.

In addition to the discomfort and dissatisfaction to patients, these effects add to the risk of decreasing the individual's productive work and social life.

In recent years, a more subtle generalized encephalopathy often without nystagmus and ataxia has been described in terms of intellectual and behavioral deterioration.[33] This phenomenon was reported at low, usual, and high plasma levels, with more pronounced effects among those with increased drug exposure (i.e., long duration of drug therapy). While this problem is regarded as under-recognized, it is acknowledged that mental deterioration of the epileptic patient could be due to underlying brain disease, the effects of seizures, genetic or psychosocial factors, as well as anticonvulsant medications. The literature in this area is growing because of the more refined monitoring that is possible using plasma levels and neuropsychological testing methods.

Specific Phenytoin-Related Effects

- Gingival hypertrophy, acne, hirsutism (irreversible)
- Acromegaly, hypocalcemia, and osteomalacia
- Folic acid deficiency can produce megaloblastic anemia that responds to folic acid therapy. If folate therapy is required, Vitamin B_{12} levels should be monitored to avoid Vitamin B_{12} deficiency. The occurrence of phenytoin-induced megaloblastic anemia is rare.
- Pseudo-lymphoma syndrome: a potentially serious, rare event that usually occurs within 4 weeks of initiating drug therapy and may present as painless lymphadenopathy. The lymphadenopathy disappears several weeks following discontinuation of phenytoin.

Specific Carbamazepine-Related Effects

- Aplastic anemia can occur early in treatment and requires monitoring of neutrophils, reticulocytes and white cell counts as previously described (see p. 189).

Specific Phenobarbital-Related Effects

- Irritability and hyperactivity especially in children, have been reported. Avoidance in elderly psychiatric patients is suggested because of the potential for similar effects on personality and behavior.

DRUG-DRUG INTERACTIONS

Oral Birth Control Pills and Anticonvulsants

In addition to published case reports of pill failure in more than 35 anticonvulsant-treated patients, a clinical study was conducted and the relative risk of pregnancy was found to be 25 times higher in women taking anticonvulsants and oral birth control pills than in the control group taking oral birth control pills alone.[80] The mechanism of the interaction is believed to be due to enzyme induction of the metabolism of the steroids by the anticonvulsants (phenytoin, phenobarbital, primidone). Consequently, to avoid pregnancy women should be advised to use alternative methods of contraception during anticonvulsant therapy.

Within-Class Interactions

There is no rationale for the combined use of phenobarbital and primidone since both are barbiturates of comparable efficacy and the variation in metabolites has no demonstrated clinical significance. Additive CNS depressant effects are produced.

Between-Class Interactions

The following between class interactions require monitoring if the use of the combination is clinically justified. Discussion of their significance is found in Hansten and Horn's textbook.[81] Excellent review articles include those of Kutt[82] and Perucca.[83]

- *Valproic Acid and Clonazepam:* Absence status has been reported with this combination.[84]
- *Phenytoin and Antitubercular Agents (Isoniazid):* Phenytoin toxicity may occur; similar effects have been reported for primidone[85] and carbamazepine.[86]
- *Phenytoin and Antipsychotics:* May increase seizure frequency; additive CNS depressant effects; may induce liver enzyme destruction.

- *Phenytoin and Sulfonylurea Antidiabetic Agents:* Possible hypoglycemia due to decreased effect of antidiabetic agent.
- *Barbiturates and Tricyclic Antidepressants:* Tricyclic effect decreased and depression may be exacerbated.
- *Phenytoin and Valproic Acid:* Birth defects.
- *Phenobarbital and Valproic Acid:* Elevated phenobarbital level by slowing its metabolism.
- *Phenytoin and Benzodiazepines:* Additive CNS toxicity.
- *Barbiturates and Benzodiazepines:* Additive CNS toxicity. The combination lacks rationale and is not recommended.
- *Barbiturates and Coumarin Anticoagulants:* Decreased anticoagulant effect that may exacerbate clotting problems.
- *Carbamazepine and Tricyclic Antidepressants:* Carbamazepine and imipramine are related compounds which should be avoided whenever possible. Until evidence of their combined safety is demonstrated, they should be used with close monitoring of serum levels and side effects.
- *Carbamazepine and Coumarin Anticoagulants:* Anticoagulant effect is decreased and may exacerbate clotting problems.
- *Carbamazepine and Macrolide Antibiotics [Erythromycin[87] and Triacetyloleandomycin[88]]:* Carbamazepine toxicity. The use of a suitable alternative antibiotic is recommended.
- *Carbamazepine and Antipsychotics or Lithium:* Carbamazepine has been reported to reduce antipsychotic plasma levels (see Chapter 1) and to increase lithium levels (see Chapter 3).

REFERENCES

1. New York State Commission of Quality on Care for the Mentally Disabled: Psychotropic Drug Usage: Rx for Improvement. August, 1983 (Unpublished)
2. New York State Office of Mental Health, Quality Assurance Survey on Anticonvulsant Medications. July, 1982 (Unpublished)
3. Friedhoff A, Craig TJ, Lehmann H, Schukla D, Haugland G, Zito JM: Final Report of the Subcommittee on Medication Documentation. Anxiolytics and Blood Level Monitoring; the NYS Office of Mental Health Committee on Therapeutics, January, 1986
4. Hauser WA: Epidemiology of epilepsy. Adv Neurol 1978; 19:313–339

5. Stevens JR: Psychiatric aspects of epilepsy. J Clin Psychiatry 1988; 49 (Suppl):49–57

6. Commission: Proposal for classification of epilepsies and epileptic syndromes. Epilepsia 1985; 26:268–278

7. Hauser WA, Anderson VE, Loewenson RB, McRoberts SM: Seizure recurrence after a first unprovoked seizure. New Eng J Med 1982; 307: 522–528

8. Gumnit RJ: The Epilepsy Handbook. New York, Raven Press, 1983

9. Eadie MJ: Anticonvulsant drugs. An update. Drugs 1984; 27:328–363

10. Coatsworth JJ: Studies on the clinical efficacy of marketed antiepileptic drugs. NINDS Monograph Nr. 12, US GPO, Washington DC, 1971

11. Rall TW, Schleifer LS: Drugs effective in the therapy of the epilepsies, in Goodman and Gilman's Pharmacological Basis of Therapeutics, 8th ed. Edited by Gilman AG, Goodman LS, Rall TW, Murad F. New York, MacMillan, 1985

12. Anon: Dilantin vs. generic phenytoin sodium. The Medical Letter on Drugs and Therapeutics 1980; 22:49–50

13. Wyllie E, Pippenger CE, Rothner D: Increased seizure frequency with generic primidone (case report). JAMA 1987; 258:1216–1217

14. Approved Drug Products with Therapeutic Equivalence Evaluations, 11th ed. Rockville, MD: US Dept HHS, PHS, FDA, Center for Drug Evaluation and Research, 1991

15. Reidenberg MM, Odar-Cederlof I, von Bahr C, Borgä O, Sjöquist F: Protein binding of diphenylhydantoin and desmethyl-imipramine in plasma from patients with poor renal function. New Eng J Med 1971; 285:264–267

16. Richens A: Clinical pharmacokinetics of phenytoin. Clin Pharmacokinetics 1979; 4:153–169

17. Allen JP, Ludden TM, Burrow SR, Clementi WA, Stavchansky SA: Phenytoin cumulation kinetics. Clin Pharmacol Therapeutics 1979; 26:445–448

18. Lott R: Epilepsy in Applied Therapeutics: The Clinical Use of Drugs. Edited by Katcher BS, Young LY, Koda-Kimble MA. Spokane, Applied Therapeutics, Inc, 1983

19. Browne TR, Penry JK: Benzodiazepines in the treatment of epilepsy. A review. Epilepsia 1973; 14:277–310

20. Leppik IE: Status Epilepticus. Neurologic Clinics 1986; 4:633–643

21. Trimble MR: Benzodiazepines in epilepsy, in Benzodiazepines Divided. Edited by Trimble MR. Chichester, Wiley and Sons Ltd, 1983

22. Schmidt RP: Benzodiazepines, in Antiepileptic Drugs. Edited by Woodbury DM, Penry JK, Schmidt RP. New York, Raven Press, 1972

23. Chien C, Keegan D: Diazepam as an oral long-term anticonvulsant for epileptic mental patients. Dis Nerv Syst 1972; 33:100–104

24. Chandra B: Clonazepam in the treatment of petit mal. Asian J Med 1973; 9:433–438

25. Mikkelsen B, Birket-Smith E, Bradt S, Holm P, Lund M, Thorn I, Vestermark S, Olsen PZ: Clonazepam in the treatment of epilepsy. Arch Neurol 1976; 33:322–325

26. Nanda RN, Johnson RH, Keogh HJ, Lambie DG, Melville ID: Treatment of epilepsy with clonazepam and its effect on other anticonvulsants. J Neurol Neurosurg Psychiatry 1977; 40:538–543

27. Wilensky AJ, Ojemann LM, Temkin NR, Troupin AS, Dodrill CB: Clorazepate and phenobarbital as antiepileptic drugs: a double-blind study. Neurology (NY) 1981; 31:1271–1276

28. Reynolds EH: Serum levels of anticonvulsant drugs. Interpretation and clinical value. Pharmacology and Therapeutics 1980; 8:217–235

29. Haigh JR, Pullar T, Gent JP, Dailley C, Feely M: N-desmethylclobazam: a possible alternative to clobazam in the treatment of refractory epilepsy? Brit J Clin Pharmacology 1987; 23:213–218

30. Anon: Drugs for Epilepsy. The Medical Letter on Drugs and Therapeutics 1986; 28:91–94

31. Mattson RH, Cramer JA, Collins JF, Smith DB, Delgado-Escueta AV, Browne TR, Williamson PD, Treiman DM, McNamara JO, McCutchen CB, Homan RW, Crill WE, Lobozynski MF, Rosenthal NP, Mayersdorf A: Comparison of carbamazepine, phenobarbital, phenytoin, and primidone, in partial and secondarily generalized tonic-clonic seizures. New Eng J Med 1985; 313:145–151

32. Trimble MR, Reynolds EH: Anticonvulsant drugs and mental symptoms: a review. Psychol Med 1976; 6:169–178

33. Reynolds EH: Chronic antiepileptic toxicity: a review. Epilepsia 1975; 16:319–352

34. Leppik IE: personal communication

35. Hart RG, Easton JD: Carbamazepine and hematological monitoring. Ann Neurol 1982; 11:309–312

36. Joffe R, Post RM, Roy-Byrne PP, Uhde TW: Hematological effects of carbamazepine in patients with affective illness. Am J Psychiatry 1985; 142:1196–1199

37. Lovett L, Watkins SE, Shaw DM: The use of alternative drug therapy in nine patients with recurrent affective disorder resistant to conventional prophylaxis. Biol Psychiatry 1986; 21:1344–1347

38. Emrich HM, Dose M, Von Zerssen D: The use of sodium valproate, carbamazepine and oxcarbazepine in patients with affective disorders. J Affective Disorders 1985; 8:243–250

39. Dreifuss FE, Santilli N, Langer DH, Sweeney KP, Moline KA, Menander KB: Valproic acid hepatic fatalities: a retrospective review. Neurology (Cleve) 1986; 37 (Suppl):379–385

40. Parker PH, Helinek GL, Ghishan FK, Greene, HL: Recurrent pancreatitis induced by valproic acid. A case report and review of the literature. Gastroenterology 1981; 80:826–828

41. Scheffner D, König S: Valproate hepatotoxicity (letter). Lancet 1987; 1:389–390

42. van Egmond H, Degomme P, deSimpel H, Dierick AM, Roels H: A suspected case of late-onset sodium valproate-induced hepatic failure. Neuropediatrics 1987; 18:96–98

43. Krall RL, Resor SJ, Jr.: Drug treatment of epilepsy. Seminars in Neurology 1987; 7:128–138

44. Shorvon SD, Chadwick D, Galbraith AW, Reynolds EH: One drug for epilepsy. Brit Med J 1978; 1:474–476

45. Shorvon SD, Reynolds EH: Unnecessary polypharmacy for epilepsy. Brit Med J 1977; 1:1635–1637

46. Wilson N, Cooper TB: Laboratory values for psychopharmacologic agents, New York State Psychiatric Institute, 1988

47. Buchthal F, Svensmakr O, Schiller PJ: Clinical and encephalographic correlations with serum levels of diphenylhydantoin. Arch Neurol 1960; 2:624–630

48. Lund L: Anticonvulsant effects of diphenylhydantoin relative to plasma levels. A prospective 3–year study in ambulant patients with generalized epileptic seizures. Arch Neurol 1974; 31:289–294

49. Kutt H, Penry JK: Usefulness of blood levels of antiepileptic drugs. Arch Neurol 1974; 31:283–288

50. Pellock JM, Willmore LJ: A rational guide to routine blood monitoring in patients receiving antiepileptic drugs. (Editorial) Neurology 1991; 41:961–964

51. Levy LL, Fenichel GM: Diphenylhydantoin-activated seizures. Neurology (Minneap.) 1965; 15:716–722

52. Lascelles PT, Kocen RS, Reynolds EH: The distribution of plasma phenytoin levels in epileptic patients. J Neurol Neurosurg Psychiatry 1970; 33:501–505

53. Troupin AS, Ojemann LM: Paradoxical intoxication: a complication of anticonvulsant administration. Epilepsia 1975; 16:753–758

54. Snead OC, Hosey LC: Exacerbation of seizures in children by carbamazepine. New Eng J Med 1985; 313:916–921

55. Bruni J: Seizure exacerbation related to antiepileptic drug treatment. (abstract) Le Journal Canadien Des Sciences Neurologiques 1987; 14:207

56. Johnsen SD, Tarby TJ, Sidell AD: Carbamazepine-induced seizures. (abstract) Annals of Neurology 1984; 16:392

57. Shields WD, Saslow E: Myoclonic, atonic, and absence seizures following institution of carbamazepine therapy in children. Neurology 1983; 33:1487–1489

58. Edwards VE: Side effects of clonazepam therapy. Proceedings of the Australian Association of Neurologists 1974; 11:199–202

59. Leppik IE, Brundage RC, Krall R, Cloyd JC, Bowman-Cloyd T, Jacobs MP: Double-blind withdrawal of phenytoin and carbamazepine in patients treated with progabide for partial seizures. Epilepsia 1986; 27:563–568

60. Reynolds EH, Shorvon SD: Monotherapy or polytherapy for epilepsy? Epilepsia 1981; 22:1–10

61. Milano Collaborative Group for studies on epilepsy: Long-term intensive monitoring in the difficult patient. Preliminary results of 16 months of observations—usefulness and limitations, in Antiepileptic Drug Monitoring. Edited by Gardner-Thorpe C, Janz D, Meinardi H, Pippenger CE. Kent, Pitman Medical, 1977

62. Callaghan N, O'Dwyer R, Keating J: Unnecessary polypharmacy in patients with frequent seizures. Acta Neurol Scand 1984; 69:15–19

63. Shorvon SD, Reynolds EH: Reduction of polypharmacy for epilepsy. Brit Med J 1979; 2:1023–1025

64. Morris JC, Dodson WE, Hatlelid JM, Ferrendelli JA: Phenytoin and carbamazepine, alone and in combination: anticonvulsant and neurotoxic effects. Neurology 1987; 37:1111–1118

65. Melmon KL, Morelli HF: Clinical Pharmacology, The MacMillan Company, 1972

66. Callaghan N, Garrett A, Goggin T: Withdrawal of anticonvulsant drugs in patients free of seizures for two years. A prospective study. New Eng J Med 1988; 318:942–946

67. Dreyfus J: A Remarkable Medicine Has Been Overlooked. New York, Simon and Schuster, 1981

68. Ballenger JC: The clinical use of carbamazepine in affective disorders. J Clin Psychiatry 1988; 49(Suppl):13–21

69. Post RM, Uhde TW: Carbamazepine in bipolar illness. Psychopharm Bull 1985; 21:10–17

70. Lerer B, Moore N, Meyendorff E, Cho SR, Gershon S: Carbamazepine versus lithium in mania: a double-blind study. J Clin Psychiatry 1987; 48:89–93

71. Leppik IE, Fisher J, Kriel R, Sawchuk RJ: Altered phenytoin clearance with febrile illness. Neurology (Cleve) 1986; 36:1367–1370

72. Nau H, Kuhnz W, Egger HJ, Rating D, Helge H: Anticonvulsants during pregnancy and lactation. Transplacental, maternal and neonatal pharmacokinetics. Clinical Pharmacokinetics 1982; 7:508–543

73. Mulder DW, Daly D: Psychiatric symptoms associated with lesions of the temporal lobe. JAMA 1952; 150:173

74. Nelson RC, Baum C: Maprotilene and seizures: an analysis of FDA's adverse reaction system. Abstracts of 1985 American Public Health Association meeting

75. Oliver AP, Luchins DJ, Wyatt RJ: Neuroleptic-induced seizures. An *in vivo* technique for assessing relative risk. Arch Gen Psychiatry 1982; 39:206–209

76. Remick RA, Fine SH: Antipsychotic drugs and seizures. J Clin Psychiatry 1979; 40:78–80

77. Logothetis J: Spontaneous epileptic seizures and electroencephalographic changes in the course of phenothiazine therapy. Neurology 1967; 17:869–877

78. Devinsky O, Honigfeld G, Patin J: Clozapine-related seizures. Neurology 1991; 41:369–371

79. Leppik IE, Cloyd JC, Sawchuk RJ, Pepin SM: Compliance and variability of plasma phenytoin levels in epileptic patients. Therapeutic Drug Monitoring 1979; 1:475–483

80. Coulam CB, Annegers JF: Do anticonvulsants reduce the efficacy of oral contraceptives? Epilepsia 1979; 20:519–525

81. Hansten PD, Horn JR: Drug Interactions and Updates, 6th ed., Philadelphia, Lea and Febiger, 1990

82. Kutt H: Interactions between anticonvulsants and other commonly prescribed drugs. Epilepsia 1984; 25(Suppl 2):S118–S131

83. Perucca E: Pharmacokinetic interactions with antiepileptic drugs. Clinical Pharmacokinetics 1982; 7:57–84

84. Watson B: Absence status and the concurrent administration of clonazepam and valproate sodium (letter). Am J Hosp Pharm 1979; 36:887

85. Sutton G, Kupferberg HJ: Isoniazid as an inhibitor of primidone metabolism. Neurology 1975; 25:1179–1181

86. Wright JM, Stokes EF, Sweeney VP: Isoniazid-induced carbamazepine toxicity and vice versa: a double drug interaction. New Eng J Med 1982; 307:1325–1327

87. Wong YY, Ludden TM, Bell RD: Effect of erythromycin on carbamazepine kinetics. Clin Pharmacol Therapeutics 1983; 33:460–464

88. Mesdjian E, Dravet C, Cenraud B, Roger J: Carbamazepine intoxication due to triacetyloleandomycin administration in epileptic patients. Epilepsia 1980; 21:489–496

CHAPTER 7

Pharmacotherapy of Child and Adolescent Psychiatric Disorders

INTRODUCTION

The goal of pharmacotherapy in children and adolescents is to make
the patient more amenable to psychosocial treatments and thus promote the development of adaptive and socially acceptable behaviors.
Many young patients can return to their normal daily functioning at

home and in school with the help of an effective and safe psychotropic drug. Drug treatment is always viewed as part of a comprehensive treatment program, and not the sole treatment modality.

Psychotropic drugs, as well as other treatment modalities, are prescribed after a careful assessment of the patient and a diagnosis have been made and after considering the benefits and risks of drug treatment in the particular patient being evaluated. The APA diagnostic manual (DSM-III-R, rev. 1987) employs operational criteria to define the psychiatric syndromes, as well as exclusion criteria and duration of symptoms. The selection of a psychotropic drug is primarily based on the patient's psychiatric diagnosis, the behavioral profile, target symptoms, and the patient's past response to medications.

The psychotropic drugs currently in use are usually effective in reducing target symptoms associated with clinical disorders in 5 areas: (1) In schizophrenia, tic disorders, mental retardation with behavioral symptoms, and pervasive developmental disorders; (2) in mood disorders such as bipolar disorder, and major depression with symptoms such as irritability, flight of ideas, depressed mood, loss of appetite and loss of energy; (3) under certain circumstances pharmacotherapy may be indicated for enuresis; (4) disruptive behavior disorders, such as attention deficit hyperactivity disorder (ADHD) and conduct disorder, solitary aggressive type, with symptoms such as hyperactivity, short attention span, distractibility, impulsivity, aggressive behavior, disorganization, tics, stereotypies, hallucinations, delusions, and thought disorders; (5) anxiety disorders that may include symptoms of anxiety, panic attacks, and school phobia.

The effects and side effects of the primary psychotropic drug should be considered in monitoring these agents for appropriate and safe use. In addition, ancillary neuroactive drugs (e.g., anticonvulsants for seizure disorder and antiparkinsonian agents or antihistamines used to treat drug-induced extrapyramidal side effects), contribute to the overall medication effects and should be considered for complete drug monitoring of psychiatric disorders in children and adolescents. Overall, the study of drug efficacy for children and adolescents is much less developed than for adults.[1] As a result, much clinical usage lacks evaluation in randomized, double-blind, controlled clinical trials and is based on information that lacks the reliability and validity that comes from more rigorous evaluation. Careful selection of a psychotropic agent is recommended as well as close clinical and laboratory monitoring.

Developmental Factors

The stage of maturation and development of the child is a major consideration in the selection of an appropriate drug and dose. Dosage guidelines are often specified according to age, weight, and severity of illness. A list of usual weights according to gender and age groups of children is provided in Table 7.1. The presence of a co-occurring central nervous system disorder can alter the response to a psychotropic drug which is being used for psychiatric symptom control. As

TABLE 7.1. Typical body weights[a] for girls and boys according to age to estimate the initial dose of a psychotropic drug from mg/kg dosing guidelines. If there is information on prior drug response in the individual, it should be considered along with these estimates.

Age (yr.)	Girls		Boys	
	Pounds	Kilograms	Pounds	Kilograms
0.5	14–19	6.4–8.6	15–19	6.8–8.6
1.0	18–25	8.2–11.3	20–25	9.1–11.3
1.5	21–28	9.5–12.7	22–29	10.0–13.2
2.0	24–32	10.9–14.5	25–32	11.3–14.5
2.5	26–34	11.8–15.4	27–35	12.2–15.9
3.0	28–36	12.7–16.3	29–37	13.2–16.8
4.0	31–41	14.1–18.6	32–43	14.5–19.5
5.0	35–48	15.9–21.8	36–48	16.3–21.8
6.0	39–53	17.7–24.0	40–54	18.1–24.5
7.0	43–60	19.5–27.2	44–62	20.0–28.1
8.0	47–68	21.3–30.8	48–70	21.8–31.8
9.0	52–78	23.6–35.4	53–80	24.0–36.3
10	57–88	25.8–39.9	60–88	27.2–39.9
11	63–99	28.6–44.9	65–100	29.5–45.4
12	70–110	31.8–49.9	71–111	32.2–50.3
13	79–125	35.8–56.7	78–126	35.4–57.2
14	90–133	40.8–60.3	90–137	40.8–62.1
15	97–138	44.0–62.6	99–148	44.9–67.1
16	101–141	45.8–64.0	111–157	50.3–71.2
17	103–143	46.7–64.9	118–165	53.5–74.8
18	104–145	47.2–65.8	120–169	54.4–76.7

[a] *Source:* RJ Baldessarini, Antipsychotics in Chemotherapy in Psychiatry: Principles and Practice. 2nd ed. Cambridge, Harvard University Press, 1985, p. 277; these estimates are adapted from WE Nelson, ed. *Textbook of Pediatrics,* 1959 based on pooled data from several studies in Massachusetts and Iowa. The ranges represent the 10th and 90th percentiles; 1 pound = 0.454 Kg; 1 Kg = 2.2 pounds. Reprinted by permission of the publishers from *Chemotherapy in Psychiatry* by Ross J. Baldessarini, Cambridge, Mass.: Harvard University Press, Copyright © 1977 by the President and Fellows of Harvard College.

in the case of adult patients, liver and kidney function must be adequate for psychotropic drug metabolism.

Pharmacodynamic Factors

The factors influencing the choice of psychotropic drug are: (1) diagnosis, (2) target symptoms, (3) duration and severity of illness, (4) age, (5) previous response to pharmacotherapy, (6) patient setting (inpatient vs. outpatient), and (7) concomitant medications, particularly neuroactive medications that pass the blood-brain barrier and produce additive, synergistic, or diminished effects in the central nervous system. The prescribing physician and those who monitor the patient's progress must be well acquainted with the range of effects, both therapeutic and unwanted, of at least 1 or 2 agents in each pharmacological class.

A review of clinical usage in children and adolescents will be considered in the following sections: (a) antipsychotics and antiparkinsonian agents for psychotic and nonpsychotic disorders; (b) lithium for the treatment of mania; (c) antidepressants for depression, obsessive-compulsive disorder, and enuresis; (d) central stimulants and disruptive disorders, attention deficit hyperactivity disorder; (e) anxiety disorders and various symptom-specific treatments such as antianxiety, hypnotics, and agents from other pharmacologic classes such as propranolol and clonidine; and (f) seizure disorder management with concomitant psychotropic agents.

Side Effect Monitoring

In general, the frequently encountered side effects of the major drug classes in children and adolescents do not differ from adults. Nevertheless, the effects of medication on the intellectual, behavioral, and physical growth of the child require intensive monitoring because of the relative lack of available information. To address the relatively poor scientific methods for monitoring psychotropic side effects once a drug has been marketed, clinical methods are emerging for more precise and regular recording of side effects. Computerized drug information profiles are useful in this regard to track dose and combination changes that occur at the same time that side effects develop. Of particular importance is monitoring to avoid behavioral toxicity[2] which, in young children, may appear *before* neurological or other types of side effects. Careful observation of the pattern of target behaviors in relation to new behavioral symptoms is necessary in order to detect the subtle personality and behavioral effects (commonly ir-ritability, aggressiveness, and altered mood and activity level) that may emerge as the patient develops and which may be produced by specific drugs, dosages or combinations of agents.

For the child or adolescent, side effect monitoring requires training and cooperation from the family or primary caregiver to gauge the effectiveness of the drug and the severity and temporal pattern of possible drug-induced effects. Educational materials in the form of printed lists of frequently encountered side effects are useful. Also, lists of typical signs and symptoms of drug intoxication due to large doses or drug combinations should be used to train the interested family in effective monitoring of their child's drug therapy.

ANTIPSYCHOTIC AGENTS

Psychotic Disorders

Antipsychotics can be helpful in alleviating symptoms associated with schizophrenic disorders, schizophreniform disorders, atypical psychosis, pervasive developmental disorders including infantile autism, and the manic phase of bipolar disorder.

Nonpsychotic Disorders

The nonpsychotic conditions for which antipsychotics are used include mental retardation *with* severe aggressiveness and/or self-injurious behavior (SIB), conduct disorder with aggressiveness, chronic tics, Tourette's disorder, and attention deficit hyperactivity disorder (ADHD) that is resistant to treatment with stimulants.

Antipsychotics are a second choice in managing ADHD after stimulants have failed. This recommendation is based on studies showing:

1. Stimulants are the drugs of first choice in ADHD.[3]
2. Double-blind comparisons of thioridazine and methylphenidate alone, in combination, and to placebo yielded superior outcome for methylphenidate *alone* compared with thioridazine. While initially superior to methylphenidate, the combined methylphenidate and thioridazine treatment lost its superiority at week 12.[4]

3. Crossover design comparisons of haloperidol and methylphenidate were both superior to placebo. However, there were some differences in the magnitude of response to drug. While antipsychotics may be as effective or nearly as effective as stimulants in the treatment of ADHD,[5] it is important to justify dyskinesias as an additional risk associated with antipsychotics in children.[6]

Drug Selection

It is widely accepted that the desired pharmacologic effects of the antipsychotics do not vary although the relative side effect profiles differ. Currently, there are less than a dozen agents frequently used in adult patients and 8 of these have manufacturer's guidelines for dosing in children. For the physician who is prescribing medication for psychiatric disorders, extensive experience with a few agents is desirable. A number of factors should be considered in the selection of the antipsychotic in order to provide the best symptom control with the lowest dose and best tolerated side effect profile. Among these factors, the following will be discussed further: the relative potency of the agents, the seizure-lowering potential, relative potential for weight gain, specific indications, long-term effects, withdrawal effects and side effect monitoring.

Relative Potency

Because they were marketed 15 years prior to the high-potency agents, the low-potency agents such as chlorpromazine and thioridazine, have accumulated greater clinical experience. Nevertheless, there is supportive evidence that haloperidol, fluphenazine, and other high-potency antipsychotics are as effective in children and adolescents as low-potency agents, such as chlorpromazine and thioridazine, when given in equivalent doses. However, the side effect profiles of the 2 groups differ. High-potency agents tend to be less sedating, hypotensive, and anticholinergic, but produce more extrapyramidal effects. Low-potency agents produce relatively more cognitive dulling, impaired arousal, and sedation. Table 7.2 lists the commonly used antipsychotics and should be consulted for the conversion factors for calculating chlorpromazine-equivalents (CPZ-EQ) of antipsychotic so that the amount of one agent relative to another is considered when switching agents. Dramatic differences in treatment response sometimes may

TABLE 7.2. Antipsychotic Drug Dosing Information for Children and Adolescents[a]

Generic Name	Age Range (years): Oral Daily Dose (mg):			Max Daily Dose (IM):			CPZ-EQ mg	CPZ-EQ Dose Multipl'r
	3–6	7–12	13–18	3–6	7–12	13–18		
Chlorpromazine	10–100	25–250	25–800	40	75	100	100	1
Thioridazine	10–100	25–250	25–800				100	1
Fluphenazine HCl	—	—	2.5–20				2	50
Fluphenazine Decanoate[b]								
Trifluoperazine	1–6	1–20	1–40				5	20
Thiothixene[c]	1–6	—	5–42				5	20
Haloperidol[c]	0.25–5	0.5–16	0.5–40				2	50
Molindone	—	1–40	1–200				10	10
Pimozide[c]	—	—	1–4				1.3[d]	77[d]

[a] Dosing in children should begin at the lower extreme of the suggested dose ranges and gradually be increased after clinical response is observed after a reasonably estimated time to achieve steady state, i.e. 5 times the average half-life (see Chapter 1, p. 7).

[b] The adult conversion rule is: Fluphenazine HCl 20 mg per day is equivalent to Fluphenazine Decanoate 25 mg every 3 weeks (1000 chlorpromazine-equivalents per day). This rule is considered by many to overestimate the relative potency of fluphenazine decanoate. The rule adapted in these guidelines is based on the suggestion of J.M. Kane, MD (personal communication): Fluphenazine HCl 13.3 mg per day is equivalent to Fluphenazine Decanoate 25 mg every 3 weeks (665 chlorpromazine equivalents per day).

[c] Suggested dosing by weight:

thiothixene	0.3 mg/kg/day	
haloperidol	0.02 mg/kg/day	low-dose strategy
	0.2 mg/kg/day	high-dose strategy
pimozide	0.2 mg/kg/day	up to 10 mg/day maximum

[d] Pimozide relative potency is estimated from reference 12.

214

be explained by the relatively greater (or lesser) dosage of one agent compared with another. This point is illustrated in a recent study of children and adolescents hospitalized in public psychiatric facilities.[7] High-potency agents were used at relative doses that were 3 times greater than the doses of low-potency agents. Furthermore, there was frequent antipsychotic usage among these patients *regardless* of diagnosis, with the average daily dosage significantly greater among long-stay (more than 90 days) compared with short-stay (discharged within 90 days).

Seizure-Threshold Lowering

The seizure-lowering potential of the antipsychotics is a poorly understood problem because of the lack of systematic study in humans. A discussion of the studies supporting the seizure-threshold lowering in adults is found in Chapter 1. In addition, in a clinical study of the mentally retarded, Tarjan et al.[8] reported that chlorpromazine lowered the seizure-threshold and increased the frequency of seizures in those with pre-existing seizure disorder. Thioridazine is often suggested as an alternative in patients with a risk of seizures, although the basis for this preference is anecdotal.

Potential for Weight Gain

Weight gain in adults is associated with most of the antipsychotics except for molindone, an indole compound that is structurally distinct from other available antipsychotics. Four studies in adults have demonstrated short-term weight loss for molindone-treated patients compared with chlorpromazine, other antipsychotics, and placebo-treated patients.[9] Presumably the findings would apply to children and adolescents as well. Several pilot studies demonstrated the effectiveness of molindone in infantile autism[10] although Campbell cautions that the wide dosage range limits the study findings' relevance to clinical practice until further support is obtained.

Specific Indications

Pimozide is a newer agent of the diphenylbutylpiperidine type marketed with a specific indication for the treatment of Tourette's disorder. Its action is similar to other dopamine-blocking agents and its side effect profile includes low-sedation, extrapyramidal side effects (EPSE) roughly comparable to haloperidol and fluphenazine, and little or no hypotensive effects.[11] It has also been shown to have efficacy at doses of 1 to 4 mg per day comparable to haloperidol at doses of 0.75–6.75 mg per day for the treatment of 3 to 16 year old psychotic patients with various diagnoses.[12] There is little that distinguishes this agent from the other antipsychotics in terms of basic pharmacologic actions. However, the relative potency concept is extremely important for smooth conversion of patients from this to other agents or vice versa. The relative potency suggested by Baldessarini[11] is the ratio of 1 mg pimozide to 100 mg chlorpromazine. From the study of Naruse et al.[12] one can derive the ratio of 1 mg pimozide to 1.5 mg haloperidol to 75 mg chlorpromazine. Electrocardiographic monitoring is suggested and when the QT interval exceeds 500 mse the drug should be discontinued.

Long-Term Exposure

Patients receiving antipsychotics continuously for a period of 3 months or longer, may develop transient withdrawal or irreversible tardive dyskinesias. The reported prevalence of this movement disorder in children and adolescents ranges from 8 to 51%, suggesting the need for further study (for a review see Campbell et al.[13]). In a prospective study, the prevalence of tardive dyskinesia in children was estimated at 29%, a figure close to the estimate for adults suggested by Kane et al.[14] The Campbell et al.[13] review indicates that, while in many cases the dyskinesias were reversible, tardive dyskinesia, defined as irreversible choreoathetotic movement disorder, also occurred. As in adults, the muscles of the mouth, tongue, and jaw are most frequently involved, although any part of the body can be affected.

The Task Force on Tardive Dyskinesia appointed by the American Psychiatric Association (1991), recommends that every patient be carefully examined for abnormal movements at baseline (i.e., *before* beginning antipsychotic drug therapy and then periodically reassessed). Careful monitoring for abnormal movements should be continued during maintenance drug treatment (for tardive dyskinesia), after dose reduction (for covert dyskinesias) or after drug withdrawal (for withdrawal dyskinesias). This is particularly important for patients who have some type of movement disorder at baseline (e.g., those with autism, mental retardation, chronic tics and Tourette's disorder). The assessments of abnormal movements should be made using the Abnormal Involuntary Movement Scale (AIMS) and the results should be carefully documented.

After reduction of symptoms when a therapeutic effect is established, efforts should be made to reduce the dose to the lowest therapeutically effective dose. Whenever possible, in general, antipsychotic administration should be discontinued, with appropriate tapering, every 6 months, for a period of at least 4 weeks in order to determine if: (1) the patient requires further antipsychotic drug treatment, and (2) if the patient develops withdrawal or tardive dyskinesia. Discontinuation of antipsychotic may not be feasible, for instance in some schizophrenic patients discontinuation would result in a return of florid psychotic symptoms or in patients with severe or unpredictable symptom control, or in those maintained on substantially high doses of antipsychotic which are supported by past history of failures at lower doses. In such instances, the rationale for not discontinuing the medication should be noted in the medical record after consultation with the clinical director or designee.

Withdrawal Protocol

Physical withdrawal symptoms [anorexia, nausea, vomiting, diarrhea, weight loss, and diaphoresis (profuse sweating)] occurred in 12% of a cohort of 41 children observed by Gualtieri et al.[15] Rebound phenomena follow drug withdrawal and are characterized by behavioral deterioration which usually resolves within a week but may take up to 8 weeks[16] or longer for long-acting products. Successful dosage reductions and complete discontinuation of an antipsychotic are increasingly recognized to vary with the length of prior history of medication exposure, the dose and the rate of reduction. To maximize the success of the withdrawal, sufficient time should be given to allow drug receptors to readjust. Dosage decrements of 25% at the upper end of the dose range every 10 to 14 days may be followed by halving the dose in 14-day intervals until the medication is discontinued.

Side Effect Monitoring

Anderson et al.[17] reported haloperidol side effects in children who were evaluated in a double-blind, randomized, controlled clinical trial. Excess sedation, acute dystonic reactions and tremor were more frequently reported than in placebo-treated patients. Increased irritability was surprisingly frequently reported among those receiving active drug which could be due to undertreatment of a target symptom but is commonly regarded in children as a side effect of medication. In another study of haloperidol for the treatment of Tourette's disorder, Mikkelsen et al.[18] reported dysphoria and school phobia as side effects.

Height and Weight Monitoring.   Children who receive medication for long periods of time should be monitored for short- and long-term growth effects. Regular charting of height and weight should be done and these should be assessed relative to age. In a study of short-term height and weight effects, there were no significant differences in comparing haloperidol and placebo phases of the treatment during a 14-week study of autistic children.[19] However, 14 weeks may have been too short a time period for perceptible growth changes to occur. Sample growth charts are reproduced in Part IV as a suggestion for monitoring height and weight beginning *before* medication is initiated (baseline) and charted regularly to monitor for long-term changes.

Behavioral Toxicity.   Attention to behavioral symptoms involves monitoring for irritability, aggressiveness, mood changes and changes in functional level (school and home activities). These symptoms may be associated with excessive dosage in children, especially the younger age group. Baseline assessments are needed and family training with written lists of behavioral symptoms would extend the monitoring beyond casual descriptive reports.

Extrapyramidal Side Effects.   These symptoms are similar to those seen in adults. Acute dystonic reactions are associated with the initial phase of treatment while parkinsonian side effects emerge after 3 or more weeks of treatment and include coarse tremor, salivation, akinesia, and rigidity. The symptoms are rare in young children but more common in the older child and adolescent.

To alleviate the acute dystonic reactions of the antipsychotics, diphenhydramine, an antihistamine with anticholinergic properties, is used in 25 mg oral or injectable doses. For the treatment of parkinsonian symptoms, dosage reduction of the antipsychotic is preferred to the addition of an anticholinergic agent because the anticholinergic can cause cognitive dulling and worsening of psychotic disorganization.[20]

LITHIUM

Indications

There is increasing use of lithium in young people for various disorders. The FDA indication for lithium in children is for the treatment of mania and maintenance therapy in bipolar disorder patients with a history of mania among children 12 years and older. Despite the increasing usage, the effectiveness of lithium is based on clinical experience rather than on rigorously designed studies in homogeneous, well-defined diagnostic groups with adequate sample size. Consequently, clinical experience has been reported as case reports and small trials in a variety of treatment-resistant disorders. The thrust of the reports concerning nearly 300 patients up to 1980 according to Jefferson[21] is toward a role for lithium in the treatment of some behaviorally disturbed children and adolescents. There is evidence that lithium is effective in some children and adolescents with a diagnosis of bipolar disorder, manic phase.[22] There is only 1 controlled study of lithium's effectiveness in conduct disorder, aggressive type.[23] There are anecdotal reports that lithium is beneficial in the treatment of mental retardation associated with a profile of explosiveness and aggressiveness directed against self or others.[24] These limited reports consist of case reports and open, unblinded studies which lack sufficient rigor in their design to permit generalizing from their findings. The circumstances of an individual treatment-resistant case must justify the use of lithium in children and adolescents who fail DSM-III-R criteria for bipolar disorder.

Factors which influence lithium's absorption, distribution, metabolism and elimination can produce changes in its therapeutic index and produce toxicity. As with adults, young patients require careful medical evaluation at baseline; this includes complete blood count (CBC) and differential counts, as well as thyroid and kidney function studies. Laboratory tests should be repeated at regular intervals. Initially a monthly review of lab values is suggested and when drug therapy is stabilized, semi-annually, when dosage is changed or when a change in physiological status is likely to alter the lithium clearance. Table 7.3 provides dosing information on lithium.

Side Effect Monitoring

Adequate fluid and electrolyte balance are influenced by diet, physical activity, and environmental temperature and must be considered in the overall monitoring of lithium. Growth changes, school sports activities and patient-initiated diet or exercise programs may dramatically alter the plasma lithium levels and lithium intoxication may result. Education of the patient and long-term monitoring may reduce some of these problems. Fine tremor, thirst, frequent urination, and

TABLE 7.3. Lithium, antidepressant and stimulant drug dosing information for children and adolescents.[a]

| | Age Range (Years): | | | |
| Class | 3–6 | 7–12 | 13–18 | Plasma Level |
		Daily Oral Dose (mg)		
Lithium Carbonate	—	600–2100	600–2100	0.5–1.2 mEq/l
Antidepressants				
Imipramine	—	25–75	25–75	(150–220 ng/ml Total: IMIP + DESIP)
Desipramine	—	25–125	25–150	
Nortriptyline	—	50–100	50–125	80–120 ng/ml
Clomipramine[b]	—		25–100[c]	—
Stimulants				
Dextro- amphetamine	—	5–40	5–40	
Methylphenidate[b]	—	20–60	20–60	
Pemoline[b]		18.75–112.5	18.75–112.5	

[a] Dosing in children should begin at the lower extreme of the suggested dose ranges and be gradually increased after clinical response is observed at a time interval reasonable to achieve steady state, i.e., approximately 5 times the average half-life of the drug.
[b] Suggested dosing by weight:
Methylphenidate 0.3–1.0 mg/kg/day
Pemoline 2.25 mg/kg/day (mean)
Clomipramine 3 mg/kg/day (maximum)
[c] Children and adolescents 10–17 years: initiate at 25 mg per day and slowly titrate up to 100 mg per day or 3 mg/kg/day, whichever is smaller; for those older than 17, dosage may be increased to 250 mg per day or 3 mg/kg/day.

reduced thyroid function are also reported. Lithium intoxication typically includes dysarthria (slurred speech), ataxia (motor incoordination), and visual disturbances.

Plasma Level Monitoring

Plasma level monitoring of lithium in young patients is similar to adult procedures (p. 69) and should be carried out every week during dose adjustments. Thereafter, plasma levels should be checked monthly until dosing is stabilized. On theoretical grounds, the higher renal function and excretion rates of young people might be expected to require higher doses to produce equivalent therapeutic serum levels[16] but there is little empirical support for differing dose-level ratios. Therapeutic levels between 0.5 and 1.2 mEq/l have been suggested in patients aged 13–18 years.[25] These levels are often achieved with doses between 600 and 1200 mg per day.

ANTIDEPRESSANTS

Childhood disorders treated with antidepressants include major depressive disorder, ADHD, separation anxiety disorders and enuresis. Similar to the psychotic disorders, there is much less systematic study of the efficacy of drugs for childhood affective disorders than in adults. This section will be divided into the 2 major drug classes commonly used in children and adolescents: tricyclic antidepressants for the treatment of depression, obsessive-compulsive disorder (OCD), ADHD, and enuresis, and monoamine oxidase (MAO) inhibitors for depression. Table 7.3 includes dosing information for the recommended agents.

Tricyclic Antidepressants

The tricyclic agents have been used in a variety of clinical syndromes involving children and adolescents, including enuresis, the treatment of school phobia, behavioral disorders that fail to respond to stimulants as well as major affective disorders. The range suggests a lack of specificity of effects and further rigorous clinical trial data is needed to establish efficacy for the lesser indications. A 5-week randomized, double-blind, controlled clinical trial of imipramine in 38 depressed children showed a *greater* placebo response.[26] This finding was attributed to dosage below an effective plasma level (150 ng/ml, total imipramine and desipramine). To correct for inadequate drug dosing, the adolescent depression study of Ryan et al.[27] used an imipramine dose titration to 5 mg/kg/day. But even at these doses, neither linear nor curvilinear relationships between total plasma levels (imipramine plus desimipramine) and clinical response were observed. Nevertheless, in individual patients favorable response may be obtained. Imipramine is recommended when psychosocial intervention alone fails.

The FDA has recommended that the dosage of imipramine in children under 12 not exceed 5 mg/kg/day due to the cardiotoxic effects. Baseline EKG patterns should be obtained before treatment is initiated and at every dose increment for those children whose dosages approximate 3.5 to 5 mg/kg/day. During the course of imipramine therapy, an EKG should be repeated monthly when the daily dose is 3.5 mg/kg/day or greater.

Nortriptyline, the secondary amine metabolite of amitriptyline, enjoys extensive use in adolescents although no controlled studies are available to support greater efficacy or fewer side effects.[28] However, the drug's usefulness may stem from the more effective clinical monitoring that is available by routine plasma levels. Possibly, the smaller absolute daily dose may be more appealing to the patient and improve compliance.

Plasma Level Monitoring

Plasma level monitoring is recommended for imipramine and nortriptyline. In monitoring children receiving imipramine, the ratio of imipramine to its secondary amine metabolite, desipramine, is reported to be greater in children than adults.[26] Practically speaking, however, the total level is used to assess the therapeutic level which is often quoted as being in the range of 180 to 220 ng/ml. There is wide interpatient variability in children reflected by the study of Weller et al.[29] in which there was a sixfold variation in steady state levels of imipramine for a fixed dose of 75 mg per day. Therefore, the utility of plasma level monitoring is within the individual patient and must always be considered in relation to clinical symptom change. Plasma level data help to rule out noncompliance or absorption problems and can pinpoint pharmacodynamic changes within the individual. Preskorn[30] has reported CNS toxicity in child patients with total imipramine plus desipramine levels greater than 250 ng/ml.

Side Effect Monitoring

The side effects of the tricyclic antidepressants include cardiotoxicity, seizure threshold-lowering, anticholinergic, and behavioral effects. These are similar to the effects observed in adults and they are generally considered dose-related. Cardiotoxicity with imipramine consists of increased heart rate and widening of the PR interval. Abrupt[31] and gradual[32] cessation of imipramine in children have been reported to produce withdrawal symptoms consisting of severe nausea, vomiting and abdominal cramps, lethargy, irritability, and a range of behavioral symptoms that are difficult to distinguish from symptoms of the illness, such as insomnia and social withdrawal. These effects were reported despite gradual tapering of high dose imipramine over a 3- to 10-day interval. Significantly more symptoms occurred during the tapering than during the treatment of depression in 6 to 12 year olds.[32]

Desipramine and Sudden Death

Since 1987, 3 sudden deaths in Northeast area children treated with desipramine for ADHD have been reported.[33] The deaths occurred after considerable drug exposure—6 months in one instance, 2 years in another, and at therapeutic or subtherapeutic plasma levels. These cases have led to a review of the possible mechanism[34] including direct cardiotoxicity, either with or without detectable pre-existing cardiac conduction defects, due to previously undetected cardiac anomalies, or on the "immature" cardiac conduction system. Until further studies establish the effectiveness to safety ratio for desipramine in the treatment of ADHD, the package insert warning should be observed that desipramine "is *not* recommended in children since safety and effectiveness in the pediatric age group have not been established."

Attention Deficit Hyperactivity Disorder (ADHD)

The effectiveness of desipramine in ADHD was reported in several small, short-term studies. These studies include a 14-day randomized double-blind trial (N = 17) in which desipramine was found to be more effective than placebo (N = 12).[35] In another study, Biederman et al.[36] reported on the efficacy of desipramine at relatively high doses for the treatment of ADD in a double-blind, placebo-controlled trial of 62 patients. The duration of the study was up to 6 weeks. Overall, a relatively small sample of children had been treated with desipramine for these indications. In the comparisons of desipramine to stimulants, the latter being the standard treatment for ADHD, there are serious limitations regarding small sample sizes and lack of comparisons to the standard treatment which preclude recommendation of desipramine for ADHD, particularly, in view of recent evidence of a possible association between sudden death and desipramine use.

Obsessive-Compulsive Disorder

Specific tricyclic agents have been evaluated for specific conditions. For example, clomipramine has been evaluated for obsessive-compulsive disorder (OCD) and found to be effective in two-thirds of a group of 21 children and adolescents (mean age, 14.5 years) after 5 weeks of treatment.[37] The researchers later reported the probable failure of the double-blind procedure as due to the obvious side effects of tricyclic antidepressants[38] and pursued further the question of clomipramine's comparative effectiveness. In this later study, a double-blind crossover comparison of clomipramine and desipramine for OCD involved 21 outpatient children and adolescents (mean age = 13.7 ± 2.9 years). Patients were assigned to successive 5-week trials of the 2 tricyclic antidepressants. The study concluded that there is a "specific antiobsessional effect" for clomipramine, based on the fact that there was a significant decrease in mean Global OCD score for clomipramine compared with desipramine. However, the lack of comparability of 3 mg/kg doses of clomipramine and desipramine was not discussed leaving the study result potentially confounded by dosage differences. The package insert for clomipramine includes efficacy findings for an 8-week study of children and adolescents 10 to 17 years of age and states the maximum dose in this group as 3 mg/kg/day. Usage beyond 10 weeks requires periodic reassessment for effectiveness. Combined studies of medication with behavioral training are discussed in Chapter 4.

Enuresis

After ruling out a physiological basis for enuresis, the treatment of functional enuresis should be behavioral or short-term pharmacologic. Children respond to 25 mg and adolescents to 50 mg of imipramine at bedtime and become dry. The theoretical basis for the action is the cholinergic inhibiting effect on smooth muscle of the bladder to decrease tone and contractility. Controlled studies indicate that bladder control is only maintained as long as the child takes the medication. Tolerance develops when some children wet again by "breaking through" their dosage and will only become dry on increased doses.[39] This tolerance to the anticholinergic bladder effect of a drug with significant other primary pharmacologic effects such as cardiac and sedating effects as well as the potential for secondary effects such as learning and memory deficits, limits the role of antidepressants in enuresis. Aside from the toxicity and tolerance problems of medication, there are reports of successful management with behavioral training methods. For example, the bell-and-pad conditioning method has been shown to be effective when compared with imipramine, amphetamine and random awakening.[40,41]

Psychosocial methods are recommended in preference to pharmacologic treatment for the management of enuresis. In specific instances pharmacologic treatment is indicated and can be very useful.

MAO Inhibitors

There are insufficient efficacy and safety data on the use of MAO inhibitors in depressed children and adolescents to recommend their usage. The dietary problems associated with these drugs, namely the hypertensive "cheese reaction" probably occurs in children and adolescents. Controlling children's diets, particularly snack foods such as pizzas, and worrying that parents inadvertently may administer the wrong medication (central stimulants), may be a difficult and insurmountable problem in assuring safe drug therapy with these agents in outpatient settings.

CENTRAL STIMULANTS AND DISRUPTIVE DISORDERS

Indications

The major central stimulants used for the control of behavioral disorders are methylphenidate, pemoline and dextroamphetamine. These drugs have been found effective in the management of Attention Deficit Hyperactivity Disorder (ADHD) by producing a reduction in motor activity, restlessness, and classroom disruptiveness while increasing the ability to concentrate on academic tasks.[42,43,44] Dosages vary with the drug being used as shown in Table 7.3. Because of the wide interpatient variability in dose response, treatment should be initiated at the low end of the dosage range and titrated to optimal response. Dosing according to body weight has been recommended for methylphenidate with target doses in the range of 0.3 to 0.6 mg/kg/day. Since this dosing mechanism has not been evaluated in a systematic study, the alternative approach of 20 to 60 mg doses in 2 divided doses, is also used.

Long-Acting Formulations

There are several long-acting stimulant preparations, namely, magnesium pemoline and methylphenidate-SR that may be selected when stabilization has occurred and the maintenance phase of treatment begins. These oral long-acting products avoid mid-day dosing during school which causes peer ridicule for many children. Magnesium pemoline should be increased slowly, in weekly increments, from 18.75 to 112 mg per day in the morning.

The long-acting methylphenidate product (SR-20) has been marketed for the past decade. This sustained-release, wax-matrix product has a duration of action of about 8 hours and is available in 20 mg tablets. The tablets should not be chewed or broken to achieve finer dosage adjustment because the enteric coating will be destroyed and the child will receive too large a dose at one time.

Anecdotal evidence suggests that the long-acting products may appear slightly less effective, mg for mg, but are also less likely to show afternoon withdrawal (rebound) effects. Rebound behavioral effects include excitability, talkativeness, overactivity, insomnia, and euphoria.[43]

The long-acting products are more costly and have not yet been evaluated for the risk of decreased stature, insomnia and growth. These concerns have led some experts to prefer standard to long-acting formulations.[44] There are more than 20 reports of the rare occurrence of drug-induced psychosis including hallucinosis and mania associated with both regular and long-acting products.[45]

Side Effect Monitoring

Stimulant side effects are of great concern to parents particularly effects on intellectual, physical, and social development. Growth effects are typically reported in age-adjusted percentiles or in rates of height and weight acquisition. There are studies reporting significant decrements in growth and others suggesting little or no impact on growth. An FDA drug advisory committee concluded that stimulants in the "high dose" range exemplified by 20+ mg/day of methylphenidate are associated with moderate suppression of weight acquisition.[46] Regular charting (every 6 months) of the height and weight in percentiles is recommended to provide long-term data on the growth changes associated with stimulant treatment. Charts for this purpose are illustrated in Part IV.

Drug-induced tics were reported in children receiving stimulants and they were shown to resolve when medication was discontinued and emerge upon rechallenge.[47] Children with family histories of Tourette's disorder or those with their own past histories of tics may show these involuntary movements of the face when treated with methylphenidate and they probably should not receive stimulants. Children who develop facial tics during treatment should be taken off their stimulants and restarted after 2 weeks on another stimulant. Behavioral toxicity, characterized by dysphoria, with signs of an acute agitated depression characterized by anxiety, pacing, hand-wringing, and self-deprecatory statements, has been seen rarely in young children treated with methylphenidate and is a reason for stopping the drug immediately. Discontinuation of methylphenidate can be accomplished quickly because of the relatively short half-life ($t_{1/2}$ = 2.5 hours).

Other Agents

Fenfluramine is a serotonin blocking agent that has been used to treat obesity and as a stimulant in the treatment of autistic children. Initially, there were a number of positive reports, but recent evidence casts doubt on the superiority of fenfluramine over placebo in this population.[48]

ANXIETY DISORDERS AND SYMPTOM-SPECIFIC TREATMENTS

Table 7.4 provides a list of agents occasionally used in the treatment of non-specific symptoms (e.g., anxiety and extrapyramidal side effects, in children and adolescents).

Antianxiety and Hypnotic Agents

Benzodiazepines

No double-blind, controlled studies have been done to demonstrate the efficacy of antianxiety agents such as the benzodiazepines in children with symptoms of anxiety and phobia. Nevertheless, benzodiazepines are used in a wide range of emotional and behavioral disorders, for

TABLE 7.4. Miscellaneous agents' dosing information for children and adolescents.[a]

Antianxiety Agents	Age Range (Years)		
	3–6	7–12	13–18
	Daily Oral Dose (mg)		
Benzodiazepines			
Diazepam	2–5	2–10	2–20
Chlordiazepoxide	—	10–20	20–30
Lorazepam	—	—	—
Oxazepam	—	10–30	30–60
Hypnotics			
Chloral Hydrate	up to 250	250–1000	500–1000
Antihistamines (For Sedative Usage)			
Diphenhydramine	1 mg/kg up to maximum of 50 mg		
Hydroxyzine	up to 50	50–100	50–100
Anticholinergics (For Extrapyramidal Effects of Antipsychotics)			
Diphenhydramine[b]	25–50	25–100	25–100

[a] Dosing in children should begin at the lower extreme of the suggested dose range and be gradually increased after clinical response is observed after a reasonably estimated time interval to permit steady state conditions to be achieved.

[b] Acute dystonic reaction is treated with 25 mg IM injection; repeat once in 24 hours if needed.

short-term relief of situational and anticipatory anxiety (e.g., premedication for dental and surgical procedures),[49] as well as for the control of seizure disorder. For psychiatric usage, chlordiazepoxide and diazepam are the commonly used agents. In reviewing the sparse study findings, there is a generally consistent set of positive findings regarding their use in sleep disorders (insomnia, night terrors (pavor nocturnus) and sleepwalking (somnambulism). There are mixed findings regarding anxiety and behavioral disorders and there are generally negative findings regarding mental retardation with behavioral disorder, depression, enuresis, severe reading retardation, attention deficit hyperactivity disorder (ADHD) and schizophrenia. In schizophrenia, there are reports of a worsening of psychotic symptoms.

Benzodiazepines vary according to the half-life of elimination, a factor which along with their lipophilicity can provide a relative index for selecting agents and choosing an appropriate administration pattern. A relative potency estimate is provided in Table 5.1 of Chapter 5. Compared with adults, the absorption of benzodiazepines in children is faster and peak levels of diazepam are reported to occur within 15 to 30 minutes.[50] Faster absorption and metabolism in children suggest greater tolerance for relatively higher dosages without side effects of drowsiness and ataxia, although the lack of a linear relationship between plasma level and clinical effects of oxazepam and diazepam makes these observations of theoretical rather than practical significance.[51] Similar to their use in adults, the dosing of benzodiazepines should be the lowest effective dosage to minimize side effects, tolerance and the risk of withdrawal effects.

Side Effect Monitoring

The benzodiazepines should be monitored for excess sedation, intoxication, and paradoxical excitation. Intoxication is dose-related and usually produces generalized central depressant effects including mental confusion and ataxia, and can progress to respiratory depression and loss of consciousness.

Paradoxical excitation typically occurs at the start of treatment or following a dose increment. These symptoms include increased psychomotor agitation, increased anxiety, rage episodes, visual hallucinations[52] and insomnia. A more extensive discussion of this problem is located in Chapter 5.

Other Agents

There are no double-blind, controlled studies of the efficacy of diphenhydramine and chloral hydrate in children and adolescents, both of which are prescribed for short intervals when the symptoms of sleep disturbance are severe enough to warrant their short-term usage.

Anticholinergic side effect monitoring is necessary when prescribing diphenhydramine, an aminoalkyl ether type of antihistamine which has substantial atropine-like activity. The drug causes drowsiness in about half of patients exposed to it. Paradoxical excitation is more often reported among children whereas sedation is the most common side effect in adults.

Discontinuation

As with adults, the short-term use of antianxiety and hypnotic agents in children and adolescents necessitates protocols for successful withdrawal of these agents. In general, dosage decrements of 25% at weekly or biweekly intervals at the start and 50% decrements at lower dosages will prevent abrupt withdrawal symptoms. Shorter half-life drugs are reported to produce more dramatic and severe withdrawal symptoms than the longer-acting agents.

Miscellaneous Agents

Various agents have been described for the treatment of rage episodes and violence in young people with mental disorders and as alternatives to stimulants for the patient with facial tics. Several are discussed below because of the need to clarify the limited information available on their usage at this time. The drugs are not recommended except in *rare* instances where the benefits clearly outweigh the risks and where adequate monitoring is assured.

Treatment of Rage and Violence

Propranolol, a beta-adrenergic blocking agent, has been widely used in adults principally as an antihypertensive and cardiac drug and in psychiatric unlabeled usage for many anxiety-associated clinical syndromes such hypertension, migraine, test and performance anxiety as well as for its cardiac antiarrhythmic effect.

In a study of treatment-resistant inpatients, propranolol was reported to control rage in children and adolescents with organic brain dysfunction.[53] This application required special high dosages (600 mg per day in children, 1500 mg per day in adolescents), so dosage adjustment was done in hospital and slowly (10 mg per dose adjustment every 3 days) with frequent vital sign monitoring (blood pressure and pulse). Withdrawal was controlled and slow to avoid rebound hypertension. There is no FDA labeled pediatric indication for this drug below the age of 12. When propranolol is added to an antipsychotic drug regimen it may exert its effect by increasing the plasma level of the antipsychotic.[54] An alternative to the addition of a second drug to alter the plasma level of the primary drug is to follow careful dose-response protocols which may achieve symptom control with a drug that was previously reported to produce a poor response. Expert consultation is recommended when propranolol is considered for addition to a drug regimen to treat rage and violent behaviors.

Propranolol is not indicated when bradycardia, congestive heart failure, cardiac conduction defects, asthma or diabetes are present.

Carbamazepine, an anticonvulsant drug, is receiving some unlabeled adult psychiatric patient usage for the treatment of affective disorders that do not respond to antidepressants and for the treatment of rage episodes and violence. In general, the anticonvulsants have not been proven effective in treating childhood behavioral disorders except for those with positive signs of seizures. Anecdotal evidence suggests that carbamazepine may decrease behavioral problems such as irritability, aggressiveness and hyperactivity, in the absence of seizure disorders as well as associated with psychomotor epilepsy, complex partial seizures and tonic clonic seizures. The FDA labeled indication for the use of carbamazepine in children 6 years or older is limited to those with seizure disorder. There are limited reports of the effectiveness of carbamazepine for the treatment of rapid cycling bipolar disorders, such as those clinical states occasionally observed in the older adolescent manic patient. Standard therapeutic dosing rules for seizure disorder might be adopted in the absence of more specific clinical data related to these newer uses. In the next section, dosage is described in greater detail and should be consulted for side effect monitoring and baseline clinical assessments.

Clonidine, a pre-synaptic alpha$_2$ agonist, has been shown to be effective in adults in the management of hypertension. In psychiatry, there are reports of its use in Tourette's disorder and possibly as an alternative to stimulants in children with facial tics who require treatment for Attention Deficit Hyperactivity Disorder.[55] Additional data to support efficacy and safety are needed before it can be recommended.[56] Clonidine requires careful medical management with dose increments of 0.05 mg every 3 days to a total dose of 3 mg. There is no FDA labeled pediatric indication for this drug below the age of 12. Equivocal effectiveness for anxiety disorders and severe side effects have been reported in adults and is discussed in Chapter 5. Based on these findings, there is a very limited role for clonidine for psychiatric usage.

SEIZURE DISORDER MANAGEMENT ALONE AND IN COMBINATION WITH PSYCHOTROPIC AGENTS

General Considerations

General principles for managing anticonvulsants in children are similar to adults. Factors that affect the drug choice and dose include: age, weight, severity of seizure disorder, presence of CNS dysfunction, and physiological factors that influence pharmacodynamics such gastrointestinal, hepatic and renal function. The anticonvulsants listed in Table 7.5 are frequently used in children and adolescents. Monotherapy is

TABLE 7.5. Frequently used anticonvulsants and their dosing for children and adolescents.[a]

Drug Name	$t_{1/2}$	Average Child Oral Dose Range[b] (mg/kg/day)	Usual Plasma Range (mcg/ml)
Carbamazepine	12 ± 6	10–30	8–12 alone
			4–8 multi-drug
Ethosuximide	30 ± 6	20–40	40–100
Phenytoin	24 ± 12	3–8	10–20
Phenobarbital (Pb)	96 ± 12	3–8	20–40
Primidone	12 ± 6	10–25	5–15
	96 ± 12(Pb)		20–40(Pb)
Valproic Acid	10 ± 6	20–60[c]	50–100

[a] Dosing information is taken from *The Epilepsy Handbook,* RJ Gumnit, Raven Press, New York 1983.
[b] Dosing should be regulated through the relationship between plasma level, seizure frequency and side effects in the individual patient.
[c] Divided dosage is recommended especially as the total dosage increases.

suggested to permit systematic monitoring of dose, plasma levels, seizure frequency and side effects. The use of more than one anticonvulsant agent or the combination of anticonvulsants and antipsychotics makes this monitoring more complicated and dose-level-side effect correlations may be unpredictable. Phenytoin and phenobarbital are the agents longest in use and consequently, they are frequently found in the drug regimens of patients hospitalized at public psychiatric facilities. Nevertheless, the barbiturates are no longer recommended as first choice agents because of behavioral toxicity in this population.

Phenytoin

Phenytoin in doses of 3 to 8 mg/kg/day is used to produce a therapeutic response in the plasma range of 10 to 20 ng/ml. Because of non-linear kinetics, a narrow range between the dose for effective seizure control and the dose that produces toxicity is expected. Dose-related side effects which may progress to frank toxicity consist of diplopia, ataxia, mental confusion, and nystagmus. Monitoring for these effects along with plasma level data is essential to guide decisions for optimal dosage. Long-term effects of phenytoin include gingival hyperplasia, a problem requiring adequate dental hygiene. Other effects include hirsutism, acromegaly, and folate deficiency. The latter problem is corrected by a daily folic acid supplement.

Barbiturates

Recent trends in clinical practice suggest avoiding the use of barbiturates in young people because of behavioral toxicity as well as the availability of alternative agents.[57] Specifically, children demonstrate hyperactivity, personality changes such as irritability and learning difficulties related to long-term exposure to barbiturates. Primidone, a chemical analogue of phenobarbital, may produce similar effects. Phenytoin, carbamazepine, and the benzodiazepines are suitable alternatives.

Carbamazepine

When the patient has not had adequate seizure control with phenytoin, a trial of carbamazepine may be indicated if appropriate hematologic monitoring is feasible. Doses of 10 to 30 mg/kg/day are used to achieve plasma levels in the range of 4 to 12 ng/ml when used alone and 4 to 8 ng/ml when combined with an agent known to increase the plasma binding of carbamazepine. While these are generally accepted therapeutic plasma level ranges, there is insufficient systematic data in large populations to validate them. Consequently, seizure control and side effects should guide dosing.

Pretreatment laboratory assessment of children and adolescents who will be given carbamazepine includes CBC (with platelet and reticulocyte counts and serum iron level). Close monitoring of white cells counts less than 4000/mm is needed and consultation with a hematologist is recommended. General adult guidelines suggest that decreased white cell counts less than 2500/mm or neutrophil counts less than 1500/mm require discontinuation. The major side effects of concern are leukopenia, aplastic anemia, agranulocytosis, and thrombocytopenia. Patients and their primary caregivers should be made aware of the early toxic signs and symptoms of a potential hematologic problem, such as fever, sore throat, ulcers in the mouth, easy bruising, petechial or purpuric hemorrhage, and should be advised to discontinue the drug and immediately report the effects.

Psychotropic and Anticonvulsant Medication Combinations

Combinations of agents which cross the blood brain barrier and produce generalized central depressant effects include most of the psychotropic and anticonvulsant classes. Additive central depressant effects are typically observed such as sedation and mental confusion, and may lead to falling episodes and impaired motor performance.

Kutt and McDowell[58] reported rare cases of reduced phenytoin metabolism produced by the addition of chlorpromazine to the drug regimen so that phenytoin intoxication resulted from the addition of the antipsychotic agent. Monitoring for additive depressant effects or diminished clinical effect is necessary when adding a psychotropic to an anticonvulsant.

On the other hand, when adding anticonvulsants to psychotropic regimens one must be alert to the possibility that phenytoin or phenobarbital would lower the plasma level of psychotropics such as chlorpromazine, haloperidol, nortriptyline or diazepam, by enzyme induction. This effect could result in a loss of effectiveness in a clinically stabilized psychiatric patient. However, there are few empirical data to support this interaction and longitudinal monitoring of dose/level and response would help to elucidate this issue.

REFERENCES

1. Simeon J: Pediatric psychopharmacology outside the USA. Dis Nerv Sys 1974; 35:7(Sec 2) 37–47

2. Campbell M, Green WH, Deutsch SI: Child and Adolescent Psychopharmacology. Beverly Hills, Sage Publications, 1985

3. Gittelman-Klein R: Pharmacotherapy of childhood hyperactivity: an update, in Psychopharmacology, The Third Generation of Progress. Edited by Meltzer HY, New York, Raven Press, 1987

4. Gittelman-Klein R, Klein DF, Katz S, Saraf K, Pollack E: Comparative effects of methylphenidate and thioridazine in hyperkinetic children. I. Clinical results. Arch Gen Psychiatry 1976; 33:1217–1231

5. Werry JS and Aman, MG: Methylphenidate and haloperidol in children. Effects on attention, memory and activity. Arch Gen Psychiatry 1975; 32:790–795

6. Campbell M, Adams P, Perry R, Spencer EK, Overall JE: Tardive and withdrawal dyskinesia in autistic children: a prospective study. Psychopharm Bull 1988; 24:251–255

7. Zito JM, Craig TJ, Wanderling, JA: Pharmacoepidemiology of 330 child and adolescent psychiatric patients. In press, J of Pharmacoepidemiology 1993; 3–4

8. Tarjan G, Lowery VE, Wright SW: Use of chlorpromazine in 278 mentally deficient patients. Am Med Archives of Diseases of Children 1957; 94:294–300

9. Gardos G, Cole JO: Weight reduction in schizophrenics by molindone. Am J Psychiatry 1977; 134:302–304

10. Campbell M, Fish B, Shapiro T, Floyd A, Jr: Study of molindone in disturbed preschool children. Current Therapeutic Research 1971; 13:28–33

11. Baldessarini RJ: Antipsychotics in Chemotherapy in Psychiatry: Principles and Practice. 2nd ed. Cambridge, Harvard U Press, 1985

12. Naruse H, Nagahata M, Nakane Y, Shirahashi K, Takesada M, Yamazaki K: A multi-center double-blind trial of pimozide (Orap), haloperidol and placebo in children with behavioral disorders, using crossover design. Acta Paedopsychiatrica 1982; 48:173–184

13. Campbell M, Grega DM, Green WH, Bennett WG: Neuroleptic-induced dyskinesias in children. Clinical Neuropharmacology 1983; 6:207–222

14. Kane JM, Smith JM: Tardive dyskinesia, prevalence and risk factors, 1959–1979. Arch Gen Psychiatry 1982; 39:473–481

15. Gualtieri CT, Quade D, Hicks RE, Mayo JP, Schroeder SR: Tardive dyskinesia and other clinical consequences of neuroleptic treatment in children and adolescents. Am J Psychiatry 1984; 141:20–23

16. Gualtieri CT, Golden R, Evans RW, Hicks RE: Blood level measurement of psychoactive drugs in pediatric psychiatry. Therapeutic Drug Monitoring 1984; 6:127–141

17. Anderson LT, Campbell M, Grega DM, Perry R, Small AM, Green WH: Haloperidol in the treatment of infantile autism: effects on learning and behavioral symptoms. Am J Psychiatry 1984; 141:1195–1202

18. Mikkelsen EJ, Detlor J, Cohen DJ: School avoidance and social phobia triggered by haloperidol in patients with Tourette's disorder. Am J Psychiatry 1981; 138:1572–1576

19. Green WH, Campbell M, Wolsky BB: Effects of short and long term haloperidol administration on growth in young autistic children, reported in Campbell M, Green WH, Deutsch SI, Child and Adolescent Psychopharmacology ibid, p. 63

20. Campbell M, Green WH, Deutsch SI: ibid p. 62

21. Jefferson JW: The use of lithium in childhood and adolescence: an overview. J Clin Psychiatry 1982; 43:174–177

22. DeLong GR: Lithium carbonate treatment of select behavior disorders in children suggesting manic-depressive illness. J Pediatrics 1978; 93: 689–694

23. Campbell M, Small AM, Green WH, Jennings SJ, Perry R, Bennett WG, Anderson L: Behavioral efficacy of haloperidol and lithium carbonate. A

comparison in hospitalized aggressive children with conduct disorder. Arch Gen Psychiatry 1984; 41:650–656

24. Goetzl U, Grunberg F, Berkowitz B: Lithium carbonate in the management of hyperactive aggressive behavior of the mentally retarded. Comprehensive Psychiatry 1977; 18:599–606

25. Campbell M, Perry R, Green WH: Use of lithium carbonate in children and adolescents. Psychosomatics 1984; 25:95–101, 105–6

26. Petti TA, Law W: Imipramine treatment of depressed children: a double-blind pilot study. J Clin Psychopharmacology 1982; 2:107–110

27. Ryan ND, Puig-Antich J, Cooper TB, Rabinovich H, Ambrosini P, Davies M, King J, Torres D, Fried J: Imipramine in adolescent major depression: plasma level and clinical response. Acta Psychiatr Scand 1986; 73:275–288

28. Geller B, Perel JM, Knitter EF, Lycaki H, Farooki ZQ: Nortriptyline in major depressive disorder in children: response, steady-state plasma levels, predictive kinetics, and pharmacokinetics. Psychopharm Bull 1983; 19:62–65

29. Weller EB, Weller RA, Preskorn SH, Glotzbach R: Steady-state plasma imipramine levels in prepubertal depressed children. Am J Psychiatry 1982; 139:506–508

30. Preskorn S, Weller E, Jerkovich G, Hughes CW, Weller R: Depression in children: concentration-dependent CNS toxicity of tricyclic antidepressants. Psychopharmacology Bulletin 1988; 24:140–142

31. Petti TA, Law W: Abrupt cessation of high-dose imipramine treatment in children. JAMA 1981; 246:768–769

32. Law W, Petti TA, Kazdin AE: Withdrawal symptoms after graduated cessation of imipramine in children. Am J Psychiatry 1981; 138:647–650

33. Anonymous: Sudden death in children treated with a tricyclic antidepressant. Medical Letter on Drugs and Therapeutics 1990; 32:53

34. Riddle MA, Nelson CJ, Kleinman CS, Rasmusson A, Leckman JF, King RA, Cohen DJ: Sudden death in children receiving Norpramin: a review of three reported cases and commentary. J Am Acad Child Adolesc Psychiatry 1991; 30:104–108

35. Donnelly M, Zametkin AJ, Rapoport JL, Ismond DR, Weingartner H, Lane E, Oliver J, Linnoila M, Potter WZ: Treatment of childhood hyperactivity with desipramine: plasma drug concentration, cardiovascular effects, plasma and urinary catecholamine levels, and clinical response. Clin Pharmacol Therapeutics 1986; 39:72–81

36. Biederman J, Baldessarini, RJ, Wright, V, Knee D, Harmatz JS: A double-blind placebo controlled study of despiramine in the treatment of ADD: I. Efficacy. J Am Acad Child Adolesc Psychiatry 1989; 28:777–784

37. Flament MF, Rapoport JL, Berg CJ, Sceery W, Kilts C, Mellström B, Linnoila, M: Clomipramine treatment of childhood obsessive-compulsive disorder. A double-blind controlled study. Arch Gen Psychiatry 1985; 42:977–983

38. Leonard HL, Swedo SE, Lenane MC, Rettew DC, Cheslow, DL, Hamburger SD, Rapoport JL: A double-blind desipramine substitution during long-term clomipramine treatment in children and adolescents with obsessive-compulsive disorder. Arch Gen Psychiatry 1991; 48: 922–927

39. Popper CW: Child and adolescent psychopharmacology, in Psychiatry. Edited by Cavenar JO, Philadelphia, JB Lippincott Co, 1985

40. McConaghy N: A controlled trial of imipramine, amphetamine, pad-and-bell conditioning and random awakening in the treatment of nocturnal enuresis. Med J Australia 1969; 2:237–239

41. Rapoport JL, Mikkelsen EJ, Zavadil A, Nee L, Gruenau C, Mendelson W, Gillin JC: Childhood enuresis, II. Psychopathology, tricyclic concentration in plasma, and antienuretic effect. Arch Gen Psychiatry 1980; 37: 1146–1152

42. Conners CK, Taylor E, Meo G, Kurtz MA, Fournier M: Magnesium pemoline and dextroamphetamine: a controlled study in children with minimal brain dysfunction. Psychopharmacologia 1972; 26:321–336

43. Rapoport JL, Buchsbaum MS, Weingarnter H, Zahn TP, Ludlow C, Mikkelsen EJ: Dextroamphetamine. Its cognitive and behavioral effects in normal and hyperactive boys and normal men. Arch Gen Psychiatry 37:933–943

44. Anonymous: Methylphenidate revisited. Medical Letter, 1988: 30:51–52

45. Bloom AS, Russell LJ, Weisskofp B, Blackerby JL: Methylphenidate-induced delusional disorder in a child with attention deficit disorder with hyperactivity. J Am Acad Child Adolesc Psychiatry 1988; 27:88–89

46. Roche AF, Lipman RA, Overall JE, Hung W: The effects of stimulant medication on the growth of hyperkinetic children. Pediatrics 1979; 63: 847–850

47. Denckla MB, Benporad JR, MacKay MC: Tics following methylphenidate administration. A report of 20 cases. JAMA 1976; 235:1349–51

48. Campbell M, Adams P, Small AM, Curren EL, Overall JE, Anderson LT, Lynch N, Perry R: Efficacy and safety of fenfluramine in autistic children. J Amer Acad Child Adolesc Psychiatry 1988; 27:434–439

49. Pfefferbaum B, Overall JE, Boren HA, Frankel LS, Sullivan MP, Johnson K: Alprazolam in the treatment of anticipatory and acute situational anxiety in children with cancer. J Amer Acad Child Adolesc Psychiatry 1987; 26:532–535

50. Baldessarini RJ: Drugs and the treatment of psychiatric disorders, in Goodman and Gilman's Pharmacological Basis of Therapeutics, 8th ed. Edited by Gilman AG, Rall TW, Nies AS, Taylor P. New York, Pergamon Press, 1986, p. 425

51. Kanto J, Iisalo EU, Hovi-Viander M, Kangas L: A comparative study on the clinical effects of oxazepam and diazepam. Relationship between plasma level and effect. Intl J Clin Pharmacol Biopharmacy 1979; 17:26–31

52. Pfefferbaum B, Butler PM, Mullins D, Copeland DR: Two cases of benzodiazepine toxicity in children. J Clin Psychiatry 1987; 48:450–452

53. Williams DT, Mehl R, Yudofsky S, Adams D, Roseman B: The effect of propranolol on uncontrolled rage outbursts in children and adolescents with organic brain dysfunction. J Am Acad Child Adolesc Psychiatry 1982; 21:129–135

54. Peet M, Middlemiss DN, Yates RA: Propranolol in schizophrenia II. Clinical and biochemical aspects of combining propranolol with chlorpromazine. Brit J Psychiatry 1981; 138:112–117

55. Cohen DJ, Leckman JF, Shaywitz BA: The Tourette syndrome and other tics, in The Clinical Guide to Child Psychiatry. Edited by Shaffer D, Eberhardt AA, Greenhill LL, New York, Free Press, 1985, pp. 3–28

56. Campbell M, Spencer EK: Psychopharmacology in child and adolescent psychiatry: a review of the past five years. J Am Acad Child Adolesc Psychiatry 1988; 27:269–279

57. Conners CK: Psychopharmacologic treatment of children in Clinical Handbook of Psychopharmacology. Edited by DiMascio A, Shader RI, New York, Science House, 1970

58. Kutt H, McDowell F: Management of epilepsy with diphenylhydantoin sodium. Dosage regulation for problem patients. JAMA 1968; 203:969–972

PART II

Monitoring the Use of Psychotherapeutic Agents

CLINICAL PRINCIPLES

1. Individualization of dosage is the standard for psychotherapeutic agents and the lowest effective dose is the goal of treatment. Thus, no low dose exception guidelines are found in this book.

2. Wherever plasma level monitoring is feasible (see individual drug sections) it should be used as a means of longitudinal evaluation of improvement in target symptoms within the individual patient. Plasma levels should not be changed unless there is dissatisfaction with symptom control. Often, therapeutic levels must be defined in terms of the individual patient's response to treatment.

3. Side effect monitoring should be performed in a systematic way for the most frequently occurring side effects. Common side effects are listed in individual drug sections of the manual. Patients' side effects and their severity should be regularly documented in the medical record along with their response on target symptoms. This review of symptoms and side effects should occur whenever a change in medication is ordered or else (at least) monthly.

4. Elderly patients are treated with one-half to one-third of adult starting doses. Intervals between increases in dosage are usually longer than for adults so that steady-state pharmacokinetics can be achieved.

5. The use of polypharmacy should be avoided. Polypharmacy is defined as the use of more than one psychotherapeutic agent in clinical situations where there is no advantage to the combination. However, the risk of adverse reactions and side effects is increased.

6. Antianxiety agents should not be prescribed continuously for more than one month. Dosage reductions and withdrawal following careful protocols should then be attempted. Only in rare instances when alternative methods have been documented as unsuccessful, should there be more than four months of continuous antianxiety treatment.

7. Once-a-day dosing of antipsychotic agents is recommended when the dose is stabilized. The dose should be given in the evening to gain the advantage of sedation at bedtime.

8. Liquid medications should be reserved for the patient who is unreliable in adhering to prescribed medication orders. The excess cost and time to administer these products is not otherwise justified.

9. Oral sustained-release antipsychotic products should not be used because of unnecessary costs and no therapeutic advantage.

10. Fixed-dose combinations are not recommended because the individual components cannot be independently titrated to optimal dose.

11. Antiparkinsonian drug use should not be initiated at the start of an antipsychotic unless the clinical situation warrants it. The criteria are discussed in Chapter 2.

12. Medications should be ordered by generic name. Clarifications can be made by consulting Part III which lists the OMH formulary alphabetically by generic name. Pharmacy personnel can further clarify any questions.

13. Nonformulary items require a medical request on an approved form with an explanation of the rationale for the request. These requests will be reviewed, summarized and discussed at regular intervals by the Pharmacy and Therapeutics Committee and ultimately by the clinical director.

14. Quarterly tardive dyskinesia rating of all patients receiving antipsychotic agents is required.

15. Annual physical examination including SMAC-20 and CBC values are the *minimum* OMH standards. The more complex the individual patient's drug regimen, the more important it is to document the patient's continuing ability to absorb, distribute, metabolize and excrete medications.

16. Explanatory progress notes should accompany all changes in drug therapy, including dosage changes.

17. Occasional use of antipsychotic PRN doses is indicated early in acute management, or to stabilize the patient later in treatment at a new, lower dose or when initiating decanoate therapy. Beyond these needs, routine PRN dosing suggests that the patient has not yet been stabilized at clinically effective dosage levels and calls for re-evaluation of the drug therapy.

18. Long-acting injectable fluphenazine antipsychotic preparations are not indicated for control of acute psychosis. They should

never be used more frequently than weekly because there is no current rationale for such usage. Dosing of haloperidol decanoate more frequently than monthly defeats the goal of the products' suggested regimen and unnecessarily complicates treatment. When these dosing intervals fail to control symptoms adequately, a review of drug therapy by an experienced psychopharmacologist is indicated.

IMPLEMENTATION OF A CLINICAL DRUG REVIEW PROCESS

The Prospective Monitoring System

During 1989, a prospective monitoring system involving computerized drug entry was implemented throughout OMH facilities. This system replaced the older retrospective review system. Figure II.1 illustrates the review process which consists of both routine facility-specific review and system-wide clinical review.

Standards for Establishing a Clinical Drug Review Process

Each facility shall establish a drug monitoring process and drug monitoring committee. *All* medication orders written for inpatients and outpatients of the facility shall be subject to the drug use evaluation process—random samples shall not be used. The exception reports will list the Severity Level 1 and 2 exceptions for a quarterly period by facility.

At the time a prescription is written, it shall be immediately reviewed for compliance with OMH prescribing guidelines. Drug orders that are not outside of OMH guidelines shall be immediately dispensed for patient use.

Severity Level 1 exceptions will not be dispensed. These exceptions represent either *imminent danger* to the patient or potentially severe reactions which will be dispensed in *exceptional* situations. These situations include IRB approved clinical studies and specific patient studies (e.g., N-of-1 studies) which have been developed with the assistance of the clinical director and outside psychopharmacology consultation. For example, if meperidine injection was ordered for a patient receiving an MAO inhibitor.

Severity Level 2 exceptions require intensive monitoring. They are of sufficient clinical concern to warrant a telephone call to the

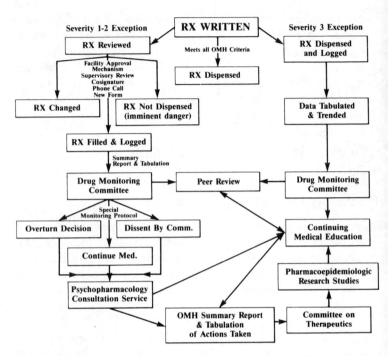

Figure II.1. Overview of prospective drug monitoring for OMH facilities.

prescriber who will seek clinical supervisory approval before proceeding. For example, when a drug for an unlabeled indication is requested. These situations include propranolol for the treatment of rage and violent behavior that has responded poorly to antipsychotic treatment. All prescriptions for propranolol should be closely monitored in order to evaluate appropriate usage of this drug. Similarly, in rare situations such as the use of medroxyprogesterone for sexual aggression, specific criteria for monitoring clinical response and side effects is needed. Written patient consent is also suggested.

Severity Level 2 exceptions may be resolved expeditiously by having the accountable supervisory individuals give verbal and then written consent. In this way, clear and accountable clinical command will facilitate good psychopharmacologic practice. A log of Severity Level 2 exceptions will be maintained and the consequent actions for each will be noted. Regular review by the Drug Monitoring Committee will be undertaken.

Severity Level 3 exceptions are of importance in regard to optimal drug regimens and dosage. These are combinations that have some published evidence of adverse events in clinical situations. There may be additional supportive animal and *in vitro* work. However, there is insufficient evidence of serious sequelae or there is only evidence of serious sequelae in rare instances which as yet do not appear to generalize to other clinical situations.

To monitor Severity Level 3 orders, the pharmacy will summarize the orders in exception and send a monthly summary of these exceptions to the Drug Monitoring Committee. The exceptions shall be tabulated and trends by type of exception, ward or physician shall be indicated for the Drug Monitoring Committee's consideration.

A listing of the criteria by severity level and subgrouped by drug class is presented in Table II.1 (pp. 248–58). Combinations are presented first with the drug classes listed in the following order: (A) Antipsychotics; (B) Lithium; (C) Antidepressants, tricyclic, and atypical antidepressants; (D) Monoamine Oxidase Inhibitors; (E) Antianxiety Agents and Hypnotics; (F) Central stimulants; (G) Anticonvulsants; (H) Anticholinergic agents; (I) Polydrug combinations; and (J) NonFDA-approved psychotherapeutic usage. To avoid duplication, the interactions are listed once.

The monitoring of medications for establishing patterns of usage, effectiveness, and safety takes place in three steps: at the facility, Central Office and Committee on Therapeutics levels.

Step 1: Facility-Level Activities

I. Overview of the Process

Reports at the facility level are reviewed by the Drug Monitoring Committee and case reviews are conducted according to the clinical significance of the topic. By reviewing individual or collective exceptional prescribing, prescribers can be made aware of current prescribing practices. The Drug Monitoring Committee may agree with the prescriber's decision, express dissent that the drug regimen reflects current psychopharmacologic practice and the best clinical decision, or overturn the original decision and request that the drug order be discontinued. If the committee allows the treatment it may request a special monitoring protocol such as periodic physical assessment, EKGs, regular drug plasma levels, target symptom response and side effects.

II. The Drug Monitoring Committee

The Drug Monitoring Committee should consist of representatives of the medical staff, such as the director of medical education, the medical director, or head of the clinical staff, senior clinicians with expertise in pharmacotherapy, the director of pharmacy or a clinical pharmacist designee and a representative from program evaluation or quality assurance to assist in record keeping and statistical analysis. Outside consultants from affiliated professional schools are encouraged. The committee should meet at intervals sufficient for their review tasks.

The Functions of the Committee are:

- Reviewing exceptions—The primary function of the Committee is to review exceptions and to resolve them in a way that ensures consensus on the standards of the statewide guidelines as detailed in the Manual.
- Recommending a clinical case review—Clinical case reviews may be appropriate to determine if the patient meets the criteria for a justified exception. The Committee should identify and have access to psychopharmacology consultants comprised of either experienced clinicians from the facility or public psychiatry psychopharmacology consultants outside of OMH. The Drug Monitoring Committee may request a psychopharmacology consultation for any drug exception or unusual therapeutic drug regimen.

  Staff to the Drug Monitoring Committee should summarize and tabulate all actions taken and prepare a quarterly report for the Office of Mental Health. This report includes the total number of Severity Level 1, 2, and 3 exceptions identified and the action taken for each: continued, changed with special monitoring protocols, discontinued, other. This summary report from the Drug Monitoring Committee should also be reported to the facility peer review committee and to the director of continuing medical education.
- Developing inservice education programs—Trends and patterns of exception rates are intended for study at the facility level and

at the statewide level so that appropriate inservice education can be developed.

- Improving the utilization of drug information—The Drug Monitoring Committee should develop methods of using the information that is available from the drug exception reporting system.

Step 2: OMH Statetwide Activities

A summary of annual psychopharmacology exception reporting should be reviewed by the Committee on Therapeutics with recommendations for follow-up actions.

Step 3: Committee on Therapeutics Follow-Up Actions

The follow-up process consists of the following steps:

- Review OMH quarterly reports from facilities for the degree of exception reporting and actions taken by severity level. Recommendation to OMH for clinical pharmacoepidemiologic studies to evaluate the effectiveness and safety of marketed medications in problem areas identified through the statewide clinical drug review process.
- Psychopharmacology consult service recommendations.
- Inclusion of topics for annual OMH continuing medical and health professional education programs.

TABLE II.1. Classification of OMH drug monitoring criteria according to severity level.

SEVERITY LEVEL 1: Potentially Severe—do not dispense; call clinical supervisor for specific review of the case.

Drug Class		Rationale/Follow-Up Action
A. Antipsychotics*		
1. Antipsychotics	+ Levodopa	Acute psychosis; lack of efficacy.
2. Antipsychotics	+ Amphetamine Methylphenidate	Exacerbates psychosis; reserve for research setting.
3. Antipsychotics	+ Epinephrine**	Augmented hypotensive effect; Epi not indicated for tx of orthostatic hypotension; use levophed or phenylepherine.
4. Clozapine	+ Bone marrow suppressants Carbamazepine Sulfonamides Captopril	Additive risk of agranulocytosis and fatality.
5. Clozapine	+ Other Antipsychotics	Multiple antipsychotics lacking efficacy and safety data.
6. Clozapine	+ Tricyclic	To avoid additive anticholinergic activity select ATD low in anticholinergic activity, e.g., doxepin.
7. Clozapine	+ Antiparkinsonian agent	Unnecessary combination with risk of anticholinergic intoxication.
8. Clozapine	+ Benzodiazepines	Severe respiratory depression, arrest and death have been reported. Chloral Hydrate is an alternative for short-term treatment of agitation at the start of clozapine treatment.
B. Lithium Severity Level 1—None		
C. Antidepressants, Tricyclic and Atypical		
1. Tricyclic	+ MAO Inhibitor	Hypertensive crisis (hyperpyrexia, muscle rigidity, convulsions, coma).
2. Tricyclic	+ Clonidine	Antagonistic to clonidine effect.
3. Tricyclic	+ Guanethidine	Antagonistic to guanethidine effect.
4. Fluoxetine	+ MAO Inhibitor	Avoid combined use; 3 fatalities reported. **N.B.** When using these drugs in sequence observe the following time intervals: Wait 2 weeks after discontinuing MAOI before starting Fluoxetine; Wait 5 weeks after discontinuing Fluoxetine before starting MAOI.

* Typical antipsychotics excluding clozapine which is listed separately.
** Epinephrine for emergency treatment of allergic reactions is justified in specific situations.

TABLE II.1. *(Continued)*

Drug Class		Rationale/Follow-Up Action
5. Bupropion	+ L-dopa Amantadine	Bupropion not recommended with agents known to produce *de novo* psychotic symptoms.
D. MAO Inhibitors		
1. See C-1		
2. MAO Inhibitor	+ Meperidine Alfaprodine	Fatal reactions.
3. MAO Inhibitor	+ Levodopa	Hypertensive crisis.
4. MAO Inhibitor	+ Tryptophan	Hypertensive crisis.
5. MAO Inhibitor	+ Amphetamine Methylphenidate	Rare but fatal hypertensive crisis.

6. MAO Inhibitor	+ Antihypertensives,
	e.g.,
	  guanethidine
	  reserpine
	  methyldopa
		Hypertensive crisis with gradual onset.

7. MAO Inhibitor	+ Sympathomimetics,
	e.g.,
	  phenylephrine
	  pseudoephedrine
	  OTC products
		Hypertensive crisis.

E. Antianxiety and Hypnotics Severity Level 1—None		
1. See A-8		
F. Central Stimulants		
1. See A-2		
2. See D-5		
G. Anticonvulsants		
1. Carbamazepine	+ Clozapine	Increased risk of agranulocytosis and fatality.
2. Carbamazepine	+ Hydrazine-type MAO Inhibitor e.g., Phenelzine	Avoid combination; non-hydrazine type MAO Inhibitor e.g., tranyl-cypromine may be an alternative but close plasma level monitoring is needed to avoid carbamazepine intoxication.
H. Antiparkinsonian Agents		
1. See A-7		
I. Miscellaneous		
1. Propranolol Atenolol	+ Clonidine	Severe arterial thrombosis, gangrene; Stop one agent at least 3 days before starting the other.

(Continued)

TABLE II.1. *(Continued)*

Drug Class		Rationale/Follow-Up Action
2. Terfenadine	+ Ketoconazole + Troleandomycin + Erythromycin	Adverse cardiac effects e.g., QT interval prolongation, ventricular tachyarrhythmias were reported at usual doses of each drug. Suspected prolongation of metabolism of terfenadine by anti-infective.

SEVERITY LEVEL 2: Moderate to severe depending on case-specific factors—dispense upon verbal or written authorization of clinical supervisor; review each case.

Drug Class		Rationale/Follow-Up Action
A. Antipsychotics		
1. Antipsychotics	+ Bromocriptine	Dose-dependent nightmares, hallucinations, paranoid delusions.
2. Antipsychotics	+ Bupropion	Insufficient effectiveness data; Not recommended for psychotic depression by manufacturer.
3. Antipsychotic (high dose)		Exceeds maximum dose.
4. See I-1, I-3		
5. Clozapine	+ Antihypertensives e.g., beta-blockers	Monitor for additive hypotensive effects, falls, dizziness.
6. Chlorpromazine or other P-450 liver metabolized psychotropic agent.	+ Cimetidine	Dosage reduction of chlorpromazine was needed after initiation of cimetidine; postulated mechanism is competitive inhibition of P-450 liver enzymes. (Br J Psychiatry 1989; 155:413).
B. Lithium		
1. Lithium	+ Thiazide diuretics Furosemide Spironolactone	Monitor lithium level and reduce dose accordingly to avoid lithium intoxication.
2. Lithium	+ Enalapril	Monitor lithium level and reduce dose accordingly to avoid lithium intoxication.
3. Lithium	+ Iodides e.g., KI	Avoid if possible; Additive hypothyroid effects.
4. Lithium	+ Succinylcholine chloride	In surgical setting: post-surgical apnea. Caution prior to ECT.
5. Lithium	+ Nonsteroidal anti-inflammatory agents e.g., piroxicam indomethacin	Monitor plasma level to prevent lithium intoxication.

TABLE II.1. (Continued)

Drug Class		Rationale/Follow-Up Action
6. Lithium	+ Methyldopa	Acute lithium intoxication has occurred *without* increase in Li level.
7. Lithium	+ Tetracycline	Increased lithium levels by interference with renal function.
8. Lithium	+ Diazepam	Acute intoxication, hypothermia was reported; monitor Li and diazepam levels for acute intoxication if continuous scheduled usage exceeds 4 months.
9. Lithium	+ Amphetamine	No established efficacy or safety data.
10. See below I-3		
11. Lithium	+ Clozapine	Additive CNS depressant effects; no established efficacy or safety.
12. Lithium (high dose)		Exceeds maximum dose and plasma level range.
C. Antidepressants, Tricyclic and Atypical		
1. Tricyclic	+ Digitalis glycosides	Monitor for increased cardiac depression and irritability.
2. Tricyclic	+ Quinidine Procainamide	Monitor for prolonged conduction delays. Avoid combination if possible. Consult with cardiologist.
3. Tricyclic	+ Norepinephrine Phenylephrine	Monitor for potentiated tricyclic cardiac effects.
4. Tricyclic	+ Epinephrine	Monitor for potentiated pressor effect; Arrhythmias.
5. Tricyclic	+ Cimetidine	Dose reduction of TCA may be needed to avoid increased plasma level of tricyclic presumed to be due to competitive inhibition (Baldessarini in Goodman and Gilman 1990, pp 403–405).
6. Tricyclic	+ Carbamazepine	Not recommended without plasma levels and close monitoring for excess stimulation, agitation. Carbamazepine may reduce plasma level of tricyclic by enzyme-induction. Not rigorously evaluated.
7. Tricyclic	+ Amphetamines Methylphenidate	Insufficient evaluation; monitor for hypertension and increased serum level of TCA.

(Continued)

TABLE II.1. *(Continued)*

Drug Class		Rationale/Follow-Up Action
8. Tricyclic	+ Anticoagulant e.g., warfarin	Monitor for increased bleeding.
9. Fluoxetine	+ Tryptophan	Avoid combination: Agitation, restlessness, GI distress has been reported.
10. Fluoxetine	+ Diazepam	Decreased metabolism of diazepam; *special caution* after 3–4 weeks. Monitor for diazepam intoxication.
11. Fluoxetine	+ Anticoagulant e.g., warfarin	Monitor for changes in free-plasma bound ratio of the drug; monitor clotting time.
	+ Digitalis glyscosides	Monitor for digitalis intoxication.
12. See below I-1, I-3		
13. Fluoxetine	+ Clozapine	No established efficacy or safety; use alternative antipsychotic agent.
14. Doxepin	+ Clozapine	Monitor for combined CNS depressant effects.
15. Fluoxetine	+ Haloperidol	Severe EPSE with low dose haloperidol (2–5mg) when fluoxetine was added. Postulated mechanism is inhibition of haloperidol metabolism.
16. TCA; Trazodone	+ Fluoxetine	Significant increase in TCA levels and trazodone response when fluoxetine was added; May be inhibition of TCA/trazodone metabolism; No established efficacy.
17. TCA; Doxepin	+ Oral sulfonylureas Insulin	Increased hypoglycemic effect by the TCA/doxepin; Monitor diabetic patients for changes in blood sugar when starting/stopping or changing dose of antidepressant.
18. Nortriptyline; TCA	+ Dimetapp or other cold preparation	Potentiated adrenergic effect; hypertensive crisis, cardiac arrhythmias. Reduce dose of adrenergic-acting compounds and monitor nortriptyline (TCA) levels.
19. Tricyclic Antidepressant (high dose)		Exceeds maximum dose and level range (if appropriate).

TABLE II.1. *(Continued)*

Drug Class		Rationale/Follow-Up Action
D. MAO Inhibitors		
1. MAO Inhibitor	+ Codeine	Observe for signs of drug intoxication.
2. MAO Inhibitor	+ Insulin	Monitor for hypoglycemia due to decreased metabolism of insulin.
3. MAO Inhibitor (low dose)	+ TCA (low dose)	Special monitoring & expert pharmacologic supervision should be instituted; potential for serious fatal adrs.
4. MAO Inhibitors (high dose)		Exceeds maximum dose.
E. Antianxiety and Hypnotics		
1. See B-8		
2. See C-10		
3. Triazolam	+ Erythromycin Triacetyloleandomycin	The antibiotics inhibit hepatic metabolism of triazolam, increase level and may cause intoxication; monitor for symptoms of increased clinical response or select alternative antibiotic.
4. Diazepam	+ Propranolol Metoprolol	Slight decrease in metabolism of diazepam; monitor for possible intoxication; alternatives are lorazepam, alprazolam.
5. Diazepam	+ Cimetidine	Delayed clearance of diazepam due to cimetidine (NEJM 1980; 302:1012).
6. Buspirone	+ Fluoxetine	Monitor for increased anxiety if fluoxetine is added to buspirone; No established efficacy or safety.
7. Antianxiety or hypnotic (high dose)		Exceeds maximum dose.

(Continued)

TABLE II.1. *(Continued)*

Drug Class	Rationale/Follow-Up Action
F. Central Stimulants	
1. See B-9	
2. See C-7	
3. Methylphenidate + Phenytoin	Plasma levels of anticonvulsants were increased to toxic levels when methylphenidate was added to treat ADHD in children (JAMA 1969; 207:2053–2056).
G. Anticonvulsants	
1. Phenobarbital + Primidone	Additive CNS depressant effects; no clinical rationale in seizure management.

2. Phenytoin   + Isoniazid
   Carbamazepine
   Primidone
	Anticonvulsant toxicity may occur; monitor levels closely.

3. Phenobarbital + Anticoagulant e.g., warfarin	May decrease anticoagulant effect; monitor clotting time.
4. Valproate + Clonazepam	Absence seizures have been reported with the combination.

5. Carbamazepine   + Macrolide Antibi-
       otics: Erythromy-
       cin, Triacetylole-
       andomycin
	Carbamazepine intoxication; switch to alternate antibiotic or close plasma level monitoring of carbamazepine.

6. Carbamazepine + Cimetidine	Reduce carbamazepine dose to avoid intoxication. Monitor for increased carbamazepine levels.
7. Carbamazepine + Propoxyphene	Monitor for increased carbamazepine levels or avoid combination.
8. Phenobarbital + Disopyramide	Metabolic clearance of disopyramide may be increased by the hepatic enzyme stimulation of phenobarbital.
9. Phenytoin + TCA; Trazodone	Monitor for increased phenytoin levels when adding antidepressant.

10. Phenytoin   + Clozapine
    Phenobarbital
    Primidone
	Monitor for additive CNS depressant effects; No established safety; medical clearance needed.

11. Anticonvulsant (high dose)	Exceeds maximum dose (and plasma level if appropriate).

TABLE II.1. *(Continued)*

Drug Class	Rationale/Follow-Up Action
H. Antiparkinsonian Agents	
1. Antiparkinsonian + Tricyclic	Additive anticholinergic effects; dose-dependent; monitor for rationale; if approved, review for continuing rationale and side effects after continuous use beyond one month.
2. Antiparkinsonian (high dose)	Exceeds maximum dose.
I. Polydrug Combinations	
1. Polydrug among *two* agents within the same class excluding anticonvulsants: example: two antipsychotics two antidepressants two benzodiazepines two antiparkinsonians	No established efficacy; risk of additive adverse effects.
2. Polydrug among *three* agents within the anticonvulsant class: example: phenytoin phenobarbital vlaproic acid	Complexity of monitoring; lack of demonstrated efficacy; risk of new seizure types or exacerbation of existing seizures.
3. Polydrug among *three* or more classes: example: antipsychotic + antiparkinson + tricyclic [exclude: antipsychotic + antiparkinson + lithium]	Additive neurotoxic effects; additive risk of adverse effects; no established efficacy.
J. Other Agents for Psychotherapeutic Use with FDA-Unapproved Indication (Prior Written Clinical Justification)	
example: Propranolol: bp, pulse, plasma level of other psychotropic e.g., antipsychotic such as haloperidol	Drug-specific effectiveness and side effect monitoring required for defined time interval e.g., 2 months, after which continuation is based on written evidence of improvement by systematic objective methods. Sample protocol: See Part IV.
Carbamazepine: baseline wbc, reticulocytes, platelets, plasma levels	
Clonidine: bp, pulse, side effects	

(Continued)

TABLE II.1. *(Continued)*

Drug Class		Rationale/Follow-Up Action
K. Miscellaneous		
1. Disulfiram	+ Theophylline	Disulfiram increases theophylline serum levels & may produce theophylline intoxication. Monitor theophylline levels if disulfiram is added/changed.

SEVERITY LEVEL 3: Minimal acute risk; little established efficacy or safety; plasma level, clinical response, side effect monitoring may be indicated; review summary data.

Drug Class		Rationale/Follow-Up Action
A. Antipsychotics		
1. Antipsychotic	+ Amantadine	Drug-induced excitation; exacerbation of psychosis; monitor closely; reserve for cases where anticholinergic agents are contraindicated.
2. Antipsychotic	+ Barbiturates Opiates Narcotic analgesics	Additive CNS effects, e.g., sedation, hypotension.
3. Antipsychotic	+ Gel type antacids containing Al, Mg, Ca salts + Cholestyramine + Kaolin, pectin	Avoid co-administration within 2 hours. Advise nurses and others who administer medication.
4. Antipsychotic	+ Lithium	Antipsychotic above 1000 CPZ-EQ/ day with lithium for greater than one month. See Protocol Part IV.
5. Antipsychotic	+ Phenytoin	Liver enzyme monitoring should occur; seizure threshold may be lowered.
6. Haloperidol	+ Carbamazepine	Monitor for changes in level of either drug.
B. Lithium		
1. Lithium	+ Theophylline	Increased lithium excretion.
2. Lithium	+ Sodium salts	Increased lithium excretion.
3. Lithium	+ Acetazolamide	Lithium effect diminished.
4. Lithium	+ Phenytoin	Increased Li levels to toxic levels can occur.

TABLE II.1. *(Continued)*

Drug Class		Rationale/Follow-Up Action
5. Lithium	+ Alprazolam	Increased Li levels in normal volunteers; monitor plasma lithium closely.
6. Lithium	+ Carbamazepine	Dose-dependent increase in Li level. Monitor both levels and side effects: ataxia, dizziness, confusion, restlessness. Neurotoxicity at normal levels of each. See Protocol Part IV.
7. Lithium	+ Hypnotics Sedatives	Additive CNS depressant effects.

C. Antidepressants, Tricyclic and Atypical

1. Tricyclic	+ Gel type antacids containing Al, Mg, Ca salts + Cholestyramine + Kaolin, pectin	Avoid co-administration within 2 hours.
2. Tricyclic	+ Barbiturates Phenytoin Narcotic analgesics Benzodiazepines	Additive CNS depressant effects; diminished effect of tricyclic; monitor plasma level of TCA for changes; increased risk of suicide.

D. MAO Inhibitors

   Severity Level 3—None

E. Central Stimulants

   Severity Level 3—None

F. Antianxiety and Hypnotics

1. See B-5		
2. Benzodiazepine	+ Phenobarbital Phenytoin	No established efficacy; additive CNS depressant effects. Monitor phenytoin level.
3. See I-3 and I-4		

G. Anticonvulsants

1. Phenobarbital Phenytoin Primione	+ Oral contraceptives	Increased risk of pregnancy; alternative contraceptive method should be employed. Educate patients regarding the issue.
2. See A-5		
3. See B-4		
4. See F-2		

(Continued)

TABLE II.1. *(Continued)*

Drug Class	Rationale/Follow-Up Action
H. Antiparkinsonian Agents	
1. Antiparkinsonian + Diphenhydramine	Additive anticholinergic effects.
I. Diagnosis-Specific Two Class Combinations	
1. Antipsychotic + Antidepressant	Additive anticholinergic, sedative, hypotensive, seizure-lowering potential. Appropriate use is symptom-, drug-, dose-, time interval-, and diagnosis-dependent.
2. Antipsychotic + Lithium	Dose and time-dependent criteria: less than 1000 CPZ-EQ/day of antipsychotic for more than one month.
3. Antipsychotic (low dose) + Benzodiazepine, scheduled	New strategy to reduce overall antipsychotic dose but as yet without sufficient rigorous evaluation.
4. Antipsychotic (low dose) + Benzodiazepine, prn	New strategy to reduce overall antipsychotic dose but as yet without sufficient rigorous evaluation.

PART III

OMH Psychopharmacology Formulary

DRUG PRODUCTS AND RECOMMENDATIONS

This alphabetic listing by generic drug name is provided for the psychotherapeutic agents and other selected agents that are important in drug interactions and drug monitoring. Brand names are listed in parentheses after the generic name. Suggested notes for prescribing and administration are also provided. IM and IV doses are listed as single doses that are generally repeated at 6-hr intervals if needed. Dosage information for adults, elderly, and children and by route of administration is provided. Plasma level data is given where appropriate. Product forms and the common dosage units available are also listed. Controlled substances are indicated by their DEA classification numbers. Footnotes with additional information are on the page where they are first mentioned.

Drug Products	Recommendations	
Aluminum & Magnesium Hydroxide and Simethicone (Mylanta) Antacids Oral suspension Tablet	Take antipsychotic drugs 1 hr. before or 2 hrs. after antacid.	
Alprazolam (Xanax) (C-IV) Antianxiety Agent (Benzodiazepines) Tablet 0.25 mg, 0.5 mg, 1 mg	Adults:	0.75–4 mg
	Elderly:	up to 2 mg
	Children:	Not established
Amantadine Dopamine Agonist Capsule 100 mg Oral liquid 50 mg/5 ml	Adults:	P.O. 100–300 mg
	Elderly:	For Epse: 100–200 mg/day in those for whom anticholinergic agents are contraindicated.
	Children:	Not established
Amitriptyline (Elavil) Antidepressants, Tertiary Amines Tablet 10 mg, 25 mg Injection 10 mg/ml	Adults:	P.O. 50–300 mg I.M. single dose 20–30 mg
	Elderly:	P.O. 25–150 mg I.M. single dose 10–20 mg
Plasma levels: 100–300 ng/ml[a] (Amitriptyline + Nortriptyline)	Children:	P.O. 25–75 mg

(Continued)

[a] Not yet accurately established. APA Task Force Report (1985) determined that additional data are needed before recommending these levels for routine clinical use.

Drug Products		Recommendations
Amobarbital (Amytal) (C-II)		
Antianxiety and Hypnotics	Adults:	PO, IM 65–500 mg
(Benzodiazepines)	Elderly:	Avoid if possible; choose
Capsules 200 mg		nonbarbiturate alternative
Injection 250 mg, 500 mg	Children:	PO, IM 2–6 mg/kg
Amoxapine (Asendin)		
Antidepressants, Secondary Amines	Adults:	PO 150–600 mg
Tablet 50 mg, 100 mg, 150 mg	Elderly:	PO 75–300 mg
	Children:	Not established

WARNING: 1. Amoxapine is chemically related to loxapine, an antipsychotic which is known to produce tardive dyskinesia. 2. Avoid use in patients with a history of seizure disorder.

Amytal (See Amobarbital)

Anafranil (See Clomipramine)

Antabuse (See Disulfiram)

Anectine (See Succinylcholine)

Antilirium (See Physostigmine)

Artane (See Trihexyphenidyl)

Ascendin (See Amoxapine)

Atarax (See Hydroxyzine)

Ativan (See Lorazepam)

Atropine sulfate		
Anticholinergic agents	Adults:	premedication for ECT
Tablets 0.4 mg, 0.6 mg		
Injection 0.4 mg/ml, 0.4 mg/0.5 ml		

Aventyl (See Nortriptyline)

Benztropine (Cogentin)		
Anticholinergics (Antiparkinson)	Adults:	PO 1–8 mg/day
Tablet 1 mg, 2 mg		IM, IV single dose 1–2 mg
Injection 1 mg/ml	Elderly:	PO 1–4 mg/day
		IM, IV 1–3 mg/day
	Acute dystonia:	1–2 mg IM/IV

Brevital (See Methohexital)

Drug Products		Recommendations
Bupropion (Wellbutrin) Antidepressant, Atypical Tablet 75 mg, 100 mg	Adult:	Beginning at 200 mg per day and increasing, after at least 3 days to 300 mg per day; max = 450 mg per day
	Elderly:	200 mg per day
	Children:	Not established
Buspirone[b] (Buspar) Antianxiety Agent (Miscellaneous)	Adults:	PO Usual 15–30 mg Extreme 30–60 mg
	Elderly:	15–30 mg
Carbamazepine (Tegretol) Anticonvulsants Tablet 100 mg, 200 mg	Adults:	400 mg–1600 mg (15 mg/kg/day)
Plasma range: 4–8 mcg/mL (multiple drug regimens) 8–12 mcg/mL (single drug regimen)		Elderly:15 mg/kg/day with the goal of achieving plasma levels of 8–12 (alone) or 4–8 mcg/mL (multi-drug regimen). Dosage should be titrated *slowly* from 100 mg/day with plasma level monitoring. Dosing increments should be weekly unless acute seizure control requires more frequent dosing.
	Children:	200–1000 mg

WARNING: Rare but serious and sometimes fatal abnormalities of blood cells have been reported following treatment with carbamazepine. Pretreatment and frequent follow-up blood counts during the first 3 months of therapy is recommended.

Catapres (See Clonidine)

Centrax (See Prazepam)

Chloral hydrate (Noctec) (C-IV) Antianxiety, Hypnotics (Miscellaneous) Capsule 500 mg Oral solution 500 mg/5 ml	Adults:	PO 500–2000 mg
	Elderly:	PO 500–1000 mg
	Children:	PO 3–6 yrs: up to 250 mg 7–12 yrs: 250–1000 mg 13–18 yrs: 500–1000 mg

(Continued)

[b] Nonformulary status

Drug Products		Recommendations
Chlordiazepoxide (Librium) (C-IV)		
Antianxiety, Hypnotics	Adults:	PO 15–60 (100) mg[c]
(Benzodiazepines)		single IV 50–100 mg
Capsule 5 mg, 10 mg, 25 mg	Elderly:	PO 10–40 mg
Injection 100 mg		single IV 10–50 mg
	Children:	PO, IV 0.5 mg/kg
Chlorpromazine (Thorazine)		
Antipsychotics, Phenothiazines	Adults:	PO 100–2000 mg
(Aliphatic)		single IM 25–50 mg
Tablet 10 mg, 25 mg, 50 mg,	Elderly:	PO up to 300 mg
100 mg, 200 mg		single IM 12.5–25 mg
Oral solution 30 mg/ml,	Children:	3–6 yrs: PO 10–100 mg
100 mg/ml		IM max of 40 mg
		7–12 yrs: PO 25–500 mg
		IM max of 75 mg
		13–18 yrs: PO 25–800 mg
		IM max of 100 mg
Clomipramine (Anafranil)		
Antidepressant, Tricyclic[d]	Adults:	Beginning at 25 mg per day, up to 100 mg per day in the first 2 weeks; after that, up to 250 mg/day.
	Children:	Beginning at 25 mg per day, up to 3 mg/kg/day or 100 mg per day, whichever is smaller, in the first 2 weeks; after that, up to 3 mg/kg/day or 200 mg, whichever is smaller.
Clonazepam (Klonopin) (C-IV)		
Antianxiety, Anticonvulsant[g]	Adults:	PO 1.0–10 mg (20 mg)[f]
(Benzodiazepine)	Elderly:	PO 0.5–10 mg
Tablet 0.5 mg, 1 mg, 2 mg	Children:	0.01–0.2 mg/kg
Plasma range: 40–60 ng/ml[e]		

[c] In exceptional cases, daily doses up to these maximum dosages have been used and require behavioral toxicity monitoring.

[d] Approved for the treatment of obsessive-compulsive disorder.

[e] Not yet accurately established for clinical monitoring purposes.

[f] In exceptional cases, daily doses up to these maximum dosages have been used and require behavioral toxicity monitoring.

[g] FDA approved indication is for anticonvulsant usage.

Drug Products	Recommendations
Clonidine (Catapres) Antihypertensive: alpha$_2$adrenergic agonist Tablet[h] 0.1 mg, 0.2 mg, 0.3 mg	Adults: PO initial: 0.1 twice a day Maintenance: 0.2–0.8 mg/ day in divided doses Elderly: PO Titrate dosage more slowly than in younger adults to prevent toxicity Children: Not established
Clorazepate (Tranxene) (C-IV) Antianxiety and Hypnotics (Benzodiapines) Capsule 3.75 mg, 7.5 mg, 15 mg	Adults: PO 15–90 mg Elderly: PO 7.5–60 mg Children: PO 7.5–60 mg
Clozapine (Clozaril)[i] Antipsychotic, Atypical Tablet 25 mg, 100 mg	Adults: PO up to 900 mg 601–900 = severity level 2 Elderly: not established[j] Children not established
Codeine Phosphate (C-II) Analgesics, Narcotic Injection 15 mg/ml	
Codeine Sulfate (C-II) Analgesics, Narcotic Tablet 15 mg, 30 mg	
Cogentin (See Benztropine)	
Cylert (See Pemoline)	
Dalmane (See Flurazepam)	
Dantrium (See Dantrolene sodium)	
Dantrolene sodium (Dantrium) Skeletal Muscle Relaxants Capsule 25 mg, 50 mg, 100 mg	
Demerol (See Meperidine)	
Depakene (See Valproic acid)	
Depakote (See Divalproex)	

(Continued)

[h] Topical Transdermal system is not recommended for psychiatric usage.
[i] Restricted to severe schizophrenia not responsive to current treatment. Requires patient's consent to weekly WBC counts.
[j] Restricted to special situations until efficacy and safety are established.

Drug Products	Recommendations		

Desipramine (Norpramin)
  Antidepressants,
  Secondary Amines
    Tablet 25 mg, 50 mg
 	
    Plasma range: 100–250 ng/mL
	Adult:
	Elderly:
	Children:
		PO 50–300 mg
		PO 25–150 mg
		7–12 yrs: 25–125 mg
		13–18 yrs: 25–150 mg	

Desyrel (See Trazodone)			
Dexedrine (See Dextro-amphetamine)			

Dextro-amphetamine (Dexedrine) (C-II)
  Cerebral Stimulants
    Tablet 5 mg
	Children:	7–18 yrs: 5–40 mg	

Diazepam (Valium) (C-IV)
  Antianxiety and Hypnotics
  (Benzodiazepines)
    Tablet 2 mg, 5 mg, 10 mg
    Injection 50 mg/ml
 	
    Plasma range: 50–200 ng/ml[c]
	Adult:
	
	Elderly:
	
	Children:
		PO 4–40 mg
		single IV 2–20 mg
		PO 2–20 mg
		single IV 2–10 mg
		3–6 yrs: PO 2–5 mg
		7–12 yrs: PO 2–10 mg
		13–18 yrs: PO 2–20 mg	

Dilantin (See Phenytoin)			

Diphenhydramine (Benadryl)
  Antihistamine
    Capsule 25 mg, 50 mg
    Injection 50 mg/ml
    Oral liquid 12.5 mg/ml
	Adult:
	
	Children:
		PO 75–200 mg
		deep IM. single IV 10–50 mg
		3–6 yrs: PO 25–50 mg/day
		7–18 yrs: PO 25–100 mg/day
		IM, IV 25 mg, may repeat
		× 1 for acute dystonia	

Disulfiram (Antabuse)
  Anti-Alcohol Abuse Agent
    Tablet 250 mg, 500 mg
	Adult:	250–500 mg	

Divalproex (Depakote)
  (Sodium valproate-valproic acid)
  Anticonvulsants
    Tablet 125 mg, 250 mg, 500 mg
    Plasma levels: 50–100 ug/ml[b]
	Adult: 15–60 mg/kg		

WARNING: Hepatic failure resulting in fatalities has occurred in patients receiving valproic acid and its derivatives. Liver function tests should be performed prior to therapy and at frequent intervals thereafter, especially during the first 6 months of therapy.

Drug Products	Recommendations	
Doxepin (Sinequan)		
Antidepressants, Tertiary Amines	Adults:	PO 50–300 mg
Capsule 25 mg, 50 mg, 75 mg,	Elderly:	PO 25–150 mg
100 mg, 150 mg	Children:	Not established
Oral liquid 10 mg/ml		
Plasma levels: 50–200 ng/ml[a]		
(includes metabolites)		

Elavil (See Amitriptyline)

Eskalith (See Lithium Carbonate)

Ethosuximide (Zarontin)		
Anticonvulsants	Children:	250 mg–1500 mg
Capsule 250 mg		
Plasma levels: 40–150 ug/ml		
Fluoxetine (Prozac)		
Antidepressant, Atypical	Adult:	usual: 20–40 mg/day
Capsule 20 mg		extreme: 5–80 mg/day
	Elderly:	10–20 mg/day
	Children:	Not established

WARNING: Dose changes should be made very slowly—not less than weekly—to adjust for the very long-half life of the drug, particularly when used in combination with other liver-metabolized drugs.

Fluphenazine (Prolixin)		
Phenothiazines, piperazines	Adult:	PO 5–40 mg
Hydrochloride		IM 1.25–40 mg
Tablet 1 mg, 2.5 mg, 5 mg, 10 mg	Elderly:	PO 1–10 mg
Oral liquid 5 mg/5 ml		IM 0.5–5 mg
Injection 2.5 mg/ml	Children:	13–18 yrs: PO 2.5–20 mg
Decanoate Maximum: 25 mg q week		
which is equivalent to approximately		
40 mg of fluphenazine hydrochloride		
daily		
Plasma levels: below 10 mcg/mL[b] (Plasma		
levels not yet accurately established		
for clinical monitoring purposes.)		
Flurazepam (Dalmane) (C-IV)		
Hypnotics	Adult:	15–30 mg
(Benzodiazepines)	Elderly:	15–30 mg
Capsule 15 mg, 30 mg		

(Continued)

Drug Products	Recommendations	

Folic Acid
  Vitamins
    Tablet 1 mg		

Halazepam (Paxipam) (C-IV)
  Antianxiety and Hypnotics
  (Benzodiazepines)
    Tablet 20 mg, 40 mg
	Adult:
	Elderly:
		60–120 mg
		20–40 mg

Halcion (See Triazolam)		
Haldol (See Haloperidol)		

Haloperidol (Haldol)
  Antipsychotic, Butyrophenones
    Tablet 0.5 mg, 1 mg, 2 mg,
      5 mg, 10 mg, 20 mg
    Oral liquid 2 mg/ml
    Injection 5 mg/ml
	Adult:
	
	Elderly:
	
	Children:
		PO 1–40 (100) mg[k]
		IM 2–5 mg
		PO 1–20 mg
		IM 0.5–2.5 mg
		7–12 yrs: PO 0.5–16 mg
		          (.25 mg/kg)
		13–18 yrs: PO 0.5–40 mg

Decanoate[l]
  Injection 50 mg/ml Conversion:
    50 mg (1 ml) Q 4 weeks = 5 mg
    haloperidol base every day		

WARNING: High dose haloperidol in combination with other neuroactive drugs requires careful monitoring and observation for toxicity, especially muscular rigidity and loss of consciousness, and changes in body temperature and cardiac function.

Imipramine (Tofranil)
  Antidepressants, Tertiary Amines
    Tablet 10 mg, 25 mg, 50 mg
    Injection 12.5 mg/ml
 	
    Plasma Levels: 150–450 ng/ml
      (Imipramine + Desipramine)
	Adult:
	
	Elderly:
	
	Children:
		PO 50–300 mg
		IM 25–120 mg
		PO 25–150 mg
		IM 10–50 mg
		7–12 yrs: PO 50–100 mg
		13–18 yrs: PO 50–125 mg

Inderal (See Propranolol)		

Kaolin/Pectin (Kaopectate)
  Antidiarrhea Agents
    Oral suspension
	Take antipsychotics 1 hr. before
	or 2 hrs. after kaolin/pectin	

Kaopectate (See Kaolin/Pectin)		
Klonopin (See Clonazepam)		

[k] Doses above 40 mg per day are associated with more side effects with no greater efficacy than lower doses.
[l] In 1993, the revised package insert increased the maximum dose from 300 to 450 mg per month. This higher maximum is intended for *maintenance* treatment where haloperidol decanoate *alone* is the maintenance treatment.

Drug Products	Recommendations

Librium (See Chlordiazepoxide)

Lithium Carbonate (Lithobid, Eskalith)

Antimanic Agents	Adults:	600–2400 mg
Tablet 300 mg	Elderly:	300–2400 mg
Capsule 300 mg	Children:	7–18 yrs: 600–2100 mg
Capsule (s.r.) 450 mg		
Oral liquid 300 mg/5 ml (citrate)		

Plasma level: 0.6–1.5 mEq/L

WARNING: Lithium toxicity is closely related to plasma lithium levels and can occur at doses close to therapeutic levels. Facilities for prompt and accurate plasma lithium determination should be available before initiating therapy. Levels above 1.2 are flagged for close monitoring.

Lithobid (See Lithium Carbonate)

Lorazepam (Ativan) (C-IV)

Antianxiety and Hypnotics	Adult:	2–6 mg
(Benzodiazepines)	Elderly:	0.5–2 mg
Tablet 1 mg, 2 mg		

Loxapine (Loxitane)

Antipsychotics,		
Dibenzoxazepines	Adult:	P.O. 20–250 mg
Capsule 5 mg, 10 mg,		I.M. 50–200 mg
25 mg, 50 mg	Elderly:	P.O. 10–100 mg
Oral liquid 25 mg/ml		I.M. 25–100 mg
Injection 50 mg/ml		

Loxitane (See Loxapine)

Ludiomil (See Maprotiline)

Maalox (See Aluminum/Magnesium Hydroxides)

Maprotiline (Ludiomil)[m]

Antidepressants, Atypical	Adult:	25–225 mg
Tablet 25 mg, 50 mg, 75 mg	Elderly:	25–75 mg

WARNING: Seizures have been associated with the use of maprotiline.

Mellaril (See Thioridazine)

Meperidine (Demerol) (C-II)

Analgesics, Narcotic	
Tablet 50 mg	
Injection 50 mg, 100 mg	

(Continued)

[m] Nonformulary status

Drug Products		Recommendations
Mesoridazine (Serentil)		
Antipsychotic, Phenothiazine,	Adult:	PO 25–400 mg
Piperidine		IM 25–200 mg
Tablet 10 mg, 25 mg, 50 mg, 100 mg	Elderly:	PO 25–200 mg
Oral liquid 25 mg/ml		IM 12.5–50 mg
Injection 25 mg/ml		
To avoid the risk of retinopathy doses		
of 400 mg/day should not be		
exceeded.		
Methohexital (Brevital) (C-IV)		
Antianxiety and Hypnotics		
(Barbiturates)		
Injection 500 mg		
Methylphenidate (Ritalin) (C-II)		
Cerebral Stimulants	Adult:	10–40 mg
Tablet 5 mg, 10 mg	Elderly:	5–20 mg
	Children:	7–18 yrs: 20–60 mg
		(0.3–1.0 mg/kg)
Milk of Magnesia		
Oral suspension		Take antipsychotics 1 hr. before
		or 2 hrs. after antacid
Moban (See Molindone)		
Molindone (Moban)		
Antipsychotics, Dihydroindolone	Adult:	20–225 mg
Tablet 5 mg, 10 mg, 25 mg,	Elderly:	10–100 mg
50 mg, 100 mg	Children:	7–12 yrs: 15–150 mg
Oral liquid 20 mg/ml		13–18 yrs: 15–200 mg
Morphine Sulfate (C-II)		
Analgesics, Narcotic		
Injection 15 mg		
Mylanta (See Al/Mg Hydroxide & Simethicone)		
Mysoline (See Primidone)		
Nardil (See Phenelzine)		
Navane (See Thiothixene)		
Noctec (See Chloral Hydrate)		
Norpramin (See Desipramine)		

Drug Products		Recommendations
Nortriptyline (Aventyl)		
Antidepressants, Secondary Amines	Adult:	PO 25–75 mg
Capsule 10 mg, 25 mg, 75 mg	Elderly:	PO 10–35 mg
Oral liquid 10 mg/5 ml		
Plasma level: 50–150 ng/ml		
Oxazepam (Serax) (C-IV)		
Antianxiety and Hypnotics	Adult:	PO 30–120 mg
(Benzodiazepines)	Elderly:	PO 10–60 mg
Capsule 15 mg	Children:	PO 7–12 yrs: 10–30 mg
		13–18 yrs: 30–60 mg
Parnate (See Tranylcypromine)		
Paxipam (See Halazepam)		
Pemoline (Cylert) (C-IV)		
Cerebral Stimulants	Children:	PO 7–18 yrs: 18.75–112.5 mg
Tablet 18.75 mg, 37.5 mg		
Perphenazine (Trilafon)		
Antipsychotics, Phenothiazines,	Adult:	PO 8–64 (96) mg
Piperazines		IM 5–30 mg
Tablet 2 mg, 4 mg, 6 mg, 8 mg,	Elderly:	PO 4–32 mg
16 mg		IM 2–12 mg
Oral liquid 16 mg/5 ml		
Injection 5 mg/ml		
Phenelzine (Nardil)		
Antidepressants (MAO Inhibitor)	Adult:	PO 15–90 mg
Tablet 15 mg	Elderly:	PO 15–60 mg
Phenobarbital (C-III)		
Anticonvulsants	Adult:	PO 30–320 mg
Tablet 15 mg, 30 mg, 100 mg		slow IV for statics
		epilepticus: 20 mg/kg or
		until seizures stop
Oral liquid 20 mg/5 ml	Children:	PO 1–20 mg/kg
Injection 130 mg/ml		IM, IV 1–20 mg/kg
Plasma levels: 20–40 ug/ml[c]		
Phenytoin (Dilantin)		
Anticonvulsants	Adults:	PO 200–600 mg
Tablet 50 mg (free base)		IV 8–15 mg/kg
Capsule 100 mg (sodium)		(IM administration is not
Oral suspension 125 mg/5 ml		recommended because of
(free base)		erratic absorption)
Injection 100 mg/2 ml (sodium)	Children:	PO 4–8 mg/kg
		IV 5 mg/kg
Plasma levels: 10–20 ug/ml		

(Continued)

Drug Products	Recommendations
Physostigmine (Antilirium) Parasympathomimetic Agents Injection 1 mg/ml	
Placebo (Non-Formulary) Unclassified Agents Tablet Capsule	
Prazepam (Centrax) (C-IV) Antianxiety and Hypnotics (Benzodiazepines) Capsule 5 mg, 10 mg, 20 mg	Adults: 20–60 mg Elderly: 10–15 mg
Primidone (Mysoline) Anticonvulsants Tablet 50 mg, 250 mg Oral suspension 250 mg/5 ml Plasma levels: 5–12 ug/ml[e]	Adults: 100–2000 mg Children: 50–750 mg
Prolixin (See Fluphenazine)	
Propranolol (Inderal) Antihypertensive Agents Unlabeled psychiatric usage only in clinically justified situations Tablet 10 mg, 40 mg Injection 1 mg/ml	
Prozac (See Fluoxetine)	
Restoril (See Temazepam)	
Ritalin (See Methylphenidate)	
Serentil (See Mesoridazine)	
Sinequan (See Doxepin)	
Stelazine (See Trifluoperazine)	
Succinlycholine (Anectine) Skeletal Muscle Relaxants Injection 20 mg/ml	
Surmontil (See Trimipramine)	
Symmetrel (See Amantadine)	
Tegretol (See Carbamazepine)	

Drug Products		Recommendations
Temazepam (Restoril) (C-IV)		
Antianxiety and Hypnotics	Adult:	15–30 mg
(Benzodiazepines)	Elderly:	15 mg
Capsule 15 mg, 30 mg		
Thiopental (C-III)		
Hypnotic and Pre-anesthetic		
Injection 1 gram		
Thioridazine (Mellaril)		
Antipsychotics, Phenothiazines	Adult:	100–800 mg
Piperidine	Elderly:	25–300 mg
Tablet 10 mg, 15 mg, 25 mg,	Children:	3–6 yrs: 10–100 mg
50 mg, 100 mg, 150 mg, 200 mg		7–12 yrs: 25–500 mg
Oral suspension 25 mg/5 ml,		13–18 yrs: 25–800 mg
100 mg/5 ml		

WARNING: To avoid the risk of retinopathy, doses of 800 mg per day should not be exceeded.

Thiothixene (Navane)		
Antipsychotics, Thioxanthenes	Adult:	PO 6–60 (90) mg
Capsule 1 mg, 2 mg, 5 mg, 10 mg,		IM 8–30 mg
20 mg	Elderly:	PO 2–30 mg
Oral liquid 5 mg/ml		IM 2–15 mg
Injection 5 mg/ml	Children:	3–6 yrs: PO 1–6 mg
		7–18 yrs: PO 5–42 mg
		(0.3 mg/kg)
Thorazine (See Chlorpromazine)		
Tofranil (See Imipramine)		
Tranxene (See Clorazepate)		
Tranylcypromine (Parnate)		
Antidepressants (MAO Inhibitor)	Adult:	PO 10–60 mg
Tablet 10 mg	Elderly:	PO 10–30 mg
Trazodone (Desyrel)		
Antidepressants (MAOI)	Adult:	PO 150–600 mg
Tablet 50 mg, 100 mg	Elderly:	PO 50–250 mg

WARNING: Trazodone has been associated with the occurrence of priapism. In these cases immediate discontinuation of the drug is recommended.

Triazolam (Halcion) (C-IV)		
Hypnotic	Adult:	PO 0.25–0.5 mg
(Benzodiazepines)	Elderly:	PO 0.125–0.25 mg
Tablet 0.25 mg, 0.5 mg		

(Continued)

Drug Products		Recommendations
Trifluoperazine (Stelazine)		
Antipsychotics, Phenothiazines,	Adult:	PO 5–60 mg
Piperazines		IM 4–30 mg
Tablet 1 mg, 2 mg, 5 mg, 10 mg	Elderly:	PO 2–20 mg
Oral liquid 10 mg/ml		IM 2–10 mg
Injection 2 mg/ml	Children:	3–6 yrs: PO 1–6 mg
		7–12 yrs: PO 1–20 mg
		13–18 yrs: PO 1–40 mg
Trihexyphenidyl (Artane)		
Anticholinergic, Antiparkinson	Adult:	2–15 mg
Tablet 2 mg, 5 mg	Elderly:	2–6 mg
Oral liquid 2 mg/5 ml		
Trilafon (See Perphenazine)		
Trimipramine (Surmontil)		
Antidepressants, Tertiary Amines	Adult:	75–300 mg
Capsule 25 mg, 50 mg, 100 mg	Elderly:	50–100 mg
Valium (See Diazepam)		
Valproic Acid (Depakene)		
Anticonvulsants	Adult:	15–60 mg/kg/day
Capsule 250 mg	Children:	20–60 mg/kg/day
Oral liquid 250 mg/5 ml		
Plasma levels: 50–100 ug/ml[c]		

WARNING: Hepatic failure resulting in fatalities has occurred in patients receiving valproic acid. Liver function tests should be performed prior to therapy and at frequent intervals thereafter, especially during the first 6 months.

Vistaril (See Hydroxyzine)

Xanax (See Alprazolam)

Zarontin (See Ethosuximide)

PSYCHOTHERAPEUTIC LISTING BY THERAPEUTIC CLASS

An alphabetized listing of the therapeutic classes and representative agents used in OMH psychiatric patients is provided below. The list includes some non-psychotropic agents because of their importance in drug interactions and monitoring of the psychotropic agents.

Analgesics, Narcotic
Codeine Phosphate
Codeine Sulfate
Meperidine
Morphine

Antacids
Aluminum and Magnesium Hydroxide and Simethicone
Aluminum Hydroxide
Milk of Magnesia

Antialcohol Abuse Agent
Disulfiram

Anticholinergics (Antiparkinson)
Benztropine
Trihexyphenidyl

Anticholinergics (For Non-Gastrointestinal Uses)
Atropine

Anticonvulsants
Carbamazepine
Divalproex
Ethosuximide
Phenytoin
Phenobarbital
Primidone
Valproic Acid

Antidepressants, Atypical
Bupropion
Fluoxetine
Trazodone

Antidepressants, MAOI
Isocarboxazid
Phenelzine
Tranylcypromine

Antidepressants, Secondary Amines
Amoxapine
Desipramine
Nortriptyline

Antidepressants, Tertiary Amines
Amitriptyline
Clomipramine
Doxepin
Imipramine
Trimipramine

Antidiarrhea Agents
Diphenoxylate/Atropine
Kaolin/Pectin

Antihistaminic Agents
Diphenhydramine

Antimanic Agents
Lithium

Antipsychotics, Butyrophenones
Haloperidol
Haloperidol Decanoate

Antipsychotics, Atypical
Clozapine
Loxapine
Pimozide

Antipsychotics, Dihydroindolones
Molindone

Antipsychotics, Phenothiazines, Aliphatic
Chlorpromazine

Antipsychotics, Phenothiazines, Piperazine
Fluphenazine
Perphenazine
Trifluoperazine

Antipsychotics, Phenothiazines, Piperidine
Mesoridazine
Thioridazine

Antipsychotics, Thioxanthines
Thiothixene

Antianxiety Agents and Hypnotics (Barbiturates)
Amobarbital
Methohexital
Thiopental

Antianxiety and Hypnotic Agents (Benzodiazepines)
Alprazolam
Chlordiazepoxide
Clorazepate
Diazepam
Flurazepam
Halazepam
Lorazepam
Prazepam
Temazepam
Triazolam

Antianxiety Agents and Hypnotics (Miscellaneous)
Buspirone
Chloral Hydrate
Hydroxyzine

Cerebral Stimulants
Dextro-amphetamine
Methylphenidate
Pemoline

Dopamine Agonists
Amantadine
Bromocriptine

Unclassified Agents
Placebo

Unlabeled Indications (Agents in other classes with some psychotherapeutic usage)
Carbamazepine
Clonidine
Propranolol

PART IV

Quick Reference Section

ADVERSE REACTION REPORT FORM (FDA 1639)

DEPARTMENT OF HEALTH AND HUMAN SERVICES PUBLIC HEALTH SERVICE FOOD AND DRUG ADMINISTRATION (HFD-730) ROCKVILLE, MD 20857 **ADVERSE REACTION REPORT** (Drugs and Biologics)	Form Approved. OMB No. 0910-0230 See OMB Statement on the Reverse							
	FDA CONTROL NO.							
	ACCESSION NO.							

I.			REACTION INFORMATION				

1. PATIENT ID / INITIALS (In Confidence)	2 AGE YRS	3 SEX	4-6 REACTION ONSET			8-12 CHECK ALL APPROPRIATE
			MO	DA	YR	☐ PATIENT DIED
7. DESCRIBE REACTION(S)						☐ REACTION TREATED WITH R_x DRUG ☐ RESULTED IN, OR PROLONGED, INPATIENT HOSPITALIZATION ☐ RESULTED IN PERMANENT DISABILITY
13. RELEVANT TESTS/LABORATORY DATA						☐ NONE OF THE ABOVE

II.	SUSPECT DRUG(S) INFORMATION	
14. SUSPECT DRUG(S) (Give manufacturer and lot no. for vaccines/biologics)	20. DID REACTION ABATE AFTER STOPPING DRUG? ☐ YES ☐ NO ☐ NA	
15. DAILY DOSE	16. ROUTE OF ADMINISTRATION	21. DID REACTION REAPPEAR AFTER REINTRODUCTION?
17. INDICATION(S) FOR USE		☐ YES ☐ NO ☐ NA
18. DATES OF ADMINISTRATION (From/To)	19. DURATION OF ADMINISTRATION	

III.	CONCOMITANT DRUGS AND HISTORY
22. CONCOMITANT DRUGS AND DATES OF ADMINISTRATION (Exclude those used to treat reaction)	
23. OTHER RELEVANT HISTORY (e.g. diagnoses, allergies, pregnancy with LMP, etc.)	

IV. ONLY FOR REPORTS SUBMITTED BY MANUFACTURER		V. INITIAL REPORTER (In confidence)	
24. NAME AND ADDRESS OF MANUFACTURER (Include Zip Code)		26.-26a. NAME AND ADDRESS OF REPORTER (Include Zip Code)	
24a. IND/NDA NO. FOR SUSPECT DRUG	24b. MFR CONTROL NO.	26b. TELEPHONE NO. (Include area code)	
24c. DATE RECEIVED BY MANUFACTURER	24d. REPORT SOURCE (Check all that apply) ☐ FOREIGN ☐ STUDY ☐ LITERATURE ☐ HEALTH PROFESSIONAL ☐ CONSUMER	26c. HAVE YOU ALSO REPORTED THIS REACTION TO THE MANUFACTURER? ☐ YES ☐ NO	
25. 15 DAY REPORT? ☐ YES ☐ NO	25a. REPORT TYPE ☐ INITIAL ☐ FOLLOWUP	26d. ARE YOU A HEALTH PROFESSIONAL? ☐ YES ☐ NO	Submission of a report does not necessarily constitute an admission that the drug caused the adverse reaction.

NOTE: Required of manufacturers by 21 CFR 314.80

FORM FDA 1639 (12/91)   PREVIOUS EDITION MAY BE USED

INSTRUCTIONS FOR COMPLETING FORM FDA - 1639

REPORTING ADVERSE REACTIONS TO FDA
   All health care providers who observe *suspect* reactions to drugs or biologics are encouraged to report these to FDA. Serious reactions, observations of events not described in the package insert, and reactions to newly marketed products are of particular importance.

GENERAL
☐ Use a separate Form FDA-1639 for each patient.
☐ Additional pages may be attached if space provided on the Form FDA-1639 is inadequate.
☐ For questions call: 301-443-4580
☐ Patient and initial reporter identification is held in confidence by the FDA.

SPECIFIC INSTRUCTIONS
I.   Reaction Information
    Item 2.   Age—For children under 5 years of age, also write date of birth (DOB) in Item 1. For congenital malformations, give the age and sex of the infant (even though the mother was exposed).
    Item 7.   Describe Reaction(s)—Give signs and/or symptoms, diagnoses, course, etc.
    Item 13.   Relevant Tests/Laboratory Data—Both pre- and post-drug values should be provided if known.
II. Suspect Drug Information
    Item 14.   Suspect Drug—The trade name is preferred. If a generically produced product is involved, the manufacturer should be identified.
    Item 15.   Dose—For pediatric patients, also give body weights.
    Item 20 and 21. NA—is defined as nonapplicable (e.g. *when only one dose given or outcome was irreversible*).
V.   Initial Reporter
    Item 26c. Have you also reported this reaction to the manufacturer? Your answer facilitates identification of duplicates in the central adverse reaction file. FDA encourages direct reporting even if a report has been submitted to the manufacturer.

NOTE TO MANUFACTURERS *(Refer to 21 CFR 314.80 and 21 CFR 310.305)*. Detailed instructions are contained in the "Guideline for Postmarketing Reporting of Adverse Drug Reactions."

Public reporting burden for this collection of information is estimated to average 5 hours per response, including the time for review instructions, searching existing data sources, gathering and maintaining the data needed, and completing and reviewing the collection of information. Send comments regarding this burden estimate or any other aspect of this collection of information, including suggestions for reducing this burden to:

Reports Clearance Officer, PHS   and to: Office of Management and Budget
Hubert H. Humphrey Building, Room 721-B   Paperwork Reduction Project (0910-0230)
200 Independence Avenue, S.W.   Washington, DC 20503
Washington, DC 20201
Attn: PRA
                        Please DO NOT RETURN your questionnaire to either of these addresses.

After completing the form on the other side of this sheet, please
triple fold, seal with tape, and mail to address shown below.
No postage is necessary.

DEPARTMENT OF
HEALTH & HUMAN SERVICES

Public Health Service
Food and Drug Administration
Rockville MD 20857

Official Business
Penalty for Private Use $300

NO POSTAGE
NECESSARY
IF MAILED
IN THE
UNITED STATES

BUSINESS REPLY MAIL
FIRST CLASS MAIL   PERMIT NO. 946   ROCKVILLE MD
POSTAGE WILL BE PAID BY ADDRESSEE

Food and Drug Administration
Division of Epidemiology and Surveillance (HFD-730)
Public Health Service
5600 Fishers Lane
Rockville MD 20852-9787

AUTOMATED CHEMISTRY—20 LABORATORY
REFERENCE VALUES

Glucose	MG/DL	65–110
BUN	MG/DL	7–18
Creatinine	MG/DL	0.9–1.5
Sodium	MEQ/L	135–148
Potassium	MEQ/L	3.5–5.3
Chloride	MEQ/L	98–106
CO_2	MEQ/L	23–32
Total Protein	G/DL	6.5–8.2
Albumin	G/DL	3.4–5.3
Albumin/Globulin	Ratio	1.1–1.8
Alkaline Phosphatase	U/L	8–76
AST (SGOT)	U/L	7–26
ALT (SGPT)	U/L	8–28
LDH	U/L	47–140
Gamma GT	U/L	1–27
Bilirubin, Total	MG/DL	0.2–1.2
Bilirubin, Direct	MG/DL	0.0–0.5
Calcium	MG/DL	8.5–10.5
Inorganic Phosphate	MG/DL	4–7
Uric Acid	MG/DL	2.0–5.5
Cholesterol	MG/DL	150–250
Triglycerides	MG/DL	44–166

CLOZAPINE EVALUATION FORM

Form 115 MED (MH) (5-90)

State of New York
OFFICE OF MENTAL HEALTH

CLOZAPINE EVALUATION

Patient's Name (Last, First, M.I.)	"C" No.

- ☐ 6 Week Evaluation   ☐ 1 Year Evaluation
- ☐ 12 week Evaluation   ☐ Discharge Evaluation   DATE

Sex   Date of Birth

Prescribing physician must complete evaluation after 6 week trial and if continued, after 12 weeks. Evaluation must also be completed at discharge (if inpatient) or at one year.

Facility Name   Unit/Ward/Residence No.

1. Patient Address	2. Facility and Facility Address

3. Date of Initiation of Clozapine	4. Current Clozapine Daily Dose

5. Side effects (Other than blood count which is monitored by CPMS)
Include presence or absence of clinial conditions or side effects listed below

0 = not present,   4 = significant

		MILD	MOD.	SEVERE	EXTREME
Seizures	0	1	2	3	4
Neuroleptic Malignant Syndrome	0	1	2	3	4
Tardive Dyskinesia *If present, AIMS Score _____*					
Acute Dystonia	0	1	2	3	4
Tremor	0	1	2	3	4
Dyskinesia *(Specify)* _____	0	1	2	3	4
Akinesia	0	1	2	3	4
Akathisia	0	1	2	3	4
Drowsiness	0	1	2	3	4
Tachycardia	0	1	2	3	4
Constipation	0	1	2	3	4
Dizziness	0	1	2	3	4
Hypotension	0	1	2	3	4
Hypertension	0	1	2	3	4
Delirium	0	1	2	3	4
Blurred Vision	0	1	2	3	4
Difficulty Urinating	0	1	2	3	4
Falling Episodes	0	1	2	3	4
Bronchia Hypersecretion	0	1	2	3	4
Fever	0	1	2	3	4
Salivation	0	1	2	3	4
Headache	0	1	2	3	4
Nausea/Vomiting	0	1	2	3	4
Dry Mouth	0	1	2	3	4
Weight Gain	0	1	2	3	4

6. Positive Symptomatology	IMPROVED	UNIMPROVED
Delusions	☐	☐
Auditory Hallucinations	☐	☐
Thought Disorder	☐	☐
Grossly Inappropriate Affect	☐	☐
Visual Hallucinations	☐	☐

7. Negative Symptomatology		
Marked Lack of Motivation	☐	☐
Marked Social Withdrawal or Isolation	☐	☐
Marked Lack of Energy, Interests	☐	☐
Anhedonia	☐	☐
Poverty of Content of Thought	☐	☐

8. Other Symptoms		
Violence Toward Others	☐	☐
Violence Toward Objects	☐	☐
Violence Toward Self	☐	☐
Other _____	☐	☐

9. BPRS Pre-Treatment Score _____

BPRS Current Score _____

10. Comments: _____

11. Recommendations:

- Definite response, continue Clozapine ☐
- Minimal response, continue Clozapine for further evaluation ☐
- No response, discontinue Clozapine ☐

12. Reason for Discontinuing Clozapine

- Patient unwilling to continue ☐
- Poor response ☐
- Blood drawing problems ☐
- Side effects problem *(Specify)* _____ ☐
- Other _____ ☐

13. Physician's Name	14. Physician's Signature
	DATE

The Following is to be Completed by the Drug Monitoring Committee

15. a. Date of Drug Monitoring Committee Review:	15. b. Comments:	15. c. Action:
		Approved ☐ Disapproved ☐ Deferred Pending Further Information *(Describe below)* ☐
	DMC CHAIRPERSON OR DESIGNEE	

CLOZAPINE SCREENING FORM

Form 114 MED (MH) (5-90)

NEW YORK STATE
OFFICE OF MENTAL HEALTH

CLOZAPINE SCREENING FORM

Patient's Name (Last, First, M.I.)	"C" No.

In order to prescribe Clozapine for an OMH patient, physicians must complete this form, along with the Clozaril Patient Management System form and forward both to the facility pharmacy for processing.

Sex	Date of Birth

Date	Patient Address

Inpatient ☐
Outpatient ☐

Facility Name	Unit/Ward/Residence No.

4. **DSMIIIR Diagnoses (All 5 Axis)**

	Primary Diagnoses	Secondary Diagnoses
Axis I		
Axis II		
Axis III		
Axis IV		
Axis V		

5. If Inpatient, Length of Current Hospitalization (include admission date)

6. Number of previous Psychiatric Hospitalization (include admission and discharge dates)

Length of Previous Psychiatric Hospitalizations (include admission and discharge dates)

a) _____ e) _____
b) _____ f) _____
c) _____ g) _____
d) _____ h) _____

7. **Treatment Refractory History**
Document patient's prior response to antipsychotic drugs which must include at least 3 periods of treatment in past 5 years with neuroleptics from at least 2 chemical classes at doses not less than 1000mg. CPZ equivalent per day for a period of 6 weeks each, without significant symptom relief

Dates of Drugs 1000mg. CPZ Equivalent

Drug	Dose	Start Date	Stop Date	Response
a)				
b)				
c)				

8. **Clinical Impression**

a Check Positive Symptoms that are Currently Present:
- Delusions ☐
- Auditory Hallucinations ☐
- Thought Disorder ☐
- Grossly Inappropriate Affect ☐
- Visual Hallucinations ☐

b. **Check Negative Symptoms that Apply:**
- Marked Lack of Motivation ☐
- Marked Social Withdrawal or Isolation ☐
- Marked Lack of Energy, Interests ☐
- Anhedonia ☐
- Poverty of Content of Thought ☐

c. **Check Other Symptoms:**
- Violence Toward Others ☐
- Violence Toward Objects ☐
- Violence Toward Self ☐
- Other ☐

d. **Brief Psychiatric Rating Scale (BPRS) Score** _____. A score of at least 45 must be demonstrated in order to meet the criteria.

e. **Medical Clearance (Check list)**

1. Conditions that are contraindications for prescribing Clozapine*

	Yes	No
myeloproliferative disease	☐	☐
granulocytopenia	☐	☐
agranulocytosis	☐	☐
severe central nervous system depression from any cause	☐	☐
concurrent medication regimen known to suppress bone marrow functions	☐	☐

* If any of these is currently present, the patient is not a candidate for Clozapine. If a patient has a history of Clozapine-induced agranulocytosis, repeat treatment with Clozapine is contraindicated.

2. Conditions that indicate special caution when prescribing Clozapine

	Yes	No
seizure disorder	☐	☐
hepatic disease	☐	☐
renal disease	☐	☐
cardiac disease	☐	☐
narrow angle-glaucoma	☐	☐
prostatic hypertrophy	☐	☐

3. Pre-existing Conditions ☐ ☐
Tardive Dyskinesia
If present, current AIMS Score _____ (within 3 months)
Note Medical Clearance ☐ ☐

9. I have informed and discussed the special requirement of weekly blood drawings with the patient. In my opinion, the patient is willing and able to comply with this special requirement. ☐ ☐

10. Other Comments/Rationale:

11. Physician's Name (Print)

12. Physician's Signature	Date

The Following to be Completed by the Drug Monitoring Committee:

13. Date of Drug Monitoring Review: _____
Comments:

Action:
- Approved ☐
- Disapproved ☐
- Deferred Pending Further Information ☐
  Describe Below:

_____
DMC Chairperson or Designee

GUIDELINES FOR DRUG MONITORING COMMITTEE (DMC)
APPROVAL PROCESS FOR CLOZAPINE TREATMENT

I.   **Diagnosis:**   The patient must have a diagnosis of schizophrenia.

II. **Age:**   The patient must be at least 16 years of age.

III. **Treatment Refractory:**

A. Patients are eligible for clozapine treatment if they are judged to be refractory to treatment by other antipsychotic medication.

B. Treatment refractoriness is determined by documentation on the OMH Clozapine Screening Form (CSF) of at least 3 periods of nonresponsive treatment in the past 5 years with antipsychotic medication of greater than or equal to 1,000 mg of chlorpromazine or its equivalent, for at least 6 weeks, at that dosage, for each period of treatment.

C. Prior treatment nonresponsiveness is based on the best clinical judgment possible, that the prior periods of antipsychotic treatment produced no, or only marginal reduction in the patient's positive or negative symptoms of schizophrenia and little or no improvement in his/her level of functioning.

IV. **Contraindications and Cautions:**

A. If a patient is judged to be treatment refractory but currently has any of the conditions listed in either 8e (1) on the Clozapine Screening Form, or a history of clozapine-induced granulocytopenia or agranulocytosis, clozapine treatment is contraindicated and the patient should be disapproved for this treatment.

B. If the patient has present or past history of any of the conditions listed in 8e (2) of the CSF, extreme caution should be exercised if clozapine is to be administered. The DMC should assess risk/benefit ratio as thoroughly as possible and, if approval is granted, alert the treating physician of any special monitoring of laboratory tests or clinical status that is recommended.

V.   **Criteria for Treatment Response:**

A. A post-treatment BPRS Score at the 6 week evaluation point must show *any* reduction from the baseline BPRS Score to be considered a minimal response and to continue clozapine treatment for further evaluation at 12 weeks.

B. A post-treatment BPRS Score at the 12 week evaluation point must show a reduction of at least 20% from the baseline BPRS or a score of 35 or lower in order to continue clozapine treatment.

NOTE: The data regarding lengths of current and past hospitalizations are for informational documentation purposes only and do not constitute a criteria for approval.

LONGITUDINAL DRUG MONITORING

Longitudinal drug monitoring for the chronic, severely ill hospitalized patient is illustrated below. The approach consists of simple graphing of various factors (y-variable) versus time (x-variable) for each drug treatment. The purpose of the method is to quantify the relationship between drug treatment and treatment outcome.

Each of the graphs illustrates one of the factors being monitored. For example, the first graph shows the daily dose of drug (mg), which in this instance is haloperidol, and is plotted on the y-axis against time in weeks on the x-axis. If the plasma level of drug is more appropriate for monitoring, e.g. in the case of lithium, then the y-axis should reflect plasma levels.

The second graph shows lithium plasma levels dropping slightly from 0.9 to 0.85 during the time that a 1200 mg per day prescribed dose was constant. To increase the validity, consumed doses (taken from the Medication Administration Form for the hospitalized patient) rather than

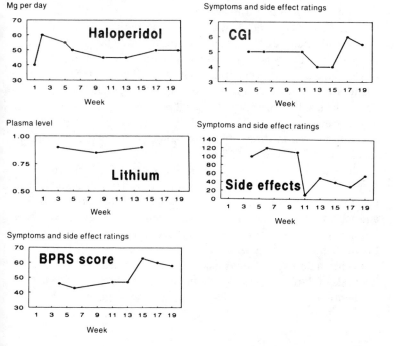

prescribed doses might be considered. The slight variation that was observed might be due to assay variation, fluctuations in metabolism, etc. and is undoubtedly too small to be clinically meaningful.

The next graph depicts the change in total symptom score according to the Brief Psychiatric Rating Scale (BPRS) and the following graph shows a global impression. The latter is based on the Clinical Global Impression (CGI) rating scale. These measures are useful for monitoring the symptoms and overall functioning of a patient. Consistency of ratings is encouraged by using scales with well-defined anchors for the various levels of severity.

The outcome measure related to drug-related adverse symptoms is shown in the last graph and involved a modified version of the Systematic Assessment of Treatment-emergent events (SAFTEE) scale. The attribution of adverse effects to a single drug is not possible with multi-drug regimens but suspicions would be raised of worsening of behavior or mental symptoms during the time a *new* agent is added to a previously monitored regimen if the side effect index increases after the new drug is started.

The case that is illustrated in this profile involved very high doses of haloperidol and an effort was being made to gradually reduce the dose. In the time period shown, doses of 45 mg per day resulted in a dramatic drop in side effects but this was followed by a corresponding increase in total symptoms and overall global impression so that a dosage increase was necessitated. Given the length of time between changes it is safe to assume that the increased psychopathology was due to the need for medication and not a temporary withdrawal effect of the previous dosage. At the end of 6 months, the patient was reduced from original doses of 90 (not shown) to 50 mg per day and was successfully managed at the lower dose.

There are several advantages to following patients in the suggested manner. First, behavioral toxicity would be recognizable when a new agent is added that is followed by increased psychopathology (BPRS) and increased dysfunctioning (CGI). Second, using several weeks as the interval between single drug changes minimizes the risk of mistaking temporary drug withdrawal effects for clinical decompensation when a dose reduction is made. If the drug is a decanoate product intervals of 2 to 4 months are not unreasonable. Acute symptom management during periods of decanoate dose adjustment for these patients requires a short-acting agent.

MINIMUM MONITORING STANDARDS

Minimum Monitoring Standards for Patients Treated with Lithium

Initial Work-Up	At 3 Months	Continuing Follow-up
CBC with Differential	yes	yearly
SMAC-20	yes	every 6 months
Urinalysis	yes	every 6 months
Thyroid Function Tests	yes	every 6 months
EKG	⸻⟶	yearly
Pregnancy test	thereafter as clinically indicated	**************** ****************
EEG	When clinically indicated	****************
Lithium levels	weekly for 1st month monthly for 1st year	every 3 months thereafter

Usual therapeutic plasma level range

ACUTE	0.8–1.4 mE/liter
MAINTENANCE	0.6–1.2 mE/liter
ELDERLY	0.8–1.0 mE/liter

Minimum Monitoring Standards for Patients Treated with Carbamazepine or Valproic Acid

Initial Work-Up	1st 3 Months	Continuing Follow-up
CBC with Differential & Platelets	monthly	every 3 months
SMAC-20	monthly	every 3 months
EKG	⸻⟶	yearly
Pregnancy test	thereafter as clinically indicated	**************** ****************
EEG	When clinically indicated	****************
Drug levels	weekly for 1st month monthly for 1st year	every 3 months thereafter

Usual therapeutic plasma level range

Carbamazepine:	Single Drug Regimen⟶	8–12 mcg/ml
	Multiple Drug Regimen ⟶	4–8 mcg/ml
Valproic Acid:	50–100 mcg/ml	(*Validity of Valproate range has not been established)

USUALLY EFFECTIVE RANGE OF PLASMA LEVELS OF FREQUENTLY USED PSYCHOTHERAPEUTIC AND NEUROACTIVE AGENTS

Generic Name	Brand Name	Plasma Range
Amitriptyline*	Elavil	100–300 ng/mL (AMT + NT = total)
Carbamazepine	Tegretol	4–8 mcg/mL multidrug regimen
		8–12 mcg/mL single drug regimen
Clonazepam*	Klonopin	40–60 ng/ml
Desipramine	Norpramin	200–250 ng/ml
Diazepam*	Valium	50–200 ng/ml
Doxepin*	Sinequan	50–200 ng/ml (includes metabolites)
Ethosuximide	Zarontin	40–150 ng/ml
Haloperidol	Haldol	5–20 ng/ml
Imipramine	Tofranil	150–450 ng/ml (IMI + DMI = total)
	Presamine	
	Various	
Nortriptyline	Aventyl	50–150 ng/ml
Phenytoin	Dilantin	10–20 mcg/ml
	Various	
Phenobarbital	Various	20–40 mcg/ml
Primidone	Mysoline	5–12 mcg/ml
Valproic Acid*	Depakene	50–100 mcg/ml

THE FOLLOWING LEVELS ARE USEFUL FOR RULING OUT TOXICITY

Chlorpromazine	Thorazine	< 1000 ng/ml (1 mcg/ml)
Fluphenazine**	Prolixin	< 10 mcg/ml
Thioridazine	Mellaril	< 1 mcg/ml

* Not yet reliably established.
** Fluphenazine decanoate frequently produces plasma levels at usually effective clinical doses that are "below detection," and reflect the *low* sensitivity of the assay rather than a measure for gauging clinical effectiveness.

SAMPLE DRUG INFORMATION SHEETS FOR PATIENTS

The following pages were reproduced with the permission of the United States Pharmacopeial Convention, Inc. Standard or personalized USP Patient Drug Education Leaflets can be ordered from the USP. To order or to obtain more information write: USP Order Processing Department, 12601 Twinbrook Parkway, Rockville, MD 20852 or call toll free 1-800-227-8772.

Benzodiazepines (Oral)—Psychiatric Use

Including Alprazolam ☐; Bromazepam ☐; Chlordiazepoxide ☐; Clonazepam ☐; Clorazepate ☐;
Diazepam ☐; Flurazepam ☐; Halazepam ☐; Ketazolam ☐; Lorazepam ☐; Nitrazepam ☐;
Oxazepam ☐; Prazepam ☐; Quazepam ☐; Temazepam ☐; Triazolam ☐.

Patient: _____ Rx No: _____

Other Drug Name: _____ Date: _____

Take _____ at the time(s) shown below

| MIDNIGHT | 1am | 2am | 3am | 4am | 5am | 6am | 7am | 8am | 9am | 10am | 11am |

| NOON | 1pm | 2pm | 3pm | 4pm | 5pm | 6pm | 7pm | 8pm | 9pm | 10pm | 11pm |

ABOUT YOUR MEDICINE

Benzodiazepines (ben-zoe-dye-AZ-e-peens) are used to relieve nervousness or tension and in the treatment of insomnia (trouble in sleeping). Some of these medicines are also used in the treatment of panic disorders.

Some benzodiazepines may also be used in the treatment of tension headaches. This use is not specifically included in approved product labeling. However, once a medicine is approved for marketing for one use, experience may show that it may also be used for other medical problems.

Benzodiazepines are also used to relax muscles or relieve muscle spasm and in the treatment of certain convulsive disorders, such as epilepsy. They may also be used for other conditions as determined by your doctor. Benzodiazepines should not be used for nervousness or tension caused by the stress of everyday life.

If any of the information in this leaflet causes you special concern or if you want additional information about your medicine and its use, check with your doctor, nurse, or pharmacist. **Remember, keep this and all other medicines out of the reach of children and never share your medicines with others.**

BEFORE USING THIS MEDICINE

Tell your doctor, nurse, and pharmacist if you . . .
- are allergic to any medicine, either prescription or nonprescription (OTC);
- are pregnant or intend to become pregnant while using this medicine;
- are breast-feeding;
- are taking any other prescription or nonprescription (OTC) medicine, especially other CNS depressants or zidovudine;
- have any other medical problems, especially asthma, bronchitis, emphysema, or other chronic lung disease; or myasthenia gravis.

PROPER USE OF THIS MEDICINE

Take this medicine only as directed by your doctor. Do not take more of it, do not take it more often, and do not take it for a longer time than your doctor ordered. If too much is taken, it may become habit-forming.

If you think this medicine is not working as well after you have taken it for a few weeks, **do not increase the dose**. Instead, check with your doctor.

If you are taking this medicine for epilepsy, it must be taken every day in regularly spaced doses in order for it to control your seizures.

Figure IV.1. Drug information sheet: Benzodiazopines (oral).

If you are taking this medicine regularly (for example, every day) and you miss
a dose, take it right away if you remember within an hour or so of the missed
dose. However, if you do not remember until later, skip the missed dose and go
back to your regular dosing schedule. Do not double doses.

PRECAUTIONS WHILE USING THIS MEDICINE

This medicine will add to the effects of alcohol and other CNS depressants (medicines that slow down the nervous system). Check with your doctor before taking
any such depressants while you are taking this medicine.

Benzodiazepines may cause some people to become drowsy. Make sure you know
how you react to this medicine before you drive, use machines, or do other
jobs that require you to be alert.

If you think you or someone else may have taken an overdose, get emergency
help at once. Some signs of an overdose are continuing slurred speech or confusion,
severe drowsiness, severe weakness, and staggering.

POSSIBLE SIDE EFFECTS OF THIS MEDICINE
Side Effects That Should Be Reported To Your Doctor

   Less common or rare—Behavior problems, including difficulty in concentrating
      and outbursts of anger; confusion or mental depression; convulsions (sei-
      zures); hallucinations; impaired memory; muscle weakness; skin rash or itch-
      ing; sore throat, fever, and chills; ulcers or sores in mouth or throat (contin-
      uing); uncontrolled movements of body, including the eyes; unusual bleeding
      or bruising; unusual excitement, nervousness, or irritability; unusual tiredness
      or weakness; yellow eyes or skin

   Signs of overdose—Confusion (continuing); drowsiness (severe); shakiness; short-
      ness of breath or troubled breathing; slow heartbeat; slow reflexes; slurred
      speech (continuing); staggering; weakness (severe)

Side Effects That Usually Do Not Require Medical Attention

These possible side effects may go away during treatment; however, if they continue
or are bothersome, check with your doctor, nurse, or pharmacist.

   More common—Clumsiness, unsteadiness, dizziness, lightheadedness, or drows-
      iness

Other side effects not listed above may also occur in some patients. If you notice
any other effects, check with your doctor, nurse, or pharmacist.

After you stop using this medicine, your body may need time to adjust. If you
took this medicine in high doses or for a long time, this may take up to 3 weeks.
During this period check with your doctor if you experience fast or pounding
heartbeat; increased sense of hearing; increased sensitivity to touch and pain; increased sweating; loss of sense of reality; mental depression; muscle or stomach
cramps; nausea or vomiting; sensitivity of eyes to light; tingling, burning or prickly
sensations; trembling; trouble in sleeping; or if you are unusually irritable, nervous,
or confused.

Figure IV.1. *(Continued)*

PSY231

Haloperidol (Oral)—Psychiatric Use

Patient: _____ Rx No: _____

Other Drug Name: _____ Date: _____

Take _____ at the time(s) shown below

MIDNIGHT	1am	2am	3am	4am	5am	6am	7am	8am	9am	10am	11am

NOON	1pm	2pm	3pm	4pm	5pm	6pm	7pm	8pm	9pm	10pm	11pm

ABOUT YOUR MEDICINE

Haloperidol (ha-loe-PER-i-dole) is used to treat nervous, mental, and emotional conditions.

Haloperidol may also be used in the treatment of early infantile autism and Huntington's disease. These uses are not specifically included in approved product labeling. However, once a medicine is approved for marketing for one use, experience may show that it may also be used for other medical problems.

Haloperidol is also used to control the effects of Tourette's disorder. It may also be used for other conditions as determined by your doctor.

If any of the information in this leaflet causes you special concern or if you want additional information about your medicine and its use, check with your doctor, nurse, or pharmacist. **Remember, keep this and all other medicines out of the reach of children and never share your medicines with others.**

BEFORE USING THIS MEDICINE

Discuss with your doctor possible side effects of this medicine. Some may be serious and/or permanent. For example, tardive dyskinesia (a movement disorder) may occur and may not go away after you stop using the medicine.

Tell your doctor, nurse, and pharmacist if you . . .
* are allergic to any medicine, either prescription or nonprescription (OTC);
* are pregnant or intend to become pregnant while using this medicine;
* are breast-feeding;
* are taking any other prescription or nonprescription (OTC) medicine, especially CNS depressants; epinephrine; levodopa; lithium; other medicines for nervous, mental, and emotional conditions; metoclopramide; metyrosine; promethazine; rauwolfia alkaloids, or trimeprazine;
* have any other medical problems, especially difficult urination, epilepsy, heart or blood vessel disease, or Parkinson's disease.

PROPER USE OF THIS MEDICINE

Do not take more of this medicine and do not take it more often than ordered. To lessen stomach upset, it may be taken with food or milk.

Sometimes haloperidol must be taken for several days to several weeks before its full effect is reached.

If you miss a dose of this medicine, take it as soon as possible. Then take any remaining doses for that day at regularly spaced intervals. Do not double doses.

PRECAUTIONS WHILE USING THIS MEDICINE

Your doctor should check your progress at regular visits, especially during the first few months of treatment with this medicine.

Figure IV.2. Drug information sheet: Hsloperidol (oral).

Do not stop taking this medicine without first checking with your doctor.

This medicine will add to the effects of alcohol and other CNS depressants (medicines that slow down the nervous system). Check with your doctor before taking any such depressants while you are taking this medicine.

Haloperidol may cause some people to become drowsy or less alert than they are normally. Even if you take this medicine at bedtime, you may feel drowsy or less alert on arising. Make sure you know how you react before you drive or do jobs that require you to be alert.

Some people who take haloperidol may become more sensitive to sunlight than they are normally. When you first begin taking this medicine, avoid too much sun and do not use a sunlamp until you see how you react to the sun, especially if you tend to burn easily. If you have a severe reaction, check with your doctor.

Use extra care not to become overheated during exercise or hot weather since overheating may result in heat stroke. Also, hot baths or saunas may make you feel dizzy or faint while you are taking this medicine.

Before having any kind of surgery or dental or emergency treatment, tell the physician or dentist in charge that you are using this medicine.

POSSIBLE SIDE EFFECTS OF THIS MEDICINE
Side Effects That Should Be Reported To Your Doctor Immediately
Stop taking this medicine and get emergency help immediately if any of the following side effects occur:

Rare—Convulsions (seizures); fast or irregular heartbeat; fever (high); increased sweating; loss of bladder control; muscle stiffness (severe); tiredness or weakness; troubled breathing; unusually pale skin

Other Side Effects That Should Be Reported To Your Doctor

More common—Difficulty in speaking or swallowing; inability to move eyes; loss of balance control; mask-like face; muscle spasms of neck and back; restlessness; shuffling walk; stiff arms and legs; trembling of hands

Less common—Difficult urination; dizziness, lightheadedness, or fainting; hallucinations; skin rash; uncontrolled movements of mouth, tongue, and jaw

Rare—Hot, dry skin, or lack of sweating; muscle weakness; sore throat and fever; unusual bleeding or bruising; yellow eyes or skin

Side Effects That Usually Do Not Require Medical Attention
These possible side effects may go away during treatment; however, if they continue or are bothersome, check with your doctor, nurse, or pharmacist.

More common—Blurred vision; changes in menstrual period; constipation; dryness of mouth; swelling or pain in breasts in females; unusual secretion of milk; weight gain

Other side effects not listed above may also occur in some patients. If you notice any other effects, check with your doctor, nurse, or pharmacist.

After you stop taking this medicine, your body may need time to adjust. Check with your doctor if you experience dizziness, stomach pain, nausea or vomiting, trembling of fingers and hands, or uncontrolled movements of mouth, tongue, and jaw.

Figure IV.2. *(Continued)*

Lithium (Oral)—Psychiatric Use

Patient: _____ Rx No: _____

Other Drug Name: _____ Date: _____

Take _____ at the time(s) shown below

MIDNIGHT	1am	2am	3am	4am	5am	6am	7am	8am	9am	10am	11am

NOON	1pm	2pm	3pm	4pm	5pm	6pm	7pm	8pm	9pm	10pm	11pm

ABOUT YOUR MEDICINE

Lithium (LITH-ee-um) is used to treat the manic stage of bipolar disorder (manic-depressive illness). It may also help reduce the frequency and severity of depression in bipolar disorder.

Lithium may also be used in the treatment of other types of mental depression, sometimes in combination with other medicines, such as monoamine oxidase (MAO) inhibitor antidepressants. Lithium is also used in the treatment of vascular headaches. These uses are not specifically included in approved product labeling. However, once a medicine is approved for marketing for one use, experience may show that it may also be used for other medical problems. Lithium may also be used for other conditions as determined by your doctor.

It is important that you and your family understand the effects of lithium. These depend on your individual condition and response and the amount of lithium you use. You also must know when to contact your doctor if there are problems.

If any of the information in this leaflet causes you special concern or if you want additional information about your medicine and its use, check with your doctor, nurse, or pharmacist. **Remember, keep this and all other medicines out of the reach of children and never share your medicines with others.**

BEFORE USING THIS MEDICINE

Tell your doctor, nurse, and pharmacist if you . . .
- are allergic to any medicine, either prescription or nonprescription (OTC);
- are pregnant or intend to become pregnant while using this medicine;
- are breast-feeding;
- are taking **any** other prescription or nonprescription (OTC) medicine;
- have any other medical problems, especially epilepsy, heart disease, kidney disease, leukemia (history of), Parkinson's disease, problems with urination, severe infections, or severe water loss.

PROPER USE OF THIS MEDICINE

During treatment with lithium, drink 2 or 3 quarts of water or other fluids each day, and use a normal amount of salt, unless otherwise directed.

Take this medicine exactly as directed. Do not take more or less of it, do not take it more or less often, and do not take it for a longer time than your doctor ordered. To do so may increase the chance of unwanted effects. **Sometimes lithium must be taken for 1 to several weeks before you begin to feel better.**

In order for lithium to work properly, it must be taken every day in regularly spaced doses as ordered by your doctor. This is necessary to keep a constant

Figure IV.3. Drug information sheet: Lithium (oral).

amount of lithium in your blood. Do not miss any doses and do not stop taking the medicine even if you feel better.

If you do miss a dose, take it as soon as possible. However, if it is within 2 hours (6 hours for the long-acting tablets or capsules) of your next dose, skip the missed dose and go back to your regular schedule. Do not double doses.

PRECAUTIONS WHILE USING THIS MEDICINE

Your doctor should check your progress at regular visits to make sure that the medicine is working properly and that possible side effects are avoided. Laboratory tests may be necessary.

Lithium may not work as well as it should if you drink large amounts of caffeine-containing coffee, tea, or colas.

Lithium may cause some people to become dizzy, drowsy, or less alert than they are normally. **Make sure you know how you react to this medicine before you drive, use machines, or do other jobs that require you to be alert.**

The loss of too much water and salt from your body may lead to serious side effects from lithium. **Use extra care in hot weather and during activities that cause you to sweat heavily, such as hot baths, saunas, or exercising. Also, check with your doctor before going on a diet to lose weight, or if you have an illness that causes sweating, vomiting, or diarrhea.**

POSSIBLE SIDE EFFECTS OF THIS MEDICINE

Side Effects That Should Be Reported To Your Doctor Immediately

> *Early signs of overdose or toxicity*—Diarrhea; drowsiness; loss of appetite; muscle weakness; nausea or vomiting; slurred speech; trembling
>
> *Late signs of overdose or toxicity*—Blurred vision; clumsiness or unsteadiness; confusion; convulsions (seizures); dizziness; trembling (severe); unusual increase in amount of urine

Other Side Effects That Should Be Reported To Your Doctor

> *Less common*—Fainting; fast, slow, or irregular heartbeat; troubled breathing (especially during hard work or exercise); unusual tiredness or weakness; weight gain
>
> *Rare*—Blue color and pain in fingers and toes; cold arms and legs; dizziness; eye pain; headache; unusual noises in the ears; vision problems
>
> *Signs of low thyroid function*—Dry, rough skin; hair loss; hoarseness; mental depression; sensitivity to cold; swelling of feet or lower legs; swelling of neck; unusual excitement

Side Effects That Usually Do Not Require Medical Attention

These possible side effects may go away during treatment; however, if they continue or are bothersome, check with your doctor, nurse, or pharmacist.

> *More common*—Increased frequency of urination or loss of bladder control—more common in women, usually beginning two to seven years after start of treatment; increased thirst; nausea (mild); trembling of hands (slight)

Other side effects not listed above may also occur in some patients. If you notice any other effects, check with your doctor, nurse, or pharmacist.

Figure IV.3 *(Continued)*

SAMPLE GROWTH CHARTS

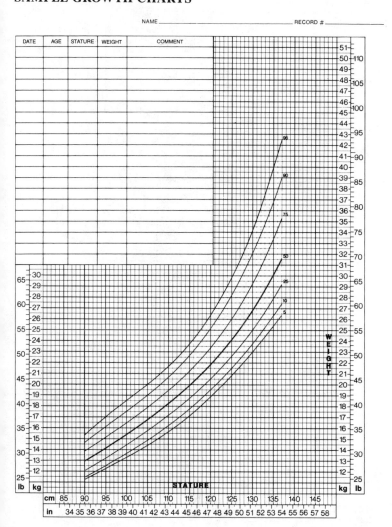

Girls: Prepubescent physical growth NCHS percentiles.
* Adapted from: Hamill PVV, Drizd TA, Johnson CL, Reed RB, Roche AF, Moore WM: Physical growth: National Center for Health Statistics percentiles. AM J CLIN NUTR 32:607–629, 1979. Data from the National Center for Health Statistics (NCHS), Hyattsville, Maryland. Reprinted with permission of Ross Laboratories, Columbus, Ohio 43216.

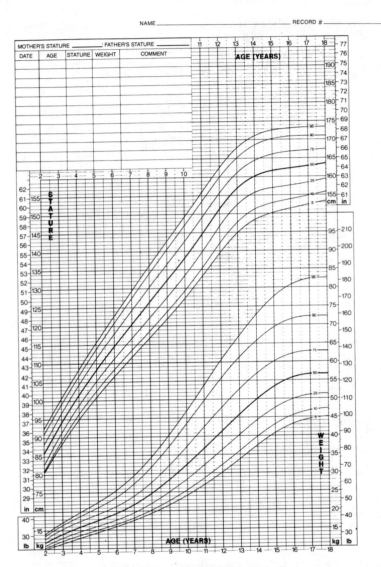

Girls: 2 to 18 years physical growth NCHS percentiles.
* Adapted from: Hamill PVV, Drizd TA, Johnson CL, Reed RB, Roche AF, Moore WM: Physical growth: National Center for Health Statistics percentiles. AM J CLIN NUTR 32:607–629, 1979. Data from the National Center for Health Statistics (NCHS), Hyattsville, Maryland. Reprinted with permission of Ross Laboratories, Columbus, Ohio 43216.

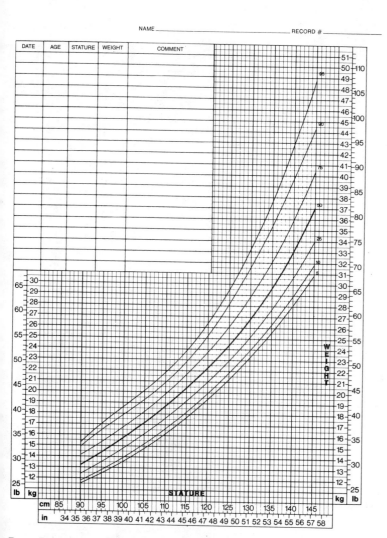

Boys: Prepubescent physical growth NCHS percentiles.

* Adapted from: Hamill PVV, Drizd TA, Johnson CL, Reed RB, Roche AF,
Moore WM: Physical growth: National Center for Health Statistics percentiles. AM J CLIN NUTR 32:607–629, 1979. Data from the National Center
for Health Statistics (NCHS), Hyattsville, Maryland. Reprinted with permission of Ross Laboratories, Columbus, Ohio 43216.

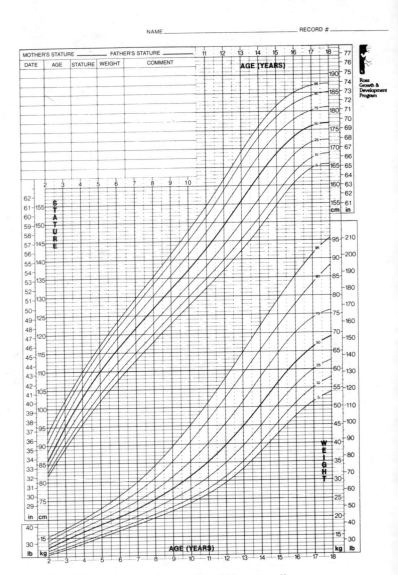

Boys: 2 to 18 years physical growth NCHS percentiles.
* Adapted from: Hamill PVV, Drizd TA, Johnson CL, Reed RB, Roche AF, Moore WM: Physical growth: National Center for Health Statistics percentiles. AM J CLIN NUTR 32:607–629, 1979. Data from the National Center for Health Statistics (NCHS), Hyattsville, Maryland. Reprinted with permission of Ross Laboratories, Columbus, Ohio 43216.

Author Index

The text reference to an author's work appears on the page number(s) listed.

Subject Index

Bupropion:
absorption of, 97
antipsychotic interaction with, 123
autonomic side effects, 99
cardiovascular effects, 100
classification of, 275
clinical trials, 96–97
cost of, 114
depression and, 96–101, 109
dosage guidelines, 97, 100, 109
drug-drug interactions, 122–123
efficacy of, 98
elderly and, 100, 109
FDA approval of, 97
half-life, 97
panic disorder treatment, 101
plasma monitoring, 97
popularity of, 101
prolactin and, 97
psychosis and, 120
recommendations for, 263
seizures and, 102, 117, 119–120
side effects, 99, 119–120
structure of, 87
tricyclic antidepressants, interaction
with, 122–123
Buspirone:
classification of, 277
fluoxetine interaction with, 123
overview, 167
recommendations for, 263
tardive dyskinesia and, 167
Butaperazine, anticholinergic agents
and, 42
Butyrophenones, psychiatric disorders
treatment, 197

Calcium channel blockers, lithium and, 75
Carbamazepine:
as anticonvulsant, 181, 183, 189–190
antipsychotics and, 32
bipolar affective disorder treatment,
196
bone marrow suppression, 18–19,
189
children/adolescent treatment,
230–231, 233
classification of, 275, 277
compliance, 198
distribution of, 185
drug-drug interactions, 195, 201
fluoxetine interaction with, 123
hematologic monitoring of, 189

imipramine and, 201
lithium, compared to, 77, 196–197
mania and, 115
monitoring standards, 289
phenytoin interaction with, 195
plasma level monitoring, 192–193
plasma ranges for, 263, 290
recommendations for, 263
seizure control, 115
side effect of, 199
tricyclic antidepressants and, 103,
121, 201
Cardiac disorders:
amitriptyline and, 102
clozapine and, 18
imipramine and, 102
Cardiac patients:
clomipramine and, 95
tricyclic antidepressants and, 102,
106, 111, 116–117
Catapres, see Clonidine
Cathecholamines, 66
Central nervous system, clomipramine
and, 118
Centrally-acting depressants, tricyclic
antidepressants interaction, 122
Centrax, see Prazepam
Cerebral stimulants:
children/adolescent disruptive
disorders treatment
fenfluramine, 227
indications, 225
long-acting formulations, 226
side effect monitoring, 226–227
tricyclic antidepressants, interaction
with, 122
Child/adolescent psychiatric disorders,
treatment of:
anticonvulsants, 231–234
antipsychotic agents, 22, 212–218
benzodiazepines, 227–229
central stimulants, 225–227
lithium, 70, 218–221
monoamine oxidase inhibitors, 225
psychotropic agents, 233–234
rage and violence, 230–231
sample growth charts, 297–300
tricyclic antidepressants, 221–225
Childhood psychoses, neuroleptics and,
21
Chloral hydrate:
anxiety treatment, 166
bupropion and, 99